NUTRITIONAL APPLICATIONS *in* EXERCISE *and* SPORT

NUTRITION in EXERCISE and SPORT

Edited by Ira Wolinsky and James F. Hickson, Jr.

Published Titles

Exercise and Disease,
Ronald R. Watson and Marianne Eisinger

Nutrients as Ergogenic Aids for Sports and Exercise,
Luke Bucci

Nutrition in Exercise and Sport, Second Edition,
Ira Wolinsky and James F. Hickson, Jr.

Nutrition Applied to Injury Rehabilitation and Sports Medicine,
Luke Bucci

Nutrition for the Recreational Athlete,
Catherine G.R. Jackson

NUTRITION in EXERCISE and SPORT

Edited by Ira Wolinsky

Published Titles

Sports Nutrition: Minerals and Electrolytes,
Constance V. Kies and Judy A. Driskell

Nutrition, Physical Activity, and Health in Early Life: Studies in Preschool Children,
Jana Parizkova

Exercise and Immune Function,
Laurie Hoffman-Goetz

Body Fluid Balance: Exercise and Sport,
E.R. Buskirk and S. Puhl

Nutrition and the Female Athlete,
Jaime S. Ruud

Sports Nutrition: Vitamins and Trace Elements,
Ira Wolinsky and Judy A. Driskell

Amino Acids and Proteins for the Athlete—The Anabolic Edge,
Mauro G. DiPasquale

Nutrition in Exercise and Sport, Third Edition,
Ira Wolinsky

Published Titles Continued

Gender Differences in Metabolism: Practical and Nutritional Implications,
Mark Tarnopolsky

Macroelements, Water, and Electrolytes in Sports Nutrition,
Judy A. Driskell and Ira Wolinsky

Sports Nutrition,
Judy A. Driskell

Energy-Yielding Macronutrients and Energy Metabolism in Sports Nutrition,
Judy A. Driskell and Ira Wolinsky

Nutrition and Exercise Immunology,
David C. Nieman and Bente Klarlund Pedersen

Sports Drinks: Basic Science and Practical Aspects,
Ronald Maughan and Robert Murry

Nutritional Applications in Exercise and Sport,
Ira Wolinsky and Judy Driskell

NUTRITION in EXERCISE and SPORT

Edited by Ira Wolinsky

Forthcoming Titles

High Performance Nutrition: Diets and Supplements for the Competitive Athlete,
Mauro DiPasquale

Nutrition and the Strength Athlete,
Catherine R. Jackson

Nutrients as Ergogenic Aids for Sports and Exercise, Second Edition,
Luke R. Bucci

NUTRITIONAL APPLICATIONS *in* EXERCISE *and* SPORT

Edited by
Ira Wolinsky and
Judy A. Driskell

CRC
CRC Press
Boca Raton London New York Washington, D.C.

Library of Congress Cataloging-in-Publication Data

Nutritional applications in exercise and sport / edited by Ira Wolinsky, Judy A. Driskell.
p. cm. --(Nutrition in exercise and sport)
Includes bibliographical references and index.
ISBN 0-8493-8199-1 (alk. paper)
1. Athletes--Nutrition. I. Wolinsky, Ira. II. Driskell, Judy A. (Judy Anne) III. Series.
TX361.A8 N89 2000
613.2′088796—dc21 00-042904
CIP

This book contains information obtained from authentic and highly regarded sources. Reprinted material is quoted with permission, and sources are indicated. A wide variety of references are listed. Reasonable efforts have been made to publish reliable data and information, but the author and the publisher cannot assume responsibility for the validity of all materials or for the consequences of their use.

Direct all inquiries to CRC Press LLC, 2000 N.W. Corporate Blvd., Boca Raton, Florida 33431.

International Standard Book Number 0-8493-8199-1
Library of Congress Card Number 00-042904
Printed in the United States of America 1 2 3 4 5 6 7 8 9 0
Printed on acid-free paper

Front Cover Photo The Legacy Statue. Courtesy of the Athletic Department of the University of Nebraska.

Preface

This book is a part of a miniseries within the CRC Series on Nutrition in Exercise and Sport, a series that publishes comprehensive books on subjects of timely interest for sports nutritionists of all walks in the expanding field of sports nutrition, written by competent editors and authors who are well known in their fields. This volume focuses on applied topics relevant to sports nutrition rather than the usual treatment of nutrient-specific metabolism. It presents, in one place, a wealth of material either not found, or difficult to find, in the open literature. Its first section deals with life-cycle nutritional concerns of athletes and group-specific nutritional concerns. This is followed by sections on sport and concludes with discussion of the nutritional knowledge of athletes. Sports nutritionists, researchers, students, health practitioners, and the educated layman will find this book useful.

Companions to this book are three other volumes we edited; *Sports Nutrition: Vitamins and Trace Elements*, 1997; *Macroelements, Water, and Electrolytes in Sports Nutrition*, 1999; and *Energy-Yielding Macronutrients and Energy Metabolism in Sports Nutrition*, 2000. Additionally useful will be the two books *Nutrition in Exercise and Sport*, Third Edition, 1998; and *Sports Nutrition*, 2000, edited by Ira Wolinsky and authored by Judy Driskell, respectively.

Ira Wolinsky, Ph.D.
University of Houston

Judy A. Driskell, Ph.D., R.D.
University of Nebraska

The Editors

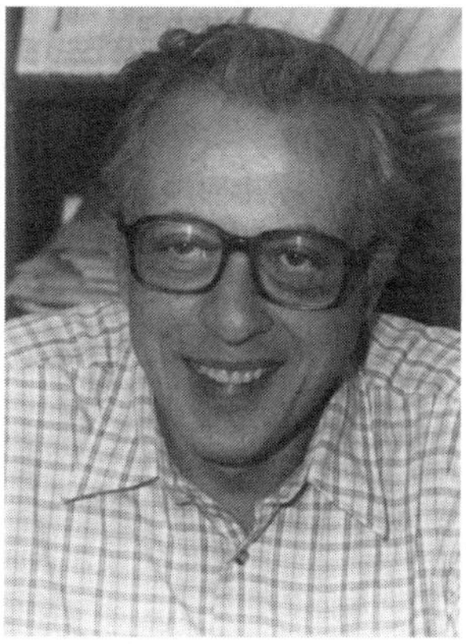

Ira Wolinsky, Ph.D., is professor of nutrition at the University of Houston. He received his B.S. degree in chemistry from the City College of New York and his M.S. and Ph.D. degrees in biochemistry from the University of Kansas. He has served in research and teaching positions at the Hebrew University (Medical School and Faculty of Agriculture), the University of Missouri, and Pennsylvania State University, as well as conducting basic research in NASA life sciences facilities.

Dr. Wolinsky is a member of the American Society of Nutritional Sciences, among other honorary and scientific organizations. He has contributed numerous nutrition research papers in the open literature. His major research interests relate to the nutrition of bone and calcium and to sports nutrition. The recipient of research grants from both public and private sources, he has also received several international research fellowships and has served in a consulting capacity in the former Soviet Union, Bulgaria, Hungary, and India. He merited a Fulbright Senior Scholar Fellowship to Greece in 1999.

Dr. Wolinsky has co-authored a book on the history of the science of nutrition, *Nutrition and Nutritional Diseases*. He co-edited *Sports Nutrition: Vitamins and Trace Elements; Macroelements; Water, and Electrolytes in Sports Nutrition; Energy-Yielding Macronutrients and Energy Metabolism in Sports Nutrition*; and the current book *Nutritional Applications in Exercise and Sport*, all with Judy Driskell. Additionally, he co-edited *Nutritional Concerns of Women* with Dorothy Klimis-Tavantzis. He edited the third edition of *Nutrition in Exercise and Sport*. He is also the editor for the CRC series Nutrition in Exercise and Sport, the CRC series Modern Nutrition, and the CRC series Exercise Physiology.

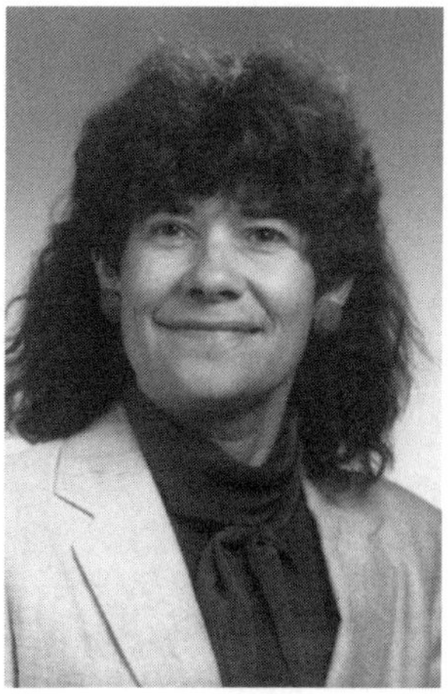

Judy Anne Driskell, Ph.D., R.D. is professor of nutritional science and dietetics at the University of Nebraska. She received her B.S. degree in biology from the University of Southern Mississippi in Hattiesburg, and her M.S. and Ph.D. degrees from Purdue University. She has served in research and teaching positions at Auburn University, Florida State University, Virginia Polytechnic Institute and State University, and the University of Nebraska. She has also served as the nutrition scientist for the U.S. Department of Agriculture/Cooperative State Research Service and as a professor of nutrition and food science at Gadjah Mada and Bogor Universities in Indonesia.

Dr. Driskell is a member of numerous professional organizations including the American Society of Nutritional Sciences, the American College of Sports Medicine, the Institute of Food Technologists, and the American Dietetic Association. In 1993 she received the Professional Scientist Award of the Food Science and Human Nutrition Section of the Southern Association of Agricultural Scientists. In addition, she was the 1987 recipient of the Borden Award for Research in Applied Fundamental Knowledge of Human Nutrition. She is listed as an expert in B-complex vitamins by the Vitamin Nutrition Information Service.

Dr. Driskell recently co-edited the CRC books *Sports Nutrition: Minerals and Electrolytes* with Constance V. Kies (deceased) and *Sports Nutrition: Vitamins and Trace Elements* with Ira Wolinsky. In addition, she authored the textbook *Sports Nutrition* and co-authored an advanced nutrition book *Nutrition: Chemistry and Biology*, both published by CRC. She has published more than100 refereed research articles and 10 book chapters as well as several publications intended for general readers, and has given numerous professional and public presentations. Her current research interests center around vitamin metabolism and requirements, including the interrelationships between exercise and water-soluble vitamin requirements.

Contributors

Jenna D. Anding, Ph.D., R.D.
Department of Animal Science
Texas A&M University
College Station, TX

Katherine A. Beals, Ph.D., R.D.
Department of Family and Consumer Sciences
Ball State University
Muncie, IN

Jacqueline R. Berning, Ph.D., R.D.
Department of Biology
University of Colorado-Colorado Springs
Colorado Springs, CO

Nancy M. Betts, Ph.D., R.D.
Department of Nutritional Sciences and Dietetics
University of Nebraska
Lincoln, NE

L. Mallory Boylan, Ph.D., R.D., L.D.
Department of Education, Nutrition, Restaurant and Hotel Management
Texas Tech University
Lubbock, TX

Samuel N. Cheuvront, M.S., R.D.
Department of Nutrition, Food, and Exercise Sciences
Florida State University
Tallahassee, FL

Kimberly E. Crawford
Department of Foods and Nutrition
University of Georgia
Athens, GA

Mauro DiPasquale, M.D., M.R.O., M.S.F.
AllProtraining.com
Austin, TX

Judy A. Driskell, Ph.D., R.D.
Department of Nutritional Science and Dietetics
University of Nebraska
Lincoln, NE

David R. Ellis, B.S., C.S.C.S., L.M.T.
Athletic Department
University of Nebraska
Lincoln, NE

Ann C. Grandjean, Ed.D.
International Center for Sports Nutrition
Omaha, NE

Jean E. Guest, B.S., R.D., L.M.N.T.
Department of Nutritional Science and Dietetics
University of Nebraska
Lincoln, NE

Patricia A. Henry, M.Ed., R.D., L.D.
Department of Nutrition
Tomball Regional Hospital
Tomball, TX

Heather B. Holden, M.Ed.
Department of Nutrition and Food Science
Auburn University
Auburn, AL

Satya S. Jonnalagadda, Ph.D.
Department of Nutrition
Georgia State University
Atlanta, GA

Jay Kandiah, Ph.D., R.D., C.D.
Department of Family and Consumer Sciences
Ball State University
Muncie, IN

Robert E. Keith, Ph.D., R.D.
Department of Nutrition and Food Science
Auburn University
Auburn, AL

Dorothea J. Klimis-Zacas, Ph.D.
Department of Food Science and Nutrition
University of Maine
Orono, ME

Nancy M. Lewis, Ph.D., R.D., F.A.D.A., L.M.N.T.
Department of Nutritional Science and Dietetics
University of Nebraska
Lincoln, NE

Richard D. Lewis, Ph.D., R.D., L.D.
Department of Foods and Nutrition
University of Georgia
Athens, GA

Jennifer A. Massoni, B.S., R.D., L.D.
Department of Foods and Nutrition
University of Georgia
Athens, GA

Lisa S. McAnulty, M.S., R.D.
Department of Nutrition and Food Science
Auburn University
Auburn, AL

Robert J. Moffatt, M.P.H., Ph.D.
Department of Nutrition, Food, and Exercise Sciences
Florida State University
Tallahassee, FL

Kristin J. Reimers, M.S., R.D.
Center for Human Nutrition
Omaha, NE

Melissa D. Ripley, B.S.
Department of Nutrition
Simmons College
Boston, MA

Jaime S. Ruud, M.S., R.D.
Sports Nutrition Consultant
Nutrition Link
Lincoln, NE

John B. Shea, Ph.D.
Department of Nutrition, Food, and Exercise Sciences
Florida State University
Tallahassee, FL

Brent J. Shriver, Ph.D.
Department of Education, Nutrition, Restaurant and Hotel Management
Texas Tech University
Lubbock, TX

Paul N. Taylor, Ph.D.
Department of Nutrition
Simmons College
Boston, MA

Ira Wolinsky, Ph.D.
Department of Human Development
University of Houston
Houston, TX

Acknowledgments

We thank the many individuals who helped, directly or indirectly, in the preparation of this volume. We thank and appreciate each of the individuals who wrote each of the chapters; without them this volume would not be possible. Special thanks go to Scott Kosatka, University of Houston, for his help and many kindnesses.

Contents

IV Eating and Addictive Disorders/Conditions

V Nutrition Knowledge of Athletes

VI Summary

CHAPTER 1

Introduction to Nutritional Applications in Exercise and Sport

Satya S. Jonnalagadda, Ph.D.

CONTENTS

I. THE FIELD OF SPORTS NUTRITION

The field of sports nutrition, although still in its infancy and not clearly defined, is a rapidly growing area of practice.[1] The training of individuals practicing in this area is quite varied, with 86% holding graduate degrees, including doctorates (33%).[2] Although nutrition is one of the most common areas of study of most individuals who are practicing in this field (47%), individuals who are trained in medicine, basic sciences (30%), education, health, or exercise physiology (23%) are also actively involved.[2] Activities that these individuals conduct may include:

- nutrition education
- counseling
- fitness assessments
- exercise physiology
- medical, physical, biochemical, and psychosocial assessments

These individuals may also need to develop care plans to meet the daily nutrition and medical needs of athletes and active individuals during training and competition, depending on the type of

0-8493-8199-1/00/$0.00+$.50

activity and on special needs such as the demands of growth and development, vegetarian dietary habits, pregnancy, and individuals with physical and mental disabilities.[3]

Over the past decade, the field of sports nutrition has grown rapidly due to an increasing number of athletes, coaches and trainers concerned about the impact of nutrition on performance.[4,5] However, nutrition misinformation is quite rampant among this group of individuals.[6–8] Clark[9] observed that information and knowledge regarding composition of meals before exercise or competition, appropriate weight gain or loss techniques, techniques for fat loss and increasing lean body mass, management of eating disorders, proper hydration strategies, and supplement use are very limited among athletes, coaches, and trainers. Pratt and Walberg,[10] in a survey of health and physical education teachers, observed that the three most important concerns of these teachers were the prescription of a balanced diet for athletes, fluid replacement, and weight maintenance. However, most of these individuals had no formal nutrition training. Likewise, Corley et al.[5] observed that the major nutritional concern of coaches was the consumption of "junk foods," poor eating habits, and consumption of unbalanced diets by their athletes. Only a third of the coaches surveyed were confident about their nutrition knowledge.[5] It is, therefore, one of several roles of the sports nutritionist to encourage and promote proper nutrition practices and food selection, to manage training table menus, to identify eating disorders, and to be a reliable source of nutrition information to these individuals. Sound nutrition practices by an athlete are typically compromised due to several factors such as:

- poor understanding of good nutrition principles and practices
- nutrition myths and misconceptions
- lack of practical nutrition knowledge and skills
- lack of understanding of individual nutrition requirements
- heavy workload that compromises intake
- inadequate finances
- frequent travel[6]

Therefore, the sports nutritionist needs to develop a well-rounded program to address these various aspects of nutrition and provide some practical guidelines to the athlete.

With the increasing popularity of sports and exercise, more individuals are actively involved in exercise programs to enhance health and well being. Increasingly, the participation in these activities is starting at an early age, as young as 5 years, and is continuing on into the later years of life, often beyond 80 years. Reaching out to individuals to make a positive impact early in life is important, not only to improve nutritional habits, but also possibly to help prevent the development of unhealthy dietary attitudes and habits.[11] Communicating positive nutrition messages to young individuals is important in promoting the practice of good nutrition. With the widening age range of active individuals, it is increasingly important to recognize the variation in the nutritional needs of these individuals to not only meet the needs of the normal physiological processes but also those of exercise and physical activity. To improve exercise capacity and performance, information about dietary intake, fluid consumption, supplements, and ergogenic aids needs to be provided to these individuals and those working with them, since these individuals are typically susceptible to erroneous information and practices with respect to nutrition and diet and are ready to try anything that will enhance performance.[5]

II. ROLE OF NUTRITION IN EXERCISE AND PERFORMANCE

Athletic and exercise performance is not only influenced by the training schedule of the athlete but is also dramatically influenced by the nutritional status of the individual. Total dietary intake not only influences training and performance, but also the strength and endurance of the individual. Additionally, the composition of dietary intake can significantly impact the metabolic responses to exercise, which, in turn, can impact performance. It is therefore important to pay close attention to the dietary and nutrient intakes of these active individuals to enhance performance and exercise capacity.

The American Dietetic Association, the Canadian Dietetic Association, and several other groups have provided recommendations on the nutritional goals for optimal performance in addition to recommendations for daily eating and dietary strategies to enhance performance.[12] Individuals undertaking daily exercise or strenuous physical activity typically have energy expenditures greater than the normal daily energy expenditures of sedentary individuals.[13] Therefore, the total energy intake of these individuals should meet the increased demands of exercise and physical activity along with the requirements for growth, muscular development, and various other components that can influence energy expenditure. Depending on the type of activity performed, the energy substrate will vary, and therefore the diet composition will play a significant role. For instance, moderate-to high-intensity exercise (>70% VO_{2max}) relies greatly on carbohydrate stores for energy, so a high carbohydrate intake is advantageous to these individuals. Therefore, food selection, timing, frequency of consumption, and composition can impact performance.

III. GENERAL DIETARY RECOMMENDATIONS FOR ACTIVE INDIVIDUALS

Because proper nutrition plays an important role in performance, it is important that athletes regularly consume a well balanced and varied diet to enhance not only their training, but also their exercise and competition capacity. Specifically, what athletes consume prior to, during, and immediately after competition or exercise can influence their performance and recovery. Pre-exercise or pre-competition meals, i.e., 4 hours prior to event, should include adequate amounts of carbohydrates, especially complex carbohydrates, and fluids.[13] Athletes should consume familiar foods and those that will not cause gastrointestinal distress (GI). Individuals who are nervous and develop GI prior to competition may benefit from liquid meal supplements that will provide not only fluids, but also the energy and nutrients needed for the actual competition.[14,15] During performance, especially endurance activities greater than 1 hour in duration, regular small carbohydrate feedings (30–60 g) in the form of sports beverages, may be beneficial in maintaining blood glucose levels during the performance.[16] Similarly, immediately after exercise or competition athletes should be encouraged to consume adequate amounts of carbohydrate-containing foods to replace muscle glycogen stores that were depleted during the performance.[14,17,18]

Children and youths who are involved in sports should be encouraged to consume adequate amounts of nutrients that are needed not only to meet the demands of the exercise activity, but also the needs of the rapidly growing and maturing individual.[19,20] Parents, coaches, trainers and other individuals closely associated with the child athlete should also be educated about their dietary needs during training and competition. Because of the high-energy needs of activity, increased frequency and number of meals may be beneficial to the athlete to enable increased energy intake and to decrease the gastric discomfort from consumption of large meals.[13] Because of the diverse nature of sports, age and gender differences, and nutrient requirements, it is rather difficult to define nutrition guidelines that cater to the needs of all active individuals. In general, all individuals involved in physical activity should be encouraged to:

- Consume sufficient energy
- Include a wide variety of foods
- Increase carbohydrate intake to at least 60% of energy
- Increase number of smaller meals and snacks
- Achieve body fat mass to optimize health, nutritional status and performance
- Achieve adequate intakes of micronutrients, especially iron and calcium
- Consume adequate amount of fluids before, during, and after activity
- Eat well when traveling or when training in specialized circumstances such as high altitudes

During both training and competition, dietary intake should provide adequate energy and nutrients to support growth, development, and maintenance of various physiological and metabolic processes. The type of activity, its physical demands, duration, intensity and frequency all can influence dietary recommendations and intake. Athletes undergoing intense training and competition have energy expenditures two to three times greater than those of sedentary individuals. Additionally, athletes might have high-energy requirements because of their larger body size, activity level, and muscular development, or a combination of these factors. Increasing energy needs also increase carbohydrate needs of the athlete, since it is one of the main energy sources during endurance activities.[16] Energy needs of highly active individuals can vary considerably from 2000 to 6000 kcal, depending on the nature and intensity of the activity. Because of the low caloric density of the high-carbohydrate, low-fat diets typically consumed by athletes, it is important that athletes use multiple strategies such as more frequent meals and planned snacks to ensure consumption of adequate energy. Liquid meal supplements may also be a viable option for highly active individuals.[6,13] Athletes with high-energy needs tend to have a "grazing" food-intake pattern (>five meals/day), which can be a practical strategy for increasing energy intake. Consumption of between-meal snacks should contribute one-third of total daily energy intake, with a significant amount of daily nutrients consumed during the exercise activity.

Individuals undertaking strenuous and prolonged training are recommended to consume diets before, during, and after exercise that contain 60–70% of energy as carbohydrate.[21,22] This high-carbohydrate intake will ensure that muscle glycogen stores are maintained. Although body fat stores can potentially provide more energy than carbohydrate stores, during exercise their use is highly regulated.[21] Long-term endurance training relies to a greater extent on the oxidation of these fat stores. However, the rate of fat oxidation in adipocytes may be limited by the regional blood flow and increased ratio of free fatty acids to albumin in the blood. Additionally, muscle uptake and utilization of free fatty acids during exercise may be limited, and carbohydrate loading, which is a common practice among active individuals, can also decrease the oxidation of free fatty acids during exercise. Consumption of medium-chain triglycerides along with carbohydrates has been shown to increase fat oxidation and decrease muscle glycogen depletion, so it may be practical for athletes to consume fluids that contain carbohydrate and medium-chain triglycerides during moderate- and high-intensity endurance activities.[21]

Although the use of amino acids and protein supplements by athletes is quite common, excessive protein intake is unnecessary, as it does not contribute to the athlete's performance. Typically, athletes may need to consume two to two and a half times more than the protein recommendations for the general population. Strength athletes may require 1.4 to 1.8 g/kg/d and endurance athletes 1.2 to 1.4 g/kg body weight/day. However, by ensuring adequate energy and carbohydrate intake, the protein needs of these active individuals can be met.[23]

Consumption of a well-balanced, high-carbohydrate, moderate-protein, low-fat diet by these active individuals typically will ensure consumption of adequate vitamin and mineral intake.[18] There is limited information on the ergogenic benefits of vitamins and mineral supplements, and inclusion of a wide variety of foods should ensure adequate intakes of these nutrients.[24] However, intakes of two nutrients that can be dramatically influenced by dietary and exercise practices, and that may need to be evaluated on a regular basis, are iron and calcium, especially among young athletes and active females of all ages.[15]

Therefore, prior to making dietary recommendations, a detailed assessment of nutritional status, optimal body weight, body composition, eating and lifestyle patterns, fitness, physiological, and psychosocial assessments should be conducted on each individual.[3] Sport- and-exercise specific targets should be developed based on type, frequency, intensity, and duration of activity and energy expended during the activity. It is also important that eating and lifestyle habits and patterns be assessed to make recommendations that, because they fit into the schedule of active individuals, are then more likely to be followed. Additionally, it is important to determine the needs of the athlete, i.e., whether the activity is being performed for a particular outcome or for enjoyment, before the appropriate dietary recommendations can be made

IV. FLUID RECOMMENDATIONS

In addition to adequate dietary and nutrient intake, fluid intake plays an important role in physical performance.[25] Dehydration by itself or along with hypothermia, which can occur as a result of dehydration, can result in decreased performance. An increase in body temperature has been shown to result in fatigue and decreased performance despite adequate glycogen stores.[25] Sweat loss during training and competition needs to be replaced with adequate amount of fluids. However, athletes typically fail to accomplish this, resulting in dehydration. The ideal rate of fluid replacement is equivalent to the rate of sweat loss. The American College of Sports Medicine[26] (ACSM) recommends that, "During exercise athletes should start drinking early and at regular intervals in an attempt to consume fluids at a rate sufficient to replace all the water lost through sweating, or consume the maximal amount that can be tolerated." Fluid consumption can be increased by keeping fluids cool, by using flavored drinks that contain carbohydrates to increase palatability and that contain sodium chloride to increase rehydration. Additionally, the composition of the fluid consumed should be such that it is emptied rapidly from the stomach and absorption is increased from the small intestine. It is the general recommendation that athletes consume 500 ml (17 oz) of fluid 2 hours before exercise and an additional 250 to 500 ml 30 to 60 min before exercise on hot days.[26] Additionally, throughout exercise activity, 4 to 6 ozs (118–176 ml) of fluids every 15 min should be consumed and thirst should not be used as an indicator of hydration status. During extreme environmental conditions, sports beverages that provide electrolytes should also be consumed. Active individuals should be educated that adequate hydration can be recognized with the passing of normal to above normal volume of light colored urine, if urine is dark yellow or small in volume or has a strong odor then it is an indicator of inadequate fluid intake and fluid intake should be increased.[25]

V. ERGOGENIC AIDS

Ergogenic aids have come under increased scrutiny mainly because of the growing popularity of several non-nutrient compounds that have been promoted for their performance-enhancing properties. Intensive athletic training and competition may be associated with increased use and reliance on ergogenic aids by athletes.[7] The frequency of intake is likely to increase during the competition season and decrease during the off season. Although the research on the effectiveness of these substances is equivocal, the perceived benefits of the various ergogenic aids used by athletes may be due more to psychological than actual physiological benefits, and these individuals need to be educated about the potential side effects and benefits if any, of these various ergogenic aids.

VI. EATING DISORDERS

Eating disorders are prevalent among athletes, especially among elite, highly competitive athletes.[27,28] Psychosocial factors, such as body image, obsession with exercise, need for control and perfection, peer, parental and coaching pressure can all influence the dietary intake of the active individual and result in disordered eating.[29] Individuals working with these athletes and active individuals should be cognizant of these factors and make appropriate referrals and recommendations. In 1991, 64% of college athletic administrators reported eating disorders among their collegiate athletes. Some 93% of disorders reported were in female athletes, especially those involved in gymnastics, cross country, swimming and track.[30] It is therefore important to identify susceptible and high-risk athletes and intervene early to prevent devastating outcomes associated with eating disorders. It is the position of the American Dietetic Association[31] that nutrition education and nutrition intervention be integrated into a multidisciplinary team in the treatment of eating disorders. Misinformation, myths, and misconceptions of athletes, trainers, coaches, and parents about diet, body weight, weight loss, body composition, and performance should be dispelled and athletes should be educated about the adverse outcomes of these disorders.[29]

REFERENCES

1. Grandjean, A. C., Diets of elite athletes: has the discipline of sports nutrition made an impact?, *J. Nutr.,* 127, 874S, 1997.
2. Grandjean, A. C., Practices and recommendations of sports nutritionists, *Intl. J. Sport Nutr.,* 3, 232, 1993.
3. Storlie, J., Nutrition assessment of athletes: a model for integrating nutrition and physical performance indicators, *Intl. J. Sport Nutr.,* 1, 192, 1991.
4. Sossin, K., Giziz, F., Marquart, L. F., and Sobal, J., Nutrition beliefs, attitudes, and resource use of high school wrestling coaches, *Intl. J. Sport Nutr.,* 7, 279, 1997.
5. Corley, G., Demarest-Litchford, M., and Bazzarre, T. L., Nutrition knowledge and dietary practices of college coaches, *J. Am. Diet. Assoc.,* 90, 705, 1990.
6. Burke, L., Practical issues in nutrition for athletes, *J. Sports Sci.,* 13, S83, 1995.
7. Clark, K. S., Sports nutrition counseling: documentation of performance, *Top. Clin. Nutr.,* 14, 34, 1999.
8. Vinci, D. M., Effective nutrition support programs for college athletes, *Intl. J. Sport Nutr.,* 8, 308, 1998.
9. Clark, K. L., Working with college athletes, coaches, and trainers at a major university, *Intl. J. Sport Nutr.,* 4, 135, 1994.
10. Pratt, C. A. and Walberg, J. L., Nutrition knowledge and concerns of health and physical education teachers, *J. Am. Diet. Assoc.,* 88, 840, 1988.
11. Berning, J., Fueling their engines for the long haul: teaching good nutrition to young athletes, *J. Am. Diet. Assoc.,* 98, 418, 1998.
12. Position of the American Dietetic Association and the Canadian Dietetic Association: Nutrition for physical fitness and athletic performance for adults, *J. Am. Diet. Assoc.,* 93, 691, 1993.
13. Hawley, J. A. and Burke, L. M., Effect of meal frequency and timing on physical performance, *Br. J. Nutr.,* 77, S91, 1997.
14. Burke, L. M. and Read, R. S. D., Sports nutrition: approaching the nineties, *Sports Med.,* 8, 80, 1989.
15. Burke, L. M. and Read, R. S. D., Dietary supplements in sport, *Sports Med.,* 15, 43, 1993.
16. Coyle, E. F. and Montain, S. J., Carbohydrate and fluid ingestion during exercise: are there trade-offs?, *Med. Sci. Sports Exerc.,* 24, 671, 1992.
17. Economos, C. D., Bortz, S. S., and Nelson, M. E., Nutritional practices of elite athletes, *Sports Med.,* 16, 381, 1993.
18. Probart, C. K., Bird, P. J., and Parker, K. A., Diet and athletic performance, *Med. Clin. N. Am.,* 77, 757, 1993.
19. Ryan-Krause, P., The score on high-tech sports nutrition for adolescents, *J. Pediatr. Health Care,* 12, 164, 1998.
20. Chapman, P., Toma, R. B., Tuveson, R. V., Jacob, M., Nutrition knowledge among adolescent high school female athletes, *Adolescence,* 32, 437, 1997.
21. Lambert, E. V., Hawley, J. A., Noakes, G. T. D., and Dennis, S. C., Nutritional strategies for promoting fat utilization and delaying the onset of fatigue during prolonged exercise, *J. Sports Sci.,* 15, 315, 1997.
22. Mullin, K., Practical nutrition education: special considerations for athletes, *Nurse Pract. Forum,* 7, 106, 1996.
23. Lemon, P. W. R., Do athletes need more dietary protein and amino acids? *Intl. J. Sport Nutr.,* 5, S39, 1995.
24. Clarkson, P. M. and Haymes, E. M., Trace mineral requirements for athletes, *Intl. J. Sport Nutr.,* 4, 104, 1994.

25. Murray, R., Dehydration, hyperthermia, and athletes: science and practice, *J. Athl. Train.,* 31, 248, 1996.
26. American College of Sports Medicine, Position stand on exercise and fluid replacement, *Med. Sci. Sports Exerc.,* 28, I, 1996.
27. Parks, P. S. and Read, M. H., Adolescent male athletes: body image, diet, and exercise, *Adolescence,* 32, 593, 1997.
28. Baer, J. T., Walker, W. F., and Grossman, J. M., Disordered eating response team's effect on nutrition practices in college athletes, *J. Athl. Train.,* 30, 315, 1995.
29. Lindeman, A. K., Self-esteem: its application to eating disorders and athletes, *Intl. J. Sport Nutr.,* 4, 237, 1994.
30. Dick, R. W., Eating disorders in NCAA athletic programs, *J. Natl. Athl. Train. Assoc.*, 26, 136, 1991.
31. Position of the American Dietetic Association: Nutrition intervention in the treatment of anorexia nervosa, bulimia nervosa, and binge eating, *J. Am. Diet. Assoc.,* 94, 902, 1994.

Part I

Nutritional Concerns of Athletes During the Life Cycle

CHAPTER 2

Nutritional Concerns of Pregnant and Lactating Athletes

Jenna D. Anding

CONTENTS

0-8493-8199-1/00/$0.00+$.50

I. INTRODUCTION

Pregnancy has been described as one of the most physically demanding events that a woman experiences during her lifetime.[1] For some women, the physiological stress of pregnancy is combined with the addition of exercise or sport.[2] The benefits of exercise are abundant and include weight control, a reduction in the risks for developing hypertension and diabetes, a promotion of psychological well-being, and maintenance of healthy bones, muscles, and joints.[3] However, the issue of exercise during pregnancy has been the subject of interest and discussion among physicians and health professionals because it not only affects the health of the mother but also may affect pregnancy outcome.[4-8] To date, research has indicated several benefits that the pregnant woman might gain from physical exercise including shortened length of labor[4] and a reduction in the need for an operative delivery.[7] From a therapeutic perspective, exercise can be an effective tool in the management of gestational diabetes.[9] In contrast, some studies have reported adverse effects of exercise on pregnancy outcome such as a reduced length of gestation and birth weight.[6,10] Other studies have not confirmed these findings[11-13] and at least one study has demonstrated a relationship between inactivity and low birth weight.[13] Nonetheless, without adequate energy and nutrition to compensate for the increased caloric needs required for pregnancy as well as physical activity, normal or exercise/sport, it is reasonable to speculate that exercise might compromise fetal growth.[14]

It is not unusual for some women to exercise during lactation.[15] Because the energy needs during lactation tend to be greater than during pregnancy,[16] it is logical to wonder what the addition of exercise does to the mother's energy and nutrient needs. Does exercise affect milk production and quality?

This chapter will address some of these questions as well as the nutritional concerns of women who exercise during pregnancy and lactation. Selected maternal and fetal responses to exercise and the proposed risks and benefits of exercise during pregnancy and lactation will be discussed briefly. Recommended guidelines for exercise during pregnancy, and the nutritional needs and concerns among women who continue their exercise regimen from pregnancy into lactation will also be addressed.

II. MATERNAL AND FETAL RESPONSES TO EXERCISE

Pregnancy brings about numerous physiological changes, including an increase in blood flow and cardiac output, an increase in basal metabolism and respiration, alterations in carbohydrate metabolism, and a relaxation in the musculoskeletal system.[17,18] These adaptations are essential for fetal development and help prepare the mother for parturition. The inclusion of exercise requires further adaptations to protect the developing fetus.[1,19-23]

A. Uterine Blood Flow

In humans, research has demonstrated that exercise results in a decreased uterine blood flow.[24-26] While the observed reduction in blood flow might not be as pronounced in physically conditioned women,[27,28] the possibility that the fetus might experience hypoxia as a result of maternal exercise has been suggested.[1,26,27] Recent research suggests that there are protective mechanisms in place that ensure that oxygen delivery to the fetus is not jeopardized.[17,28] The rise in maternal blood volume during pregnancy allows for an increase in its oxygen-carrying capacity, regardless of activity level.[17] In addition, the maternal body is thought to respond to the stress of exercise by redirecting blood flow[25] and altering placental development in a manner that protects the fetus.[29,30]

B. Maternal Body Temperature

Maternal body temperature is hypothesized to be the major predictor of fetal temperature.[31] Body temperature increases during exercise[2] and studies in animals have demonstrated a relationship between hyperthermia and reduced birth weight, reduced placental weight, and neural tube defects.[32-34] These findings, along with research in humans,[35-39] have led investigators to question whether maternal hyperthermia increases the risk of fetal abnormalities.

Human studies have confirmed an increase in maternal body temperature following bouts of exercise, but this increase does not appear to approach levels that would be considered teratogenic.[40-42] Researchers have suggested that the increase in maternal blood volume acts to transfer heat away from the fetus.[43] In addition, the demonstrated rise in maternal skin temperature[44] is thought to serve as a thermoregulatory response that protects the fetus from extreme temperatures.

A prospective study has investigated the association between maternal hyperthermia and fetal malformation risk during the first trimester of pregnancy. The results of this study, which involved 165 women, failed to confirm hyperthermia as a teratogen.[45] While this is encouraging, the existing animal evidence and limited human data make it impossible to dismiss any possible risk. The risk of teratogenesis due to hyperthermia appears to be highest during the first trimester;[19] therefore, pregnant women are encouraged to avoid strenuous exercise in hot environments, especially during the first trimester.[19,46]

C. Alterations in Carbohydrate Metabolism

During pregnancy, the maternal blood glucose supplies the fetus with a constant supply of energy necessary for growth and development.[47] Late in pregnancy, under resting conditions, hyperinsulinemia, glucose intolerance, and increased fasting plasma glucose levels occur.[48,49] Because the rate of fetal growth begins to increase after the 9th week of gestation,[50] these changes help ensure that the fetus has the continuous supply of glucose necessary for fat and protein synthesis.[48]

In humans, strenuous exercise during the latter stages of gestation has been shown to decrease maternal blood glucose levels,[51-53] raising the concern that glucose availability to the fetus might be compromised. In animals, Treadway and Young[54] found that fetal glucose uptake was reduce by 40% when sedentary pregnant rats were exercised for 50 minutes. However, when Mottola et al.[55] exercised trained pregnant rats, the reduced fetal uptake of glucose was not observed, leading the researchers to suggest that the training allowed for the utilization of lactate and other alternate energy sources, sparing the glucose for the fetus. Although the effects of strenuous maternal exercise on fetal glucose uptake in humans is unknown, it has been hypothesized that chronic maternal hypoglycemia could result in fetal malnutrition, intrauterine growth retardation and reduced birth weight.[52]

III. EXERCISE DURING PREGNANCY: THEORETICAL RISKS AND POSSIBLE BENEFITS

The physiological adaptations that occur during pregnancy serve to protect the fetus and foster an environment conducive to optimal growth and development. In contrast, exercise during pregnancy helps maintain maternal homeostasis.[1] Whether these adaptations conflict or complement each other is uncertain. Based on available research, exercising during pregnancy may be associated with a number of theoretical risks and possible benefits.[1,19,20,46,56]

A. Theoretical Fetal Risks

In addition to the possible fetal risks previously identified (hypoxia, hyperthermia, and reduced carbohydrate availability), some research has proposed a relationship between maternal exercise and fetal distress[22,44,57,58] and decreased birth weight.[4,6,10] Other studies, however, have failed to confirm these findings.[11,59-62]

Normal fetal heart rate (FHR), an indicator of fetal well-being, ranges from 120 to 160 beats per minute.[19] Depending on the intensity and duration, strenuous exercise commonly results in an increase in FHR by 5 to 25 beats per minute[19] but returns to baseline levels 10 to 30 minutes after the exercise has ended.[19,63] The etiology behind the change in FHR is unclear, but appears to be a protective response.[64]

Episodes of fetal bradycardia (FHR < 120 beats per minute for 2 minutes) as a result of maternal exercise have been demonstrated in some laboratories.[22,44,57,58] Since fetal bradycardia is a sign of fetal distress,[19] this is a concern. However, not all studies have reported fetal bradycardia following maternal exercise.[59-61] The lack of consistent criteria for identifying bradycardia along with difficulties in obtaining artifact-free data during vigorous maternal exercise makes it difficult to interpret the true occurrence of exercise-induced bradycardia.[19] Because most of the reported episodes appear to be transient in nature and in normal pregnancies,[46] there does not appear to be adverse effects of exercise-induced fetal bradycardia.[22,46,63] Long-term effects on the fetus, however, are unknown.[46]

Infant birth weight is a known predictor of morbidity and mortality.[65] Animal and human investigations have theorized that strenuous exercise might be linked to reduced birth weights.[4,6,10,66,67] Treadway et al.[66] found that pregnant rats, both trained and untrained, had decreased fetal birth weights when subjected to strenuous exercise. Picarro et al.[67] found that untrained pregnant rats that were exercised at 70 to 90% VO_{2max} delivered newborns with birth weights that were less than sedentary rats and rats that were exercised at 60% VO_{2max}. This prompted the suggestion that high-intensity exercise without training prior to pregnancy might compromise fetal development.[67] In contrast, when pre-pregnancy-trained rats were subjected to exercise during pregnancy, Mottola et al.[68] and Courant and Barr[69] found that their offspring had birth weights that were no different from the control groups. Furthermore, when the exercise is voluntary, there appears to be no adverse effect on birth weight.[70]

A limited body of research has suggested that human infant birth weights may be reduced when women continue regular, vigorous, and sustained exercise throughout their pregnancies.[71] Birth weights are increased when exercise is discontinued late in the pregnancy.[71] In a study of 336 women, Clapp and Capeless[10] found that women who exercised for 30 minutes at least three times a week at an intensity greater than 50% of their maximum heart rate had a shorter gestation period, experienced less gestational weight gain, and gave birth to infants who weighed an average of 500 grams less than the infants of women who were sedentary or reduced their exercise during pregnancy. In a second study, Clapp and Dickstein[6] reported that women who exercised prior to conception and during their pregnancy at an intensity greater than 50% of their maximum heart rate delivered infants that weighed 310 grams less than those born to matched controls who did not maintain their preconceptional exercise. In contrast, Sternfeld and colleagues[62] found that women who participated in aerobic exercise (excluding vigorous walking) for at least 20 minutes at least three times a week delivered infants who were similar to those born to women who exercised at lower intensities. Hatch et al.[11] reported that women who expended at least 1,000 kilocalories a week in recreational activities throughout their pregnancies delivered babies who were heavier than those born to women who did not exercise. One study observed an increased likelihood of very low infant birth weights among women who did not participate in vigorous physical activity during pregnancy.[13] These findings, along with a meta-analysis of 18 observational and interventional studies indicate that normal, healthy, pregnant women can participate in exercise without placing either herself or her unborn child at risk.[72] This conclusion may not hold true, however, if exercise is combined with an inadequate diet.[46]

B. Potential Maternal Risks

In addition to hypoglycemia[51-53], investigators have cited musculoskeletal injuries.[46,56,73] and premature labor[31] as possible risks for women who exercise during pregnancy. During pregnancy, a woman's posture begins to change. The increase in lumbar lordosis and the forward tilt of the pelvis combined with the increase in body weight often result in low back pain.[64] In addition, the center of gravity changes, making balance more difficult,[64] and altered hormone levels increase joint laxity.[73] These changes would seem to increase the incidence of exercise-related injuries during pregnancy. Fortunately, this has not been confirmed,[2,74,75] and the incidence may actually decrease[62] because women are generally more cautious when exercising during pregnancy.[71] While the lack of increased injuries is encouraging, women are encouraged to limit exercise that requires quick changes in body position and highly coordinated movements.[64]

In the pregnant and non-pregnant state, exercise promotes a release of adrenaline (epinephrine) and noradrenaline (norepinephrine).[76] Since noradrenaline is a uterine stimulant,[77] exercise could theoretically cause uterine contractions and premature delivery.[1] Women who engage in strenuous exercise throughout pregnancy have been shown to deliver significantly earlier than their estimated date of confinement,[71] but there is no conclusive evidence to suggest that exercise causes premature labor.[2,11,72,78-80]

C. Possible Maternal Benefits

For non-pregnant women, exercise offers a number of well-recognized benefits, including improvements in cardiovascular function, blood pressure, blood cholesterol, and blood glucose levels. In addition, exercise strengthens bones, facilitates weight management and helps reduce stress.[81,82] For a normal, healthy woman, exercise may also offer additional benefits during pregnancy.[56,64,71,73]

Weight gain and an increase in subcutaneous fat deposition are expected during a normal pregnancy.[83] Inadequate weight gain may compromise fetal growth and development.[84] On the other hand, excessive maternal weight gain has been associated with an increased risk of fetopelvic disproportion and operative delivery, although these associations seem to be more common in women whose height is less than 157 cm (62 inches).[84]

The extent to which weight gain occurs depends on a number of factors including maternal age, ethnicity, parity, pre-pregnancy body weight, energy intake, metabolism, and physical work.[83] Previous investigations studying the effects of physical work during pregnancy on maternal weight gain have suggested that the caloric needs required for regular physical activity might compromise maternal weight gain as well as fetal growth.[14,85,86] Clapp and Little[83] compared the amount of weight gain and fat deposition between women who continued their level of pre-conceptual exercised throughout their pregnancies and those who discontinued or reduced the intensity of exercise early in pregnancy. The rate of weight gain was similar for both groups until after the 15th week of pregnancy, when the rate decreased in the women who continued to exercise. Subjects who continued to exercise at their preconception levels gained less weight than their less active counterparts (13.0 ± 0.5 kg versus 16.3 ± 0.7 kg). Sum of skinfolds also was less in the exercise group (22 ± 2 mm versus 31 ± 2 mm for the control group). Weight gain was considered normal for both groups and both groups delivered healthy infants, although the infant birth weights among the women who exercised were significantly lower.[83] These findings were similar to an earlier study by Clapp and Dickstein,[6] who found that women who maintained their preconception level of endurance exercise into the late stages of pregnancy gained an average of 4.6 kg less than women who discontinued their exercise before the 28th week of gestation. From this perspective, exercise during pregnancy might be viewed by some as a possible risk. However, Sternfeld et al.[62] did not report any significant differences in maternal weight gain among women who exercised during their pregnancies at varying levels of intensity, a finding that is in agreement with other studies.[12,72] Furthermore, participating in exercise during pregnancy might be of benefit to women who are prone to excessive weight gain.[18,31]

The noted reports of maternal hypoglycemia[51-53] following exercise cannot be discounted. However, for the percentage (1.4% to 12.3%) of women who develop gestational diabetes[85], the use of exercise may help lower blood glucose to an acceptable level.[9] Although more research is needed in this area, there is some evidence that exercise may help some gestational diabetics avoid insulin therapy when properly prescribed and monitored.[9]

Other possible benefits of exercise include a reduction in the symptoms of pregnancy such as nausea, heartburn and leg cramps,[62,87] reduced anxiety, and increased self esteem.[88,89] There have also been reports that women who exercise during pregnancy perceived that labor was easier,[88,90] and were able to endure prolong labors.[6,91,92] The continuation of exercise throughout pregnancy may also reduce the incidence of caesarean section and operative vaginal delivery.[7,71] Being physically fit has been linked to shorter labors in some studies,[4,92-95] but not in others.[7,72,96]

IV. RECOMMENDATIONS FOR EXERCISE DURING PREGNANCY

The lack of consistent results surrounding the risks and benefits of exercise during pregnancy can be attributed to a number of factors including population size, subject characteristics, level of physical activity, and methods used to define preconception exercise habits and fitness. As a result, caution must be used when attempting to extrapolate research findings to general populations. Still, it is generally viewed that a normal, healthy, pregnant woman can participate in physical activity during her pregnancy without jeopardizing the health of her unborn child.[1,46,97,98] Women who are physically trained prior to conception can also continue their exercise regimen, although it is possible that the levels of intensity and duration will be modified because of the common symptoms of pregnancy.[1,69,70] Recommendations for exercise during pregnancy have been developed by The American College of Obstetricians and Gynecologists[99] (Table 2.1).

Table 2.1 Recommendations for Exercise in Pregnancy

1. During pregnancy, women can continue to exercise and derive health benefits from even mild to moderate exercise routines. Regular exercise (at least three times per week) is preferable to intermittent activity.
2. Women should avoid exercise in the supine position after the first trimester. Such a position is associated with decreased cardiac output in most pregnant women; because the remaining cardiac output will be preferentially distributed away from splanchnic beds (including the uterus) during vigorous exercise; such regimens are best avoided during pregnancy. Prolonged periods of motionless standing should also be avoided.
3. Women should be aware of the decreased oxygen available for aerobic exercise during pregnancy. They should be encouraged to modify the intensity of their exercise according to maternal symptoms. Pregnant women should stop exercising when fatigued and not exercise to exhaustion. Weight-bearing exercises can, under some circumstances, be continued at intensities similar to those prior to pregnancy throughout pregnancy. Non-weight-bearing exercises such as cycling or swimming will minimize the risk of injury and facilitate the continuation of exercise during pregnancy.
4. Morphologic changes in pregnancy should serve as a relative contraindication to types of exercise in which loss of balance could be detrimental to maternal or fetal well-being, especially in the third trimester. Further, any type of exercise involving the potential for even minor abdominal trauma should be avoided.
5. Pregnancy requires an additional 300 kcal/d to maintain metabolic homeostasis. Thus, women who exercise during pregnancy should be particularly careful to ensure an adequate diet.
6. Pregnant women who exercise in the first trimester should augment heat dissipation by ensuring adequate hydration, appropriate clothing, and optimal environmental surroundings during exercise.

Reproduced with permission of The American College of Obstetricians and Gynecologists. *Exercise During Pregnancy and the Postpartum Period,* (Technical Bulletin 189). Washington, DC; ©ACOG; 1994.

It should be noted that, despite its potential benefits, exercise is not for every pregnant woman. According to the American College of Obstetricians and Gynecologists,[99] the presence of the following conditions should be considered contraindications to exercise during pregnancy:

- pregnancy-induced hypertension
- preterm rupture of membranes
- preterm labor during the prior or current pregnancy or both
- incompetent cervix/cerclage
- persistent second- or third-trimester bleeding
- intrauterine growth retardation

In addition, women with chronic medical conditions such as hypertension, cardiovascular or pulmonary disease should be carefully evaluated by their physician to determine the appropriateness of an exercise program.[99]

V. RECOMMENDED WEIGHT GAIN AND ESTIMATED ENERGY AND NUTRIENT NEEDS DURING PREGNANCY

A. Weight Gain

As mentioned earlier, the very nature of pregnancy requires that a woman increase her body weight and subcutaneous body fat. The Institute of Medicine's[84] recommended ranges for weight gain, based on prepregnancy body weight, are outlined in Table 2.2. Weight gain studies among women carrying multiple fetuses are limited, but those pregnant with twins should strive to gain 16 to 20 kg (35 to 45 pounds).[84]

Table 2.2 Recommended Total Weight Gain Ranges for Pregnant Women,[a] by Prepregnancy Body Mass Index (BMI)[b]

	Total Weight Gain		1st Trimester Gain		2nd and 3rd Trimester Weekly Gain	
BMI Category	kg	lb	kg	lb	kg	lb
Low (BMI < 19.8)	12.5–18	28–40	2.3	5	0.49	1.07
Normal (BMI = 19.8–26)	11.5–16	25–35	1.6	3.5	0.44	0.97
High (BMI >26.0–29.0)	7–11.5	15–25	0.9	2	0.3	0.67
Obese (BMI > 29.0)	6.0	15				

[a] Young adolescents and black women should strive for gains at the upper end of the recommended range. Short women (< 157 cm or 62 inches) should strive for gains at the lower end of the range.

[b] BMI may be calculated by 1) weight (kilograms)/height (meters^2) or 2) weight (pounds) x 703/height (inches^2)[99]

Reprinted with permission from *Nutrition During Pregnancy, Part 1: Weight Gain*, Copyright 1990, Washington, D.C.: National Academy of Sciences. Courtesy of the National Academy Press, Washington, D.C. and *Krause's Food, Nutrition, and Diet Therapy*, L. Kathleen Mahan and Sylvia Escott-Stump, Eds., WB Saunders, Philadelphia, 1996.

B. Energy

Many of the physiological changes that occur during pregnancy require additional energy. Early studies[101,102] estimated that the caloric cost of pregnancy ranged from 68,000 and 83,000 kcal, respectively. Based on these estimates, a woman would have to increase her daily caloric intake by 250 to 280 kcal per day to achieve this increase over the course of a normal pregnancy.[101,102]

Durnin and colleagues[103] found that estimated energy needs for pregnancy were approximately 69,000 kcal based on changes in body composition, energy intake and metabolism, and normal activity during the course of pregnancy among women residing in Scotland and Holland. They concluded that sedentary pregnant women living in industrialized countries could meet the estimated needs for pregnancy by consuming an additional 100 to 150 kcal during the second and third trimesters[103], a recommendation that is slightly lower than the 150 to 200 kcal recommended by the Institute of Medicine[84] and less than previously suggested by Hytten and colleagues.[101,102] Durnin and others[104] later reduced their recommendations to 100 to 150 additional calories in the third trimester only, based on a review of several longitudinal studies and other published data. By comparison, the 1989 Recommended Dietary Allowances (RDA) has more liberal guidelines, suggesting an increase in 300 kcal per day during the second and third trimester.[16]

Cross-sectional studies in developed countries suggest that pregnant women, on average, consume about 210 kcal more per day than their non-pregnant, non-lactating counterparts.[105] In contrast, longitudinal studies have found that the energy intakes among pregnant women can range from 95 kcal/day to 190 kcal/day.[106–108] Based on these reports, it would appear that women consume less energy than recommended. There is a possibility that cross-sectional studies tend to over-report caloric intake.[105] Measurement fatigue and under-reporting could influence longitudinal studies of caloric intake.[105] Other factors are believed to determine the amount of energy required by a woman during pregnancy and may help explain why estimated energy intakes of pregnant women tend to be lower than recommended. For example, women in industrialized nations are generally believed to be less active than women who live in developing countries.[84] In addition, obese women generally have more lean muscle mass and body fat than women whose weight is within a normal range.[84] Since the amount of lean muscle tissue present influences basal metabolism[84], it is reasonable to expect that obese women would require more energy to maintain their current body composition than women who are of a normal weight. Increases in maternal and fetal tissues will also increase basal metabolism,[105] although this seems to be more prominent in women residing in developed countries than those in developing countries.[105] Sustaining pregnancy under less-than-desirable conditions may result in specific alterations in energy metabolism to produce an energy-sparing effect.[105] While this could result in lower energy requirements for basal metabolism, Prentice and colleagues[105] have suggested that they might also lead to inadequate weight gain during pregnancy

C. Estimating Energy Needs for the Exercising Pregnant Woman

If energy recommendations for pregnancy seem inconclusive for sedentary women, taking into account regular physical exercise only makes the issue more challenging. During pregnancy, it is reasonable to expect that the energy requirements necessary to perform a specific activity might increase due to the increase in the mother's weight.[105] However, the extent to which regular physical activity increases energy needs during pregnancy may depend on the type of exercise carried out by the mother.

In an extensive review of studies of pregnant women in both developed and undeveloped countries, Prentice and colleagues[105] concluded that the caloric cost of non-weight-bearing exercises such as cycling increases by about 10% during the final stages of pregnancy. The net cost of weight-bearing exercises such as treadmill walking or stepping up and down from a bench (step test) appears to stay the same during the first half of pregnancy but then increase by about 20% by the end of gestation.[105] A self-paced activity like walking may also increase energy needs if the pace of walking stays constant throughout pregnancy.[105]

The lack of conclusive energy requirements for physically active pregnant women is of little comfort to the dietitian or health care provider who is asked by an expectant mother, "How many calories do I need?" While no single recommendation can be applied to all pregnant women, estimating energy needs can be accomplished using a variety of methods. Increasing pre-pregnancy energy intake by up to 300 kcal during the second and third trimesters is probably one of the simplest methods. Another method, proposed by the American College of Obstetricians and Gynecologists, allows 35 kcal per kilogram of optimal body weight plus an additional 300 kcal.[109] More recently, Allen and colleagues[110] have proposed two other estimates of additional energy requirements during pregnancy. These estimates not only account for the existence of physical activity, but also the noted changes in energy requirements as pregnancy progresses. The first method estimates energy needs using the basal metabolic rate (BMR) x physical activity level (PAL) ratio, which is defined as total daily energy expenditure divided by BMR. Using this method suggests that the increased energy needs for pregnancy are 1.1 MJ (264 kcal) per day throughout the pregnancy.[110] Women who reduce their physical activity may require an additional 0.7 MJ (168 kcal) per day. The second method proposed is based on a compilation of data from well-nourished females.[106] Energy needs for maintenance, the increase in body fat stores, diet-induced thermogenesis, and the noted rise in the energy needs to participate in weight-bearing activities were considered. Based on their review of these studies, a pregnant woman requires a caloric increase of 0.3 MJ (72 kcal) per day during her pregnancy.[110]

Regardless of which method is used for estimating increased energy needs, it is important to monitor the expecting mother's weight to ensure that adequate weight gain is in progress (Table 2.2), especially since some female athletes may begin their pregnancies underweight.[46] Regular monitoring of this anthropometric measurement is probably the simplest way to evaluate the adequacy of caloric intake. Adjustments can be made to increase or decrease energy intake based on changes in weight or the rate of weight gain.

D. Nutrient Requirements During Pregnancy

Nutrient needs for vitamins and minerals increase during pregnancy to compensate for the growth and development of the fetus and supporting maternal tissues.[84] Because the increase in energy is small, the expecting mother must choose nutrient-dense foods to meet her nutrient needs without consuming excess energy.

In the United States, expressing the nutrient needs for pregnant and lactating women involves the use of Dietary Reference Intakes (DRIs).[111] Currently, DRIs are composed of four types of values: Recommended Dietary Allowance (RDA), Estimated Average Requirement (EAR), Adequate Intake (AI) and Tolerable Upper Intake Level (UL). Briefly, the RDA of a given nutrient is defined as the amount needed to meet the needs of practically all healthy people in a given population.[16] The AI of a nutrient is an estimated intake of a nutrient in observational or experimental studies of healthy people. It is used when an RDA cannot be identified. A nutrient's UL is considered the highest amount of a nutrient that a healthy person in a general population can ingest without experiencing adverse health effects. The EAR of a nutrient is considered the amount of a specific nutrient that will meet 50% of healthy people within a population. The RDIs for selected nutrients are found in Tables 2.3 and 2.4. The evaluation and development of DRIs for vitamins C, E, A, K as well as other nutrients are currently under way.[111]

E. Nutrient Intakes of Women During Pregnancy

Dietary intake studies suggest that pregnant women in the United States consume diets that contain less than recommended levels of vitamins B_6, D, E, and folate, as well as the minerals calcium, iron, and zinc.[84,112] Inadequate intakes of these and other nutrients have been documented in pregnant women in other countries as well.[113–117] Non-pregnant female athletes have demonstrated dietary intakes that lack vitamin B_6, calcium, iron, zinc, folate, vitamin E, and vitamin B_{12}.[118] Dietary evaluations among physically active pregnant women are limited, but it would not be unreasonable to find athletes who enter pregnancy consuming less-than-desirable diets, based on separate reports of pregnant women's and non-pregnant athletes' dietary habits. The physiological significance, along with food sources of selected nutrients is shown in Table 2.5.

Life-stage group	Calcium (mg/d)	Phosphorus (mg/d)	Magnesium (mg/d)	Vitamin D[bc] (µg/d)	Fluoride (mg/d)	Thiamin (mg/d)	Rioflavin (mg/d)	Niacin[d] (mg/d)	Vitamin B-6 (mg/d)	Folate[e] (µg/d)	Vitamin B-12 (µg/d)	Pantothenic Acid (mg/d)	Biotin (µg/d)	Choline[f] (mg/d)
Infants														
0-6 mo	210*	100*	30*	5*	0.01*	0.2*	0.3*	2*	0.1*	65*	0.4*	1.7*	5*	125*
7-12 mo	270*	275*	75*	5*	0.5*	0.3*	0.4*	4*	0.3*	80*	0.5*	1.8*	6*	150*
Children														
1-3 y	500*	**460**	**80**	5*	0.7*	**0.5**	**0.5**	**6**	**0.5**	**150**	**0.9**	2*	8*	200*
4-8 y	800*	**500**	**130**	5*	1.0*	**0.6**	**0.6**	**8**	**0.6**	**200**	**1.2**	3*	12*	250*
Males														
9-13 y	1,300*	**1,250**	**240**	5*	2*	**0.9**	**0.9**	**12**	**1.0**	**300**	**1.8**	4*	20*	375*
14-18 y	1,300*	**1,250**	**410**	5*	3*	**1.2**	**1.3**	**16**	**1.3**	**400**	**2.4**	5*	25*	550*
19-30 y	1,000*	**700**	**400**	5*	4*	**1.2**	**1.3**	**16**	**1.3**	**400**	**2.4**	5*	30*	550*
31-50 y	1,000*	**700**	**420**	5*	4*	**1.2**	**1.3**	**16**	**1.3**	**400**	**2.4**	5*	30*	550*
51-70 y	1,200*	**700**	**420**	10*	4*	**1.2**	**1.3**	**16**	**1.7**	**400**	**2.4[g]**	5*	30*	550*
> 70 y	1,200*	**700**	**420**	15*	4*	**1.2**	**1.3**	**16**	**1.7**	**400**	**2.4[g]**	5*	30*	550*
Females														
9-13 y	1,300*	**1,250**	**240**	5*	2*	**0.9**	**0.9**	**12**	**1.0**	**300**	**1.8**	4*	20*	375*
14-18 y	1,300*	**1,250**	**360**	5*	3*	**1.0**	**1.0**	**14**	**1.2**	**400[h]**	**2.4**	5*	25*	400*
19-30 y	1,000*	**700**	**310**	5*	3*	**1.1**	**1.1**	**14**	**1.3**	**400[h]**	**2.4**	5*	30*	425*
31-50 y	1,000*	**700**	**320**	5*	3*	**1.1**	**1.1**	**14**	**1.3**	**400[h]**	**2.4**	5*	30*	425*
51-70 y	1,200*	**700**	**320**	10*	3*	**1.1**	**1.1**	**14**	**1.5**	**400**	**2.4[g]**	5*	30*	425*
> 70 y	1,200*	**700**	**320**	15*	3*	**1.1**	**1.1**	**14**	**1.5**	**400**	**2.4[g]**	5*	30*	425*
Pregnancy														
≤ 18 y	1,300*	**1,250**	**400**	5*	3*	**1.4**	**1.4**	**18**	**1.9**	**600[i]**	**2.6**	6*	30*	450*
19-30 y	1,000*	**700**	**350**	5*	3*	**1.4**	**1.4**	**18**	**1.9**	**600[i]**	**2.6**	6*	30*	450*
31-50 y	1,000*	**700**	**360**	5*	3*	**1.4**	**1.4**	**18**	**1.9**	**600[i]**	**2.6**	6*	30*	450*
Lactation														
≤ 18 y	1,300*	**1,250**	**360**	5*	3*	**1.5**	**1.6**	**17**	**2.0**	**500**	**2.8**	7*	35*	550*
19-30 y	1,000*	**700**	**310**	5*	3*	**1.5**	**1.6**	**17**	**2.0**	**500**	**2.8**	7*	35*	550*
31-50 y	1,000*	**700**	**320**	5*	3*	**1.5**	**1.6**	**17**	**2.0**	**500**	**2.8**	7*	35*	550*

[a] Recommended Dietary Allowances (RDAs) are presented in bold type and Adequate Intakes (AIs) in ordinary type followed by an asterisk (*). RDAs and AIs may both be used as goals for individual intake. RDAs are set to meet the needs of almost all (97% to 98%) individuals in a group. For healthy breast-fed infants, the AI is the mean intake. The AI for other life-stage and gender groups is believed to cover needs of all individuals in the group, but lack of data or uncertainty in the data prevent being able to specify with confidence the percentage of persons covered by this intake. Source: The National Academy of Sciences. © 1998.
[b] As cholecalciferol. 1 µg cholecalciferol = 40 IU vitamin D. [c] In the absence of adequate exposure to sunlight.
[d] As niacin equivalents (NE). 1 mg niacin = 60 mg tryptophan; 0 to 6 mo = preformed niacin (not NE).
[e] As dietary folate equivalent (DFE). 1 DFE = 1 µg food folate = 0.6 µg folic acid (from fortified food or supplement) consumed with food = 0.5 µg synthetic (supplemental) folic acid taken on an empty stomach.
[f] Although AIs have been set for choline, there are few data to assess whether a dietary supply of choline is needed at all stages of the life cycle, and it may be that the choline requirement can be met by endogenous synthesis at some of these stages. [g] Because 10% to 30% of older people may malabsorb food-bound vitamin B-12, it is advisable for those older than 50 years to meet their RDA mainly by consuming foods fortified with vitamin B-12 or a supplement containing vitamin B-12. [h] In view of evidence linking folate intake with neural tube defects in the fetus, it is recommended that all women capable of becoming pregnant consume 400 µg synthetic folic acid from fortified foods and/or supplements in addition to intake of food folate from a varied diet. [i] It is assumed that women will continue consuming 400 µg folic acid until their pregnancy is confirmed and they enter prenatal care, which ordinarily occurs after the end of the periconceptional period – the critical time for formation of the neural tube.

Yates, A., Schlicker, S., Suitor, C. Dietary Reference Intakes: The new basis for recommendations for calcium and related nutrients, B vitamins, and choline. Copyright, The American Dietetic Association. Reprinted with permission from JOURNAL OF THE AMERICAN DIETETIC ASSOCIATION, 1998, Vol. 98, 699-706.

Table 2.3 Food and Nutrition Board, Institute of Medicine—National Academy of Sciences—Dietary Reference Intakes: Recommended

Table 2. 4 Tolerable Upper Intake Levels[a] (ULs) for certain nutrients[b]

Life-Stage Group	Calcium (g/d)	Phosphorus (g/d)	Magnesium[c] (mg/d)	Vitamin D (μg/d)	Fluoride (mg/d)	Niacin[d] (mg/d)	Vitamin B6 (mg/d)	Synthetic Folic Acid[d] (μg/d)	Choline (g/d)
0–6 mo	ND[e]	ND	ND	25	0.7	ND	ND	ND	ND
7–12 mo	ND	ND	ND	25	0.9	ND	ND	ND	ND
1–3 y	2.5	3	65	50	1.3	10	30	300	1.0
4–8 y	2.5	3	110	50	2.2	15	40	400	1.0
9–13 y	2.5	4	350	50	10	20	60	600	2.0
14–18 y	2.5	4	350	50	10	30	80	800	3.0
19–70 y	2.5	4	350	50	10	35	100	1000	3.5
> 70 y	2.5	3	350	50	10	35	100	1000	3.5

Yates, A., Schlicker, S., Suitor, C. Dietary Reference Intakes: The new basis for recommendations for calcium and related nutrients, B vitamins, and choline. Copyright, The American Dietetic Association. Reprinted with permission from *JOURNAL OF THE AMERICAN DIETETIC ASSOCIATION*, 1998, Vol. 98, 699-706.

F. Nutrient Supplementation

Most experts agree that a pregnant woman can obtain the recommended amounts of most nutrients, with the exception of iron, to support pregnancy by consuming a nutritious diet alone[84] but many do not.[119] Consequently, it is not surprising that as many as 90% of women in the United States take prenatal vitamin and mineral supplements during pregnancy.[84] Keen and Zidenberg-Cherr[120] have identified some potential benefits of vitamin and mineral supplementation during pregnancy, which include a reduced risk of selected birth defects, improved immune systems, and an improved nutrient intake.[120] On the other hand, concerns have been raised about the use of such supplements.[120] For example, individuals might assume that if they take a supplement, they don't need to worry about eating a healthy diet, leading to a reduction in the intakes of food with potential disease-preventing properties beyond the recognized vitamins and minerals. Another concern is that vitamin- and mineral-supplement usage could lead to excessive intakes of some nutrients, resulting in toxicities, birth defects, or reduced absorption of competing nutrients.[120]

G. Nutrient Needs — General Recommendations

Any woman who is contemplating pregnancy should visit with her health care provider and adopt nutritious dietary habits prior to conception to help ensure the delivery of a normal, healthy infant.[84] Given the published reports linking folic acid deficiency with neural tube defects [121–123] women of childbearing age, regardless of their plans for pregnancy, are encouraged to consume an additional 400 micrograms of synthetic folic acid either through the use of a supplement or the inclusion of fortified foods.[111] Synthetic folic acid appears to be absorbed in greater amounts than the folate naturally found in foods.[111] Since not all pregnancies are planned, adhering to these recommendations is likely not possible for all women.

Recommendations of the B-vitamins, thiamin, niacin, and riboflavin are tied to energy intake.[16] Consequently, an increase in energy needs would result in an increased need for these nutrients. However, in the United States, deficiencies of these nutrients are not common due, at least in part, to the enrichment of specific foods.[16] A woman who increases her caloric intake will most likely consume adequate amounts of these nutrients necessary for proper energy metabolism. If iron deficiency anemia is present, then supplemental iron will often be necessary. In male athletes, particularly distance runners, iron deficiency has been observed and may be due to a number of factors including increased iron loss in sweat and urine, gastrointestinal blood loss, and poor iron absorption.[124] Whether this holds true for females is unclear, but it does raise the possibility that some pregnant athletes might require more iron than their sedentary counterparts, especially if they continue to participate in endurance-type activities.

Table 2.5 Functions and Food Sources of Selected Vitamins and Minerals

Nutrient	Functions/Significance	Food Sources
Vitamin A	vision (photochemical reactions with rhodopsin) cellular growth and differentiation aids in glycoprotein synthesis antioxidant (vitamin A precursor beta-carotene)	preformed vitamin A (retinol) is found in liver, fortified milk and margarine, cheese, butter, cream and eggs. Beta-carotene is found in dark green leafy vegetables (spinach), broccoli, cantaloupe, carrots, sweet potatoes, and pumpkin
Vitamin B_6	component of the coenzymes pyridoxal phosphate and pyridoxamine phosphate which are utilized in the metabolism of amino acids and fatty acids; required for erythrocyte, immune, and hormonal functions; some speculation that it may be beneficial in relieving nausea and vomiting, although most research suggests otherwise	whole grains, legumes, green and leafy vegetables, potatoes, bananas, watermelon, chicken, meat, and fish
Folate	component of the coenzymes tetrahydrofolate (THF) and dihydrofolate (DHF), which are needed for DNA synthesis; plays a vital role in the formation of new cells; during pregnancy, there is evidence of a link to neural tube defects	dark green leafy vegetables (spinach), broccoli, asparagus, okra, legumes (beans and peas), seeds, and fortified foods
Vitamin C	antioxidant; plays role in collagen synthesis (a component important for wound healing, bone growth and the walls of blood vessels); aids in thyroxin synthesis, the metabolism of amino acids, and immune responses; aids in iron absorption	spinach, broccoli, sweet potatoes, tomatoes, red bell peppers, orange, grapefruit, kiwi fruit, mango, strawberries, and watermelon
Vitamin D	required for the formation of the skeleton (increases calcium absorption); essential for mineral homeostasis	eggs (yolk), butter, fortified milk and margarine, liver, fatty fish; with sunlight, vitamin is synthesized by the body from cholesterol
Vitamin E	antioxidant; helps stabilize cell membranes	vegetable oils and products made from them (margarine, salad dressing, shortening), egg yolks, nuts, seeds, liver
Calcium	major mineral in bones and teeth; also needed for muscle contraction and relaxation, blood clotting, and nerve conduction	dairy products (milk, cheese, yogurt), tofu, sardines with bones, broccoli, spinach, bok choy (Chinese cabbage), chard (cooked), and fortified foods
Iron	component of hemoglobin and myoglobin, (oxygen transport); component of the electron-transport-chain (energy production)	meat, fish, poultry, eggs, legumes, whole grains and enriched breads and cereals, dried fruits, dark greens; heme iron found in the flesh of meat, poultry, and fish is absorbed more readily than nonheme iron, which includes vegetables, fruits, grains, and eggs; vitamin C increases the absorption of nonheme iron
Zinc	component of numerous enzymes including those that function in nucleic acid and protein metabolism; functions in immune reactions, wound healing, vitamin A transport, taste perception, and spermatogenesis	meat, poultry, liver, eggs, seafood; lesser amounts in whole grains
Magnesium	essential for all biosynthetic processes, energy formation, nerve impulse transmission, muscle contraction, and bone mineralization	nuts, legumes, unmilled grains, halibut; lesser amounts found in vegetables, seafood, chocolate, yogurt, milk, and bananas

Women who exercise during pregnancy should consume diets that are rich in complex carbohydrates to replace muscle glycogen lost and ensure an adequate energy supply for the fetus.[46] Daily protein needs are increased during pregnancy by approximately 10 grams and that requirement may be higher among women who continue their exercise regimens during pregnancy.[125] For women in the U.S., this should not be a serious concern, since protein intake tends to exceed recommended amounts.[16,124] Good sources of protein include eggs; meat; fish and shellfish; dairy products such as milk, cheese, and yogurt; and legumes.

A sedentary pregnant woman needs to consume a minimum of 8 cups (1.9 L) of fluids daily.[125] More fluid is needed if the woman participates in physical activities. During exercise, a pregnant woman should consume at least 4 to 8 ounces (120 to 240 ml) of a rapidly absorbed fluid such as water or sports beverage every 15 minutes.[125]

With respect to the remaining nutrients, there is no conclusive evidence to suggest that pregnant women who continue to exercise during pregnancy will have higher nutritional needs than their more sedentary counterparts as a result of their exercise regimen.

Regardless of their activity level, women who do not consume calcium-rich foods, whether due to lactose intolerance or for other reasons, can benefit from calcium supplementation to reduce maternal calcium losses, especially during the last trimester when the fetal skeleton is forming.[126] However, consuming megadoses of vitamin and mineral supplements may reduce the absorption of other nutrients and, in the case of vitamins A and D, may cause more harm than good to the developing fetus.[84] For this reason, pregnant women should refrain from consuming levels of calcium, phosphorus, magnesium, vitamin D, fluoride, niacin, vitamin B_6, synthetic folic acid and choline in excess of the UL (Table 2.4).[111] If there is any doubt as to the adequacy of the maternal diet, a prenatal vitamin and mineral supplement can help ensure that sufficient amounts of nutrients are consumed. Supplements, however, are no substitute for a nutritious diet.

H. Non-Nutrients — Caffeine and Alcohol

Caffeine and alcohol are viewed as sources of fluid by some individuals, but caffeine intake has been associated with intrauterine growth retardation[127,128] and reduced infant birth weight.[129,130] Cook and others[131] found that caffeine intake was inversely related to infant birth weight only in the presence of smokers, but this could be related to the finding that smokers consumed more caffeine than nonsmokers. Other studies have no reported adverse side effects when caffeine is consumed in moderation.[132,133] Because safe levels of caffeine consumption have not been determined, it is prudent for pregnant women to consume caffeine in moderation, if at all. Alcohol should also be avoided completely because of its adverse effects, including fetal alcohol syndrome, on the fetus.[134–136]

I. Ergogenic Aids

In some situations, athletes may use more than just vitamin and mineral supplements,[137] although the extent of this among female athletes is not known. A female athlete should fully disclose to her physician or health care provider all supplements being used, including multivitamins and minerals and ergogenic aids — preferably before conception or, at the very latest, during the first prenatal visit. Any doubt about a supplement's safety during pregnancy should result in its immediate discontinuation.

VI. EXERCISE DURING LACTATION

Although published research is limited, there is evidence that suggests that resuming or beginning physical activity 6 to 8 weeks postpartum may improve maternal cardiovascular fitness.[138]

Lovelady and colleagues [138] randomly assigned 33 sedentary, healthy, nonsmoking women, 6 weeks postpartum, to either a control (n = 15) or an exercising group (n =18). Both groups of women exclusively breastfed their infants during the study period. Subjects in the exercise group participated in self-selected aerobic exercises (walking, jogging, biking) and increased their length of exercise from 20 minutes up to 45 minutes for an average of 4.5 times per week for 12 weeks. Heart rate, $V0_{2max}$ dietary intake, body composition, and metabolic response to a meal also were assessed during the study period, which lasted 20 weeks post partum. At the end of the study period, the women in the exercise group demonstrated a significantly improved $V0_{2max,}$ suggesting an improvement in cardiovascular fitness. Women who exercised consumed more energy, but also expended more energy. All subjects reduced weight and body fat, but there were no significant differences between the two groups, suggesting that exercise alone is probably not sufficient to achieve weight loss during lactation. [138]

A. Effect of Exercise on Milk Quantity

Human milk is believed by experts to be nutritionally complete for infants during their first 6 months of life, provided that the woman is healthy and well-nourished.[139] Women who desire to nurse their infants may want to resume their previous regimens of physical activity but may be concerned that exercise might affect the quality or quantity of breast milk. In early studies investigating the effects of exercise on the reproductive outcome and production of milk among dairy heifers, researchers found that heifers exercised prior to and for 10 days following parturition produced significantly less milk than controls.[140] In a second trial, however, heifers that were exercised following parturition demonstrated a significant increase in milk production as well as feed efficiency in comparison with controls that were not exercised.[140] In humans, lactating women who exercise at maximum intensities have been shown to significantly increase the lactic acid (LA) concentration in breast milk both 10 and 30 minutes after the exercise has ended.[141] Lactic acid produces a sour taste[142], and a significant inverse correlation has been reported between LA concentration in the breast milk and the mother's perception of how readily her infant accepted the breast milk.[141] There does not appear to be a consistent pattern to the noted increase in LA[141] and some research[143] suggests that the level of LA concentration in breast milk may be influenced more by the state of fullness of milk in the breast than by the level of exercise intensity. Carey and others[144] also reported that exercising at maximum intensity increases the LA content of breast milk, but moderate levels of activity do not.[144,145] These early studies have raised the concern that exercising at high intensities might result in reduced milk quantity or quality but subsequent studies in animals[146] and humans [147–150] have not validated this concern. Dewey et al. [147] compared milk volume and composition between a group of sedentary women, and women who participated in aerobic exercise for up to 20 weeks postpartum. Protein concentration was higher in the breast milk of women in the exercise groups; otherwise, there were no significant differences in milk composition (lipid, lactose, and energy density) between the two groups.[147] In addition, there was no significant differences between the study groups with respect to the amount of breast milk consumed by the infants, the energy output in the breast milk, or in the body weight of the infants during the study period.[147] Fly et al.[148] found that maximal exercise did not affect breast-milk concentrations of calcium, phosphorus, potassium, magnesium, or sodium. These findings, along with others,[149,150] suggest that women can participate in moderate levels of physical activity four or five times a week starting 6 to 8 weeks postpartum without adversely affecting lactation.

B. Exercise and its Effects on Selected Immunological Properties of Breast Milk

Human breast milk contains immunoglobulins that help fight disease. Immunoglobulin A (IgA), the major immunoglobulin isotype found in human milk,[151] is believed to be the first line of defense against most infection-causing agents.[152,153] In a recent study investigating the effects of maximal exercise on IgA concentrations in human milk, Gregory and colleagues[153] found that maximal exercise resulted in a decrease in total milk IgA concentrations 10 and 30 minutes following exercise. Milk IgA levels returned to normal levels within 60 minutes. Interesting was the finding that when the breasts were emptied, IgA concentrations increased in both the exercising and control groups, suggesting that IgA production may be in this manner.[153] Recognizing the previous associations between exercising at maximum intensities and the reported increases in LA concentrations in breast milk, it is possible that the rejection of milk containing LA concentrations might serve as a means to prevent infants from consuming milk that has reduced immune properties.[153] Exercising at a level to reduce LA build-up and discarding breast milk produced during the first 30 minutes following exercise have been suggested as measures that might alleviate this concern.[153]

One cannot ignore findings that maximal exercise might increase the concentration of LA in the milk, decrease immune properties, and possibly decrease an infant's acceptance of the mother's milk. However, typical workouts are usually not at maximal intensity.[154] Furthermore, when exercise is at a moderate level of intensity, the LA concentrations in breast milk will not likely be increased.[144,145] If a woman has concerns that her exercise regimen might influence the acceptance of her milk by her infant, it has been suggested that the mother could nurse prior to exercising or collect her milk prior to exercising and feed it to her infant later.[141] Other experts have stated that problems with an infant's rejecting breast milk due to high LA concentrations following maternal exercise are not common and warn that such recommendations could imply that there are disadvantages to exercising during lactation.[154] This could inadvertently discourage women from breast feeding.[154] The reported changes in breast milk's immunological properties following maximum-intensity exercise are interesting, but they are far from conclusive. Clearly, more research with respect to exercise and its effect on milk composition is needed. However, there does not appear to be any reason that a healthy, well-nourished woman cannot continue to exercise at moderate levels without fear that her milk will be nutritionally inadequate or rejected by her infant.

VII. ENERGY, WEIGHT LOSS, AND NUTRIENT NEEDS FOR WOMEN DURING LACTATION

A. Energy

The energy needs of lactating women are based on several factors including the energy cost of milk production, energy expended during lactation (basal metabolism, diet-induced thermogenesis, and physical activity), and the amount of maternal energy reserves available.[155] Research has estimated that lactating women expend 2100 to 2600 kcal per day.[107,156-158] The amount of additional energy needed by lactating women ranges from 369 to 670 kcal,[155] depending on whether she exclusively breastfeeds her infant and the extent to which she desires to lose body fat acquired during pregnancy. The National Research Council's recommendation of 500 additional kcal per day[16] falls within this suggested range. At the very least, the diets of lactating women should contain 1800 kcal per day,[159] although they may be as high as 2800 kcal.[160] Under no circumstances, should energy intakes be less than 1500 kcal.[159] Presently, there are no clear recommendations for energy targeted toward women who are participating in physical activities during the lactation period.

B. Weight Loss During Lactation — Is It Safe?

Activity levels vary during lactation among women. In addition, the number of well-controlled studies that have investigated the safety of weight loss during lactation are limited. Therefore, it is unrealistic to assign specific energy needs to women who are trying to return to their pre-pregnancy weight.[155] In a short-term (11 days) study using exercise and a 35% reduction in caloric intake, McCrory and colleagues[150] demonstrated that healthy, well-nourished women could safely lose weight without compromising the volume of milk produced provided that the rate of weight loss did not exceed 1 kg per week. Previous studies in humans[161,162] and baboons[163] have found similar findings, although the duration of the McCrory et al. study[150] was shorter than other investigations.[161–163] For women who are initially overweight, weight reduction is thought to be safe provided that the rate of weight loss does not exceed 2 kg per month.[155] Rapid weight loss as well as the use of liquid diets (defined as > 2 kg/month) is not advised.[159] There is very little information on the effects of weight loss among women who are already lean but it is likely that their lactation performance will be decreased if energy intake is restricted.[155]

C. Nutrient Requirements

Like pregnancy, lactation requires an increase in specific nutrients.[16,111] The National Research Council[16] has suggested that protein needs are increased by 15 grams daily, but metabolic studies suggest that the additional needs may be closer to 20 grams.[155] Lactating women who are exercising on a regular basis may require more protein than women who abstain from exercise, but protein needs can be met through diet alone, and should not be a concern for most women. Other nutrients that are increased during lactation, regardless of activity level, include calcium, phosphorus, B-vitamins, vitamin C, zinc, iodine, and selenium.[16,111]

Recommended nutrients for lactation can be met through the consumption of a varied diet. In most cases, vitamin and mineral supplements are not required unless the maternal consumption of key nutrients such as calcium, magnesium, zinc, folate and vitamin B_6 is inadequate.[159]

Lactating women are encouraged to consume adequate amounts of fluids to prevent thirst. Beverages such as milk, juice, water, and soup are excellent sources.[164] Caffeine consumption should be kept to no more than two servings per day; alcohol should be avoided as much as possible, as it does not contribute to successful lactation.[164] For women who are continuing to exercise during lactation, it is probably best to follow hydration guidelines outlined for pregnancy earlier in this chapter. Excessive intakes beyond what is needed to avoid thirst and to compensate for fluids lost during exercise have not been shown to increase milk production and are most likely not indicated.[160]

In a number of studies,[165–168] lactation has been shown to reduce maternal bone mineral density, stimulating an interest as to whether calcium supplements could be of benefit. Exercise has not been proven to be beneficial in retarding bone density loss[169] and the effects of calcium supplementation are inconclusive.[170,171] Presently, intakes of calcium beyond the upper limits of the DRI (Table 2.4) are not advised. Bone mineral density does appear to rebound upon the cessation of lactation.[167,169,171]

VIII. SUMMARY

For healthy women experiencing normal pregnancies, regular exercise is not contraindicated, except under specific circumstances. Women who plan to exercise during pregnancy should discuss their plans with their physician and be aware of both the potential risks and benefits that may be experienced. While athletes may suffer poor performances if dietary intakes are inadequate, the consequences of consuming a poor diet while exercising during pregnancy could be far greater. Clearly, nutrient needs are increased during pregnancy, but most of these needs can be met through the consumption of a well-balanced diet. The exception, recognized by most experts, is iron. A multivitamin and mineral supplement may be necessary during pregnancy, but excessive intake of specific nutrients might be harmful and are not indicated, even for athletes. All supplement use should be discussed with the physician — preferably before conception, since the safety of many supplements during pregnancy is unknown.

Resuming physical activity as soon as 6 weeks postpartum has been shown to be beneficial to women. Although there may be some concern that exercise might alter breast milk production and quality, available research suggests that exercising at moderate intensities will not affect milk production or quality. A limited body of research has shown that weight loss can be achieved in overweight and well-nourished women without compromising lactation, but long-term studies are needed before any conclusions can be made. Athletes who are lean and continuing lactation may compromise milk production if caloric intake is restricted.

As with pregnancy, specific nutrient needs are increased, but not to levels that would require supplementation unless usual dietary intake patterns are shown to be inadequate. Women will likely experience a decrease in bone mineral density during pregnancy, but bone mass will likely rebound when lactation ceases.

REFERENCES

1. Sternfeld, B. Physical activity and pregnancy outcome: review and recommendations, *Sports Med.*, 23,33,1997.
2. Clapp III, J. F., Exercise in pregnancy: good, bad, or indifferent?, in *Current Obstetric Medicine*, volume 2, Lee, R. V., Cotton, D. B., and Barron, W., Eds., Mosby, Chicago, 1993.
3. U.S. Department of Health and Human Services, *Physical activity and health: a report of the Surgeon General*, National Center for Chronic Disease Prevention and Health Promotion, Atlanta, 1996.
4. Clapp III, J. F., The course of labor after endurance exercise during pregnancy, *Am. J. Obstet. Gynecol.*, 163,1799,1990.
5. Bell, R. J., Palma, S. M., Lumley, J. M., The effect of vigorous exercise during pregnancy on birth weight. *Aust. N. Z. Obstet. Gynaecol.*, 35, 46, 1995.
6. Clapp III, J. F., Dickstein, S. Endurance exercise and pregnancy outcome, *Med Sci Sports Exerc*, 16, 556, 1984.
7. Hall, D. C., Kaufmann, D. A., Effects of aerobic and strength conditioning on pregnancy outcomes, *Am. J. Obstet. Gynecol.*, 157, 1199, 1987.
8. Pivarnik, J. M., Potential effects of maternal physical activity on birth weight: brief review. *Med. Sci. Sports. Exerc.*, 30, 400, 1997.
9. Bung, P., Artal, R. Gestational diabetes and exercise: a survey, *Seminars in Perinatology*, 20, 328, 1996.
10. Clapp III J. F., Capeless, E. L., Neonatal morphometrics after endurance exercise during pregnancy, *Am. J. Obstet. Gynecol.* 163, 1605, 1990.
11. Hatch, M. C., Shu, X. O., McLean, D. E., Levin, B., Begg, M., Reuss, L., Susser, M. Maternal exercise during pregnancy, physical fitness, and fetal growth, *Am. J. Epidemiol*, 137, 1105, 1993.
12. Hatch, M., Levin, B., Shu, X. O., Susser, M., Maternal leisure-time exercise and timely delivery, *Am. J. Public Health*, 88, 1528, 1998.
13. Schramm, W. F., Stockbauer, J. W., Hoffman, H. J., Exercise, employment, other daily activities, and adverse pregnancy outcomes, *Am. J. Epidemiol.*, 143,211,1996.
14. Tafari, N., Naeye, R. L., Gobzie, A., Effects of maternal undernutrition and heavy physical work during pregnancy on birth weight, *Br. J. Obstet Gynaecol.*, 87, 222 1980.
15. Prentice, A., Should lactating women exercise? *Nutr. Rev.*, 52, 358, 1994.
16. Food and Nutrition Board, *Recommended Dietary Allowances,* 10th ed., National Academy Press, Washington, DC, 1989.
17. Guyton, A.C., *Textbook of Medical Physiology*, 8th ed., W. B. Saunders, Philadelphia, 1991.
18. Margolis, R. S., Exercise and pregnancy. *Maryland Medical Journal*, 45, 637, 1996.
19. Wolfe, L. A., Brenner, I. K. M., Mottola, M. F., Maternal exercise, fetal well-being and pregnancy outcome, in *Exercise and Sport Sciences Reviews*, volume 22, Holloszy, J. O., Ed., 1994, pp. 145-194.
20. Bell, R., O'Neill, M., Exercise and pregnancy: a review, *Birth*, 21, 85, 1994.
21. Pivarnik, J. M., Cardiovascular responses to aerobic exercise during pregnancy and post partum. *Semin. Perinat.*, 20, 242, 1996.
22. McMurray, R. G., Mottola, M. F., Wolfe, L. A., Artal, R., Millar, L., Pivarnik, M. M., Recent advances in understanding maternal and fetal responses to exercise, *Med. Sci. Sports Exerc.*, 25, 1305, 1993.
23. Wolfe, L. A., Mottola, M. F., Aerobic exercise in pregnancy: an update. *Can. J. Appl. Physiol.*, 18, 119, 1993.

24. Morris, N., Osborn, S., Wright, H. et al. Effective uterine blood flow during exercise in normal and pre-eclamptic pregnancies, *Lancet*, 271, 481, 1956.
25. Rauramo, I., Forss, M., Effect of exercise on maternal hemodynamics and placental blood flow in healthy women, *Acta. Obstet. Gynecol. Scand.*, 67, 271, 1988.
26. Anderson, T. D., Exercise and sport in pregnancy, *Midwife Health Visit Commun. Nurse*, 22, 275, 1986.
27. Morton, M. J., Paul, M. S., Metcalfe, J., Exercise during pregnancy, *Med. Clin. North Am*, 69, 97, 1985.
28. Winder, W. W., Hickson, R. C., Hagberg, J.M., Ehsani A., A., McLane J. A., Training-induced changes in hormonal and metabolic responses to submaximal exercise, *J. Appl. Physiol.*, 45,766,1979.
29. Jackson, M. R., Gott, P., Lye, S. J., Ritchie, J. W., Clapp III, J. F., The effects of maternal aerobic exercise on human placental development: placental volumetric composition and surface areas. *Placenta*, 16, 179, 1995.
30. Clapp III, J. F., Rizk, K. H., Effect of recreational exercise on midtrimester placental growth, *Am J. Obstet. Gynecol.*, 167, 1518, 1990.
31. Snyder, J. L., Aerobic exercise during pregnancy, *J. Am. Board. Fam. Pract.*, 3, 50, 1990.
32. Dreiling, C. E., Carman, F. S., Brown, D. E., Maternal endocrine and fetal responses to heat stress, *J. Dairy Sci.*, 74, 312, 1991.
33. Mottola, M. F., Fitzgerald, H. M., Wilson, N. C., Taylor, A. W., Effect of water temperature on exercise-induced maternal hyperthermia on fetal development in rats, *Int. J. Sports. Med.*, 14, 248, 1993.
34. Chernoff, G. F., Golden, J. A., Hyperthermia-induced exencephaly in mice: effect of multiple exposures, *Teratology*, 37, 37, 1988.
35. Edwards, M. J., Hyperthermia as a teratoagen, *Teratogenesis Carcinog Mutagen.*, 6, 563, 1986.
36. Milunsky, A., Ulcickas, M., Rothman, K. J., Willett, W., Jick, S. S., Jick, H., Maternal heat exposure and neural tube defects, *JAMA*, 268, 882, 1991.
37. Harvey M. A. S., McRorie, M. M., Smith, D. W., Suggested limits to the use of hot tubs and saunas by pregnant women, *Can. Med. Assoc. J.*, 125, 50, 1981.
38. Miller, P., Smith, D. W., Shepard, T. H., Maternal hyperthermia as a possible cause of anencephaly, *Lancet*, 1, 519, 1978.
39. Shiota, K., Neural tube defects and maternal hyperthermia in early pregnancy. Epidemiology in a human embryonic population, *Am J. Med. Genet.*, 12, 281, 1982.
40. Lotgering, F. K., Gilbert, R. D., Longo, L. D., The interactions of exercise and pregnancy: a review. *Am. J. Obstet. Gynecol.*, 149, 560, 1984.
41. Jones R. J., Botti, J., Anderson, W. M., Bennett, N. L., Thermoregulation during aerobic exercise in pregnancy, *Obstet. Gynecol.*, 65, 340, 1985.
42. Hauth, J. C., Gilstrap III, L. C., Widmer, L., Fetal heart rate reactivity before and after maternal jogging during the third trimester, *Am. J. Obstet. Gynecol.* 142, 545, 1982.
43. Artal-Mittlemark R., Posner, M. D., Fetal responses to maternal exercise, in: *Exercise in Pregnancy* 2nd ed., Artal-Mittlemark, R, Wiswell, A., Drinkwater, B. L., Eds. Williams and Wilkins, Baltimore, 1991, pp 213-224.
44. Artal R., Rutherford S., Romen, Y., Kammula, R. K., Dorey, F. J., Wiswell, R. A. Fetal heart rate responses to maternal exercise, *Am. J. Obstet. Gynecol.*, 155, 729, 1986.
45. Clarren, S. K., Smith, D. W., Harvey, M. A. S., Hyperthermia: a prospective evaluation of a possible teratoagenic agent in man, *J. Pediatr.* 95, 81, 1979.
46. Artal, R., Exercise and pregnancy, *Clin. Sports Med.*, 11, 363, 1992.
47. Jones C. T., Control of glucose metabolism in the perinatal period, *J. Dev. Physiol.* 15, 81, 1991.
48. Zaidise I., Artal, R., Bessman, S. P., Fuel metabolism in pregnancy, In: *Exercise in Pregnancy*, Artal, R. Wiswell R.A., Eds., Williams and Wilkins, Baltimore, 1986, pp. 83-98.
49. Falk, P. Body fuel metabolism and diabetes mellitus in pregnancy, *Med. Clin. North Am.*, 61, 43, 1977.
50. Kretchmer, N., Zimmerman, M. *Developmental Nutrition*, Allyn and Bacon, Needham Heights, MA, 1997, chapter 2.
51. Bonen A., Campagna, P., Gilchrist, L. Young, D., Beresford, P., Substrate and endocrine responses during exercise at selected stages of pregnancy, *J. Appl, Physiol.*, 73, 134, 1992.
52. Clapp III, J. F., Wesley, M., Sleamaker, R. H., Thermoregularory and metabolic responses prior to and during pregnancy, *Med. Sci. Sports Exerc.*, 19, 124, 1987.
53. Clapp III, J. F., Capeless, E. L., The changing glycemic response to exercise during pregnancy, *Am. J. Obstet. Gynecol.*, 165, 1678, 1991.

54. Treadway, J. L., Young, J. C., Decreased glucose uptake in the fetus after maternal exercise, *Med. Sci. Sports Exerc.*, 21, 140, 1989.
55. Mottola, M. F., Mezzapelli, J., Schachter, L. L., McKenzie, K., Training effects on maternal and fetal glucose uptake following acute exercise in the rat., *Med. Sci. Sports Exerc.*, 25, 841, 12993.
56. Jarski, R. W., Trippett, D. L., The risks and benefits of exercise during pregnancy, *J. Fam. Pract.*, 30, 185, 1990.
57. Carpenter, M. W., Sady, S. B., Hoegsberag, B., Sady, M. A., Haydon, B., Cullinane, E. M., Coustan, D. R., Thompson, P. D., Fetal response to maternal exertion, *JAMA*, 259, 3006, 1988.
58. Dale E., Mullinax, M. Bryan, D. H., Exercise during pregnancy: effects on the fetus, *Can. J. Appl. Sport Sci.*, 7,98,1982.
59. Brenner, I. K. M., Wolfe, L. A., Monga, M. Dumas, G. A., McGrath, M. J., *Effects of Maternal Exercise and Physical Conditioning on Fetal Well-Being*. Proceedings of the International Conference on Physical Activity, Fitness and Health. May 10-13, Toronto, 1992.
60. Katz, W.V. L., McMurray, R., Goodwin, W. E., and Cefalo, R. C., Non-weight-bearing exercise during pregnancy on land and during immersion: a comparative study. *Am. J. Perinatol.* 7, 281, 1990.
61. Sorensen, K. E., Borlum, K., Heart function in response to short-term maternal exercise, *Br. J. Obstet. Gynaecol.*, 93, 310, 1986.
62. Sternfeld, B., Quesenberry, C. P. J., Eskenazi, B., Newman, L. A., Exercise during pregnancy and pregnancy outcome, *Med. Sci. Sports Exerc.* 27, 634, 1995.
63. Webb, K. A., Wolfe, L. A., McGrath, M. J., Effects of acute and chronic maternal exercise on fetal heart rate, *J. Appl. Physiol.*, 77, 22207, 1994.
64. Stevenson, L., Exercise in pregnancy. Part 1: Update on pathophysiology, *Can. Fam. Physician*, 43, 97, 1997.
65. McCormick, M. C., The contribution of low birth weight to infant mortality and childhood morbidity, *N. Engl. J. Med.*, 312, 82, 1985.
66. Treadway, J., Dover, E. V., Morse, W., Newcomer, L., Craig, B. W., Influence of exercise training on maternal and fetal morphological characteristics in the rat, *J. Appl. Physiol.*, 60, 1700, 1986.
67. Piccaro, I. C., Turecki, G. X., Barros-Neto, T. L., Russo, A. K., Silva, A. C., Tarasantchi, J., Effect of exercise training during pregnancy: maternal and fetal responses of the rat, *Braz. J. Med. Biol. Res.*, 22, 1535, 1989.
68. Mottola, M. F., Bagnall, K. M., Belcastro, A. N., Effects of strenuous maternal exercise on fetal organ weights and skeletal muscle development in rats, *J. Dev. Physiol.*, 11, 111, 1989.
69. Courant, G. T., Barr, S. I., Exercise during rat pregnancy and lactation: maternal effects and offspring growth, *Physiol. Behav.*, 47, 427, 1990.
70. Jones, M. T., Norton, K. I., Black, D. M., Graham, R. E., Armstrong, R. B., Effect of regular voluntary exercise on resting cardiovascular responses in SHR and WKY pregnancy rats, *J. Appl. Physiol.*, 73, 713, 1992.
71. Clapp III, J. F., Little K. D., The interaction between regular exercise and selected aspects of women's health, *Am. J. Obstet. Gynecol.*, 173, 2, 1995.
72. Lokey E. A., Tran, Z. V., Wells, C. L., Myers, B. C., Tran A. C., Effects of physical exercise on pregnancy outcomes: a meta-analytic review, *Med. Sci. Sports Exerc.*, 23, 1234, 1991.
73. Wang, T. W., Apgar, B. S., Exercise during pregnancy, *Am. Fam. Phys.*, 57, 1846, 1998.
74. Sherer, D. M., Schenker, J. G., Accidental injury during pregnancy, *Obstet. Gynecol. Surv.*, 44, 330, 1989.
75. McNitt-Gray, J. L., Biomechanics related to exercise in pregnancy, in: *Exercise in Pregnancy*, Mittlemark R. A., Wiswell, R. A., Drinkwater, B. L., Eds. Williams and Wilkins, Baltimore, 1991, pp. 133-140.
76. Artal R., Hormonal responses to exercise in pregnancy, in: *Exercise in Pregnancy*, Artal R., Wiswell, R. A., Eds., Williams and Wilkins, Baltimore, 1986, pp 139-146.
77. Rauramo, I., Andersson, B., Laatikainen, T., Pettersson, J., Stress hormones and placental steroids in physical exercise during pregnancy, *Br. J. Obstet. Gynecol.*, 89, 921, 1982.
78. Durak, E. P., Jovanovic-Peterson L., Peterson, C. M., Comparative evaluation of uterine response to exercise on five aerobic machines, *Am. J. Obstet. Gynecol.*, 162, 754, 1990.
79. Grisso, J. A., Main, D. M., Chiu G., Synder, E. S., Holmes, J. H., Effects of physical activity and life-style factors on uterine contraction frequency, *Am. J. Perinat.* 9, 489, 1992.

80. Veille, J. C., Hohimer, A. R., Burry, K., Speroff, L., The effect of exercise on uterine activity in the last eight weeks of pregnancy, *Am. J. Obstet. Gynecol.*, 151, 727, 1985.
81. McArdle, W. D., Katch, F. I., Katch, V. L. *Exercise Physiology: Energy, Nutrition, and Human Performance,* 4th ed., Williams and Wilkins, Baltimore, 1996.
82. Snow-Harter, C., Marcus, R., Exercise, bone mineral density, and osteoporosis, *Exerc. Sports Sci. Rev.*, 19, 351, 1991.
83. Clapp III, J. F., Little, K. D., Effect of recreational exercise on pregnancy weight gain and subcutaneous fat deposition, *Med. Sci. Sports. Exerc.,* 27, 170, 1995.
84. Institute of Medicine, *Nutrition During Pregnancy, Part 1: Weight Gain*, National Academy Press, Washington, DC, 1990.
85. Naeye, R. L., Peters, E. C., Working during pregnancy: effects on the fetus, *Pediatrics*, 69, 724, 1982.
86. Magee, M. S., Walden, C. E., Benedetti, T. J., Influence of diagnostic criteria on the incidence of gestational diabetes and perinatal morbidity, *JAMA,* 270, 1993.
87. Horns, P. N., Leggett, J. C., Pregnancy outcomes among active and sedentary primiparous women, *J. Obstet. Gynecol. Neonatal Nurs.*, 25, 49, 1996.
88. Wolfe L. A., Hall, P., Webb, K. A., Goodman, L., Monga, M., McGrath, M. J., Prescription of aerobic exercise during pregnancy, *Sports Med.*, 8, 273, 1989.
89. Clapp III, J. F., Rokey R, Treadway, J. L., Carpenter, M. W., Artal, R. M., Warrnes, C., Exercise in pregnancy, *Med. Sci. Sports Exerc.* 24, S2294, 1992.
90. Rice, P. L., Fort, I. L., The relationship of maternal exercise on labor, delivery, and health of the newborn, *J. Sports Med. Phys. Fitness.*, 31, 95, 1991.
91. Pomerance, J. J., Gluck, L., Lynch, V. A., Physical fitness in pregnancy: its effect on pregnancy outcome, *Am. J. Obstet. Gynecol.*, 119, 867, 1974.
92. Erkkola, R., The physical work capacity of the expectant mother and its effect on pregnancy, labor, and the newborn, *Int. J. Gynaecol. Obstet.*, 14, 153, 1976.
93. Zaharieva, E., Olympic participation by women: effects on pregnancy and childbirth, *JAMA*, 221, 992, 1972.
94. Dibblee, L., Graham, T. E., A longitudinal study of changes in aerobic fitness, body composition and energy intake in primigravid patients, *Am. J. Obstet. Gynecol.*, 147, 908, 1983.
95. Wong, S. C., McKenzie, D. C., Cardiorespiratory fitness during pregnancy and its effect on outcome, *Int. J. Sports Med.*, 8, 79, 1987.
96. Collins, C. A., Curet, L. B., Mullin, J. P., Maternal and fetal responses to a maternal aerobic exercise program, *Am. J. Obstet. Gynecol.*, 145, 702,1983.
97. Fishbein, E. G., Phillips, M., How safe is exercise duriang pregnancy? *J. Obstet. Gynecol. Neonatal Nurs*, 19, 45, 1990.
98. Stevenson L., Exercise in pregnancy. Part 2: recommendations for individuals*, Can. Fam. Physician*, 43, 107, 1997.
99. The American College of Obstetricians and Gynecologists*, Exercise During Pregnancy and The Postpartum Period*, Technical Bulletin #189, ACOG, Washington, DC, 1994.
100. Lee, R. D., Nieman, D. C., Nutritional Assessment, Wm. C. Brown, Dubuque, 1993.
101. Hytten, F. E., Leitch, I., *The Physiology of Human Pregnancy,* 2nd ed., Blackwell Scientific Publications, Oxford, 1971.
102. Hytten, F. E., Chamberlain, G. V. P., *Clinical Physiology in Obstetrics*, Blackwell Scientific Publications, Oxford, 1980.
103. Durnin J. V. G. A., Energy requirements of pregnancy, *Acta. Paediatr. Scand. Suppl.* 373, 33, 1991.
104. Durnin J. V., Energy requirements in human pregnancy, in human nutrition and parasitic infection, *Parasitology*, 107, S169,1993.
105. Prentice, A. M., Spaaig, C. J., Goldberg, G. R., Poppitt, S. D., van Raaij, J. M., Totton, M., Swann, D., Black, A. E., Energy requirements of pregnant and lactating women, *Eur. J. Clin. Nutr.*, 50, S82, 1996.
106. Black A. E., Wiles, S. J., Paul, A. A. The nutrient intakes of pregnant and lactating mothers of good socioeconomic status in Cambridge, UK: some implications for recommended daily allowances of minor nutrients, *J. Nutr.*, 56, 59, 1986.

107. Goldberg, G. R., Prentice, A. M., Coward, W. A., Davies, H. L., Murgatroyd, P. R., Sawyer, M. B., Ashford, J., Black, A. E., Longitudinal assessment of the components of energy balance in well-nourished lactating women. *Am. J. Clin. Nutr.* 54, 788, 1991.
108. King J. C., Cohenour, S. H., Calloway, D. H., Jacobson, H. N., Assessment of nutritional status of pregnant girls. I. Nutrient intake and pregnancy, *Am. J. Clin. Nutr.* 25, 916, 1972.
109. Nutrition During Pregnancy. ACOG Technical Bulletin Number 179, April 1993, *Int. J. Gynaecol. Obstet.*, 43, 67, 1993.
110. Allen, L. H., Hautvast, J. G. A. J., Prentice, A. M., Report of the working group on energy requirements for pregnancy and lactation, *Eur. J. Clin. Nutr.*, 50, S190, 1996.
111. Yates, A. A., Schlicker, S. A., Suitor, C. W., Dietary Reference Intakes: The new basis for recommendations for calcium and related nutrients, B vitamins, and choline. *J. Am. Diet. Assoc.*, 98, 699, 1998.
112. Block, G., Abrams, B., Vitamin and mineral status of women of childbearing potential, *Ann. N. Y. Acad. Sci.*, 678, 244, 1993.
113. McKenzie-Parnell, J. M., Wilson, P. D., Parnell, W. R., Spears, G. F., Robinson, M. F., Nutrient intake of Dunedin women curing pregnancy, *N. Z. Med. J.* 106, 273, 1993.
114. Huddle, J. M., Gibson, R. S., Cullinan, T. R., Is zinc a limiting nutrient in the diets of rural pregnant Malawian women? *Br. J. Nutr.*, 79, 257, 1998.
115. Rogers, I., Emmett, P., Diet during pregnancy in a population of pregnant women in southwest England. ALSPAC Study Team. Avon Longitudinal Study of Pregnancy and Childhood, *Eur. J. Clin. Nutr.* 52, 246, 1998.
116. Erkkola, M., Karppinen, M., Jarvinen, A., Knip, M., Virtanen, S. M., Folate vitamin D and iron intakes are low among pregnant Finnish women, *Eur. J. Clin. Nutr.* 52, 742, 1998.
117. Panwar, B., Punia, D., Nutrient intake of rural pregnant women of Haryana State, northern India: relationship between income and education. *Int. J. Food Sci. Nutr.*, 49, 391, 1998.
118. Wolinsky, I. Ed. *Nutrition in Exercise and Sport,* 3rd. ed., CRC Press, Boca Raton, 1998.
119. Menard, M. K., Vitamin and mineral supplement prior to and during pregnancy, *Obstetrics and Gynecology Clinics of North America*, 24, 479, 1997.
120. Keen, C. L., Zidenberg-Cherr, S. Should vitamin-mineral supplements be recommended for all women with childbearing potential? *Am. J. Clin. Nutr.*, 59, 532S, 1994.
121. Eskes, T. K., Folates and the fetus, *Eur. J. Obstet. Gynecol. Reprod. Biol.*, 71, 105, 1997.
122. Werler, M. M., Shapiro, S., Mitchell, A. A., Periconceptional folic acid exposure and risk of occurrent neural tube defects, *JAMA*, 269, 1257, 1993.
123. Gordon, N. Folate metabolism and neural tube defects. *Brain Dev.* 17, 307, 1995.
124. Nielsen, P., Nachtigall, D., Iron supplementation in athletes: current recommendations, *Sports Med.*, 26, 207, 1998.
125. Coleman, E., Steen, S. N., *The Ultimate Sports Nutrition Handbook*, Bull Publishing, Palo Alto, 1996, pp. 143-145.
126. Widdowson, E. M., Growth and composition of the fetus and newborn, in: Assali, N. E., Ed. *Biology of Gestation,* vol. 2, Academic Press, New York, 1968.
127. Fenster, L., Eskenazi, B., Windham, G. C., Swan, S. H., Caffeine consumption during pregnancy and fetal growth, *Am. J. Public Health*, 1991, 81, 458.
128. Fortier, I., Marcoux, S., Beaulac-Baillargeon, L. Relation of caffeine intake during pregnancy to intrauterine growth retardation and preterm birth, *Am. J. Epidemiol.*, 137, 931, 1993.
129. Vlajinac, H. D., Petrovic, R. R., Marinkovic, J. M., Sipetic, S. B., Adanja, B. J., Effect of caffeine intake during pregnancy on birth weight, *Am. J. Epidemiol.*, 145, 335, 1997.
130. Santos, I. S., Victora, C. G., Huttly, S., Morris, S., Caffeine intake and pregnancy outcomes: a meta-analytic review, *Cad. Saude. Publica.*, 14, 523, 1998.
131. Cook, D. G., Peacock, J. L., Feyerabend, C., Carey, I. M., Jarvis, M. J., Anderson, H. R., Bland, J. M., Relation of caffeine intake and blood caffeine concentrations during pregnancy to fetal growth: prospective population based study, *Brit. Med. J.*, 313, 1358, 1996.
132. Santos, I. S., Victora C. G., Huttly, S., Carvalhal J. B., Caffeine intake and low birth weight: a population-based case-control study, *Am. J. Epidemiol.*, 147, 620, 1998.
133. Shu, X. O., Hatch, M. C., Mills, J., Clemens, J., Susser, M., Maternal smoking, alcohol drinking, caffeine consumption, and fetal growth: results from a prospective study, *Epidemiology*, 6, 115, 1995.

134. Henderson, G. I., Chen, J. J., Schenker, S., Ethanol, oxidative stress, reactive aldehydes, and the fetus, *Front Biosci.* 15, D541, 1999.
135. Shaw, G. M., Lammer, E. J., Maternal periconceptional alcohol consumption and risk for orofacial clefts, *J. Pediatr.* 134, 298, 1999.
136. Bagheri, M. M., Burd, L., Martsolf, J. T., Klug, M. G., Fetal alcohol syndrome: maternal and neonatal characteristics, *J. Perinat. Med.* 26, 263, 1998.
137. National Collegiate Athletic Association: *NCAA Study of Substance Use and Abuse Habits of College Student-Athletes.* NCAA Committee on Medical Safeguards and Medical Aspects of Sports, September, 1997.
138. Lovelady, C. A., Nommsen-Rivers, L. A., McCrory, M. A., Dewey, K. G., Effects of exercise on plasma lipids and metabolism of lactating women. *Med. Sci. Sports Exerc.*, 27, 22, 1995.
139. Kunz, C., Rodriguez-Palmero, M., Koletzko, B., Jensen, R., Nutritional and biochemical properties of human milk, Part I: General aspects, proteins, and carbohydrates, *Clin Perinatol.*, 26, 307, 1999.
140. Lamb, R. C., Barker, B. O., Anderson, M. J., Walters, J. C., Effects of forced exercise on 2-year-old Holstein heifers, *J. Dairy Sci.*, 62, 1791, 1979.
141. Wallace, J. P., Inbar, G., Ernsthausen, K., Infant acceptance of postexercise breast milk, *Pediatrics*, 89, 1245, 1992.
142. Guyton A., *Textbook of Medical Physiology*, W. B. Saunders, Philadelphia, 1976.
143. Wallace, J. P., Ernsthausen, K., Inbar, G., The influence of the fullness of milk in the breast on the concentration of lactic acid in post exercise breast milk, *Int. J. Sports Med.*, 13, 395, 1992.
144. Carey, G. B., Quinn, T. J., Goodwin, S. E., Breast milk composition after exercise of different intensities, *J. Hum. Lact.* 13, 115, 1997.
145. Quinn, T. J., Carey, G. B., Does exercise intensity or diet influence lactic acid accumulation in breast milk? *Med. Sci. Sports Exerc.*, 31, 105, 1999.
146. Karasawa, K., Suwa, J., Kimura, S., Voluntary exercise during pregnancy and lactation and its effects on lactational performance in mice, *J. Nutr. Sci. Vitam.*, 27, 333, 1981.
147. Dewey, K. G., Lovelady, C. A., Nommsen-Rivers, L. A., McCrory, M. A., Lonnerdal, B., A randomized study of the effects of aerobic exercise by lactating women on breast-milk volume and composition, *N. Engl. J. Med.*, 330, 449, 1994.
148. Fly, A. D., Uhlin, L. K., Wallace, J. P., Major mineral concentrations in human milk do not change after maximal exercise testing, *Am. J. Clin. Nutr.*, 68, 345, 1998.
149. Lovelady, C. A., Lonnerdal, B., Dewey, K. G., Lactation performance of exercising women, *Am. J. Clin. Nutr.*, 52, 103, 1990.
150. McCrory, M. A., Nommsen-Rivers, L. A., Mole, P. A., Lonnerdal, B., Dewey, K. G., Randomized trial of the short-term effects of dieting compared with dieting plus aerobic exercise on lactation performance, *Am. J. Clin. Nutr.*, 69, 959, 1999.
151. Mestecky, J. Russell, M. W., Jackson, S., Brown, T. A., The human IgA system: a reassessment, *Clin. Immunol. Immunopathol.*, 40, 105, 1986.
152. Gregory, R. L., The biological role and clinical implications of IgA, *Lab. Med.*, 25, 724, 1994.
153. Gregory, R. L., Wallace, J. P., Gfell, L. E., Marks, J., King, B. A., Effect of exercise on milk immunoglobulin A, *Med. Sci. Sports Exerc.*, 29, 1596, 1997.
154. Dewey, K. G., Lovelady, C., Exercise and breast-feeding: a different experience, *Pediatrics*, 91, 514, 1993.
155. Dewey, K. G., Energy and protein requirements during lactation, *Annu. Rev. Nutr.*, 17, 19, 1997.
156. Forsum, E., Kabir, N., Sadurskis, A., Westerterp, K., Total energy expenditure of healthy Swedish women during pregnancy and lactation, *Am. J. Clin. Nutr.* 56, 334, 1992.
157. Lovelady, C. A., Meredith, C. N., McCrory, M. A., Nommsen, L. A., Joseph, L. J., Dewey, K. G., Energy expenditure in lactating women: a comparison of doubly-labeled water and heart-rate-monitoring methods, *Am. J. Clin. Nutr.*, 57, 512, 1993.
158. Singh, J., Prentice, A. M., Diaz, E., Coward, W. A., Ashford, J., Sawyer, M., Whitehead, R. G., Energy expenditure of Gambian women during peak agricultural activity measured by the doubly-labelled water method, *Br. J. Nutr.* 62, 315, 1989.
159. Institute of Medicine, *Nutrition During Lactation*, National Academy Press, Washington, D.C., 1990.
160. Duerbeck, N., Breast-feeding: what you should know so you can talk to your patients, *Comp. Ther.*, 24, 310, 1998.

161. Dusdieker, L. B., Hemmingway, D. L., Stumbo, P. J., Is milk production impaired by dieting during lactation? *Am. J. Clin. Nutr.* 59, 833, 1994.
162. Strode, M. A., Dewey, K. G., Lonnerdal, B., Effects of short-term caloric restriction on lactational performance of well-nourished women, *Acta. Paediatr. Scand.* 75, 222, 1986.,
163. Roberts, S. B., Cole, T. J., Coward, W. A., Lactational performance in relation to energy intake in the baboon, *Am. J. Clin. Nutr.*, 41, 1270, 1985.
164. Institute of Medicine, *Nutrition During Pregnancy and Lactation: An Implementation Guide*, National Academy Press, Washington, DC, 1992.
165. Kalkwarf, H. J., Specker, B. L., Bone mineral loss during lactation and recovery after weaning, *Obstet. Gynecol.* 86, 26, 1995.
166. Honda, A., Kurabayashi, T., Yahata, T., Tomita, M., Takakuwa, K., Tanaka, K., Lumbar bone mineral density changes during pregnancy and lactation, *Int. J. Gynaecol. Obstet.* 63, 253, 1998.
167. Hayslip, C. C., Klein, T. A., Wray, L., Duncan, W. E., The effects of lactation on bone mineral content in healthy postpartum women, *Obstet. Gynecol.* 73, 588, 1989.
168. Sowers, M., Corton, G., Shapiro, B., Jannausch, M. L., Crutchfield, M., Smith, M. L., Randolph, J.F., Hollis, B., Changes in bone density with lactation, *JAMA*, 269, 3130, 1993.
169. Little, K. D., Clapp III, J. F., Self-selected recreational exercise has no impact on early postpartum lactation-induced bone loss, *Med. Sci. Sports Exerc.*, 30, 831, 1998.
170. Polatti, F., Capuzzo, E., Viazzo, F., Colleoni, R., Klersy, C., Bone mineral changes during and after lactation, *Obste. Gynecol.*, 94, 52, 1999.
171. Kalkwarf, H. J., Specker, B. L., Bianchi, D. C., Ranz, J., Ho, M., The effect of calcium supplementation on bone density during lactation and after weaning, *N. Engl. J. Med.*, 337, 523, 1997.

CHAPTER 3

Nutritional Concerns of Child Athletes

Nancy Lewis and Jean E. Guest

CONTENTS

0-8493-8199-?/00/$0.00+$.50

I. INTRODUCTION

Regular physical activity (PA) in childhood is positively associated with improved strength, maintenance of healthy body weight (BW) and composition, and cardiorespiratory fitness.[1] The development of habitual PA patterns in childhood may persist into adulthood,[2] laying the foundation for a healthier life. However, growth needs and considerations unique to childhood require special attention. This chapter will explore some of these considerations in children 5 to 13 years of age, although some overlap into adolescence (>13 years) is unavoidable.

II. EXERCISE

A. Sports

Lifestyle changes in the United States over the second half of the 20th century have led to a curious dichotomy between activity and inactivity. Expanded use of technology to ease the burdens of daily life has resulted in a sedentary lifestyle for many adults and children. The incorporation of PA into a lifestyle must be a conscious and continuing commitment.

Physical education (PE) is available for children in most public schools. However, it is unclear if these experiences and lessons lead to PA and healthier lifestyles in adulthood. Participation in sports is one way to incorporate PA into a lifestyle.

1. Organized Physical Activity

Sports activity in past generations consisted of spontaneous game playing among neighborhood children. However, in today's environment, children participating in organized sports join teams originating from school, civic, private, or public organizations. These are highly competitive teams that limit participation to only the most talented and highly trained children. Preadolescent or childhood participation in organized sports presents special demands both physically and emotionally.

Sports activity has been classified by the Joint Committee on Sports Medicine of the American Academy of Pediatrics (AAP), American Academy of Family Physicians, American Orthopedic Society for Sports Medicine, American Medical Society for Sports Medicine, and the American Osteopathic Academy of Sports Medicine into contact and non contact sports.[3] These two categories are further delineated into contact/collision and limited contact/impact, and strenuous, moderately strenuous, and non strenuous sports. These classifications provide a guide for the type of physical conditioning as well as energy expenditure (EE) required for participation. Table 3.1 provides classification of selected organized sports for children (not all sporting activities are listed).

2. Informal Physical Activity

Establishing a lifestyle that includes daily PA is central to maintaining good health. Participation in organized sports or PE classes are not the only means by which children can obtain PA. Another important component to individual daily PA is informal athletic activity. Although informal athletic activity and PA are not synonymous terms, their results may be similar.

Table 3.1 Classification of Selected Childhood Sports

Contact		Noncontact		
High Contact	**Limited Contact**	**Strenuous**	**Moderately Strenuous**	**Nonstrenuous**
Boxing	Baseball	Aerobic dance	Badminton	Archery
Field and ice hockey	Basketball	Jogging	Curling	Golf
Football	Cycling	Swimming	Table tennis	Riflery
Lacrosse	Diving	Tennis		
Marital arts	Gymnastics	Weight lifting		
Rodeo	Horseback riding			
Soccer	Skating			
Wrestling	Skiing			
Softball				
Racketball				
Volleyball				

Adapted from Reference 3.

a. *Effect on Physical Activity in Adulthood*

Telama et al.[4] conducted a 12-year longitudinal study of PA in 1687 children. This study was part of a "Cardiovascular (CV) Risk in Young Finns" national research program. A physical activity index (PAI) questionnaire was used to measure intensity of PA, frequency of intensive PA, hours/week of intensive PA, and membership in a sports club. The children and adolescents were 9, 12, 15, and 18 years of age in 1980 when the study was initiated.

The objective of the study was to explore to what extent leisure time PA at these ages predicts PA 9 and 12 years later. A secondary goal was to analyze the relationship of participation in organized sport, the intensity of PA, and some other relationships of PA in childhood and adolescence with later PA.

Telama et al.[4] reported that PA and participation in sports at 9, 12, 15, and 18 years of age was significantly, but weakly, correlated with PA measured 9 and 12 years later. Frequency of PA decreases considerably between ages 12 and 21 years. In this period, the number of children participating in PA at least twice a week decreased from 81% to 49% in males, and from 69% to 49% in females. Although participation in PA decreased, the number of children participating in intense PA over the same time period increased from 13% to 34% in males, and from 6% to 25% in females. These findings indicate that the number of children who participate regularly in PA decreases in puberty and thereafter while the intensity of PA increases. The authors concluded that the correlation between PA and sports participation before and during puberty increases the probability of a physically active lifestyle in early adulthood.

PA among multiethnic third graders was studied by Simons-Morton et al.[5] in California, Texas, Louisiana, and Minnesota. Their study was part of the Child and Adolescent Trial for Cardiovascular Health (CATCH). In all, 2410 children were screened between September 1991 and January 1992. Data collected included total cholesterol (TC), blood pressure (BP), body mass index (BMI), skinfolds, 9-minute timed run for distance, PA interview, dietary recall, and a health behavior questionnaire.

Mean daily PA for all children was 90 minutes for moderate–vigorous activity, 35 minutes for vigorous activity, and 120 minutes for sedentary behaviors. Less than 60 minutes of moderate–vigorous PA per day was reported by 37% of the children. Males, Caucasians, and children in California reported the most activity, while children in Louisiana reported the least. Half of the mean daily sedentary activity reported was spent playing video games, watching TV, and sitting listening to music. The other half was spent doing schoolwork, homework, lying down resting, and artwork. More sedentary activity was reported by males ($p = 0.0001$) than females, and children in Louisiana ($p<0.05$) than in the other states. Ethnicity was not a significant factor in predicting time spent in sedentary activity.

Lower TC was positively associated with more minutes of moderate–vigorous, and vigorous minutes (r# 0.1) of PA. BP, BMI, and CV fitness were not significantly associated with PA in this study. The authors concluded that PA in these children did meet the Healthy People Year 2000[6] objectives, but attention should be paid to the number of children who are physically inactive.

Although the number of children included in Simons-Morton et al.[5] study is large, the study does have limitations. First, data for each child was a sample of one day. PA varies from day to day. Second, the association between high density lipoprotein cholesterol (HDL-C) and PA was not explored, since only TC was measured. Third, CV fitness was assessed by a 9-minute run, which may not be a sensitive measure in third graders.

In children, fitness as a measure of health can be more difficult to measure than in adults. Fitness measures such as appropriate weight for height (Wt/Ht), BMI, and skinfold measures[7] are tools recommended for use in the pediatric population. PA is recommended as a method of impacting these fitness measures.

Physical fitness tests are routinely administered as part of traditional public school PE courses. A component of these tests is a 1-mile [1.6 kilometer (km)] run as an indicator of endurance [measured by maximal oxygen consumption ($\dot{V}O_{2max}$)]. To examine the validity of this practice, Rowland et al.[8] studied 36 healthy males with a mean age of 12.2 years. All males were Tanner[9] Stage I (61%) or II (39%). Data collection included maximum cycle ergometer testing, height (Ht), BW, percent body fat (%BF) (estimated from scapular and triceps skinfolds by Slaughter et al.[10] equations), heart rate (electrocardiogram), $\dot{V}O_{2max}$ (standard open circuit spirometry), and a timed 1-mile (1.6km) run.

Rowland et al.[8] reported significant ($p<0.05$) correlations between %BF ($r = -0.56$), maximum cardiac index ($r = 0.41$), and stroke index [a component of $\dot{V}O_{2max}$ ($r = 0.39$)]. A negative correlation was observed between %BF and $\dot{V}O_{2max}$ per kilogram (kg) ($r = -0.73$). Together %BF (31%) and $\dot{V}O_{2max}$/kg (28%) accounted for approximately 60% of the variance in 1-mile (1.6km)-run velocity. Consequently, 40% of variance in 1-mile-run velocity can be attributed to nonaerobic factors (nonaerobic capacity, skill, and muscle strength). True CV fitness ($\dot{V}O_{2max}$/kg) and body composition (%BF) account for the majority of variance in 1-mile-run velocity, indicating their significance as a measure of endurance when testing physical fitness. Therefore, inadequate performance on such tests may identify children at risk for health problems associated with poor CV fitness or excessive body fat (BF).

Do physical fitness tests in childhood predict PA in adulthood? Dennison et al.[11] investigated this question in a nonconcurrent prospective study of 453 males aged 23 to 25 years. As children in the Baltimore County public school system, they had taken the Youth Fitness Test[12] between ages 10 and 11 years or 15 and 18. The questionnaire was designed to assess PA and evaluate other variables including current Ht, BW, perceived general health status, history of CV disease or smoking, hypertension, organized sports participation, individual and parental education level, perceived encouragement by parents or spouse of individual's exercise habits, and family history of CV disease.

Dennison et al.[11] divided respondents into two groups — physically active or physically inactive — based on minimum exercise criteria (2 days per week for at least 20 to 30 minutes). Current PA and Youth Fitness Test[12] scores of the two groups were compared. Statistical analysis indicated an association between childhood fitness test scores and current adult PA. The best predictors of physical inactivity in adulthood were low scores on the 600-yard (548.6 meter run) ($p<0.001$), maximum number of sit ups (<0.005), and shuttle run ($p<0.005$) tests. Stepwise multivariate discriminant analysis of adult inactivity demonstrated the best predictor was the 600-yard (548.6 m) run. Respondents scoring ≤ 20% on the 600-yard run as children were 42% more likely to be physically inactive adults than respondents who scored higher on this run as children.

Parental encouragement of exercise ($p<0.001$), level of education ($p<0.001$), participation in organized sports after high school ($p<0.001$), and spousal encouragement of exercise ($p<0.01$) were also significant factors contributing to the ability to predict physical inactivity in adulthood.

Sensitivity and specificity of these factors were 65% and 63%, respectively. Establishing PA and exercise habits during childhood may decrease the risk of physical inactivity in adulthood.

b. Effect on Childhood Fitness Levels

Health risks associated with physical inactivity in adulthood include coronary artery disease (CAD), hypertension, type 2 diabetes, osteoporosis, and obesity.[13,14] Childhood obesity is also associated with an increased incidence of type 2 diabetes.[15] Establishing and maintaining physical activity patterns that continue into adulthood may decrease health risks associated with inactivity.

The effectiveness of PA as an adjunct in weight control or loss programs in children has been mixed.[16-18] Studies in adults [19,20] indicate females do not compensate for increased PA by decreasing normal daily activities. On the other hand, lean males increased their spontaneous PA during non-exercise hours.

Blaak et al.[21] examined the effect of training on ten obese males ages 10 to 11 years with 30% to 40% BF. Training consisted of five cycling sessions per week over a 4-week period on electronic cycle ergometer. Data collection included average daily metabolic rate (MR), sleeping metabolic rate (SMR), body composition, and $\dot{V}O_{2max}$). The goal was to increase MR by 10% over 5 hours of exercise per week. Each 1-hour session included bouts of 20, 15, and 10 minutes, respectively, on the cycle ergometer. Training intensity for each subject was determined by $\dot{V}O_{2max}$) and peak mechanical power (PP). PP was defined as the highest power maintained for 1 minute by the subject on a progressive-continuous cycling test.

Maximal heart rate, $\dot{V}O_{2max}$, and $\dot{V}CO_{2max}$), were continuously monitored during each exercise session. Body composition was measured at the beginning and end of the study by collecting BW, body density (hydrostatic weighing with simultaneous lung-volume measurement), total body water (doubly labeled water), and %BF using Lohman's[21] equation, which corrects for differences in gender and age. Resting metabolic rate (RMR) was measured by open circuit ventilated-hood at weeks 0, 2, 4, and 6 after at least a 12-hour overnight fast.

Blaak et al.[21] reported no change in BW, % BF, SMR, RMR, heart rate, or oxygen consumption. There was a significant increase in fat-free mass (FFM) ($p<0.05$), PP ($p<0.01$), and average daily MR (12%). No increase in spontaneous PA was seen. Half of the increased average daily MR can be explained by cost of energy for training, and the remaining half by increased EE outside training hours. Increased diet-induced thermogenesis (DIT) was surmised to be responsible for > 60% of the increased EE outside training hours. The authors concluded that training stimulated increased EE during nonexercise parts of the day. However, the authors caution that this information should not be extrapolated to obese young females or children of different ethnic origin or socioeconomic backgrounds, as they may respond differently to training programs.

Do prepubertal overweight females have lower PA, EE, and fitness levels than their non-overweight counterparts? Trueth et al.[23] examined this question in 24 healthy prepubertal females aged 7 to 10 years. They were equally divided into two groups classified as overweight (OW) and nonoverweight (NOW). Females in the OW group were > 95% Wt/Ht, while females in the NOW group were between 10% and 95% Wt/Ht. Basal metabolic rate (BMR), total energy expenditure (TEE), SMR and 24-hour sedentary EE (SEE), body composition by dual-energy X-ray absorptiometry (DEXA), and $\dot{V}O_2$) peak were measured. Physical activity EE and physical activity level were calculated according to Coward et al.[24] Twenty-four-hour dietary intake was collected.

Trueth et al.[23] demonstrated that the OW group compared to the NOW group had significantly higher ($p<0.001$) BW (46.5 ± 9.0 kg vs. 28.5 ± 3.5 kg), %BF (39.3 ± 6.4% vs. 27.6 ± 5.0%), fat mass (FM) (18.1 ± 6,5 kg vs. 7.7 ± 2.0 kg), and FFM (26.9 ± 3.2 kg vs. 19.9 ± 2.3 kg). BMR, SMR, SEE, and TEE were higher ($p<0.001$) in the OW group until adjustment for FFM rendered the two groups the same. Physical activity EE, physical activity level, and $\dot{V}O_2$ peak (fitness level) were not significantly different between OW and NOW groups. Dietary intake was not significantly different between OW and NOW groups in respect to energy intake (2146 ± 480 kcal/d vs. 2389

± 615 kcal/d) and percent of total calories from carbohydrate (CHO) (63 ± 1% vs. 61 ± 1%), protein (PRO) (12 ± 1% vs. 14 ± 1%), and fat (27 ± 1% vs. 27 ± 1%), respectively.

The authors concluded that OW prepubertal females do not have lower physical activity EE or fitness levels than NOW prepubertal females. However, they question if the high %BF observed in the NOW group might have precluded finding any differences between the two groups.

Goran et al.[25] examined whether BF content in prepubertal children is influenced by PA related EE or more qualitative aspects of PA. Their study consisted of two parts. In the first part, 101 children with a mean age of 5.3 ± 0.9 years and mean BW of 20.2 ± 3.6 kg were examined. These children were of Caucasian (36 females and 38 males) and Mohawk (17 females and 10 boys) ethnic backgrounds. In the second part of the study, 68 of the original Caucasian children were re-examined after 1 year. Their mean age was 6.3 ± 0.9 years and mean BW 23.6 ± 5.0 kg. Measurements collected included FM by electrical impedance, FFM by skinfolds, post-prandial RMR by indirect calorimetry, TEE by doubly labeled water, and PA by questionnaire. The PA questionnaire was designed to collect qualitative (time and intensity) information of PA patterns, and assess hours per day of sleeping, television viewing, and recreational physical activities.

Results demonstrated that the children in the first study spent a mean of 5.2 ± 2.4 hours per day (hr/d) playing, 2.1 ± 1.3 hr/d watching television, and 6.1 ± 4.4 hours per week (hr/wk) in recreational activities. Children in the second study spent a mean of 4.3 ± 2.2 hr/d playing, 1.8 ± 0.8 hr/d watching television, and 6.3 ± 5.0 hr/wk in recreational activities. None of these variables were significantly correlated to PA related EE in either the first or second study. PA-related EE was significantly correlated to FFM ($P<0.05$), and BW ($p<0.05$) in both studies. A significantly and inversely partial correlation was seen after adjustment for FFM, gender, and age between PA related to EE and recreational activities (study 1 partial $r = -0.27$, $p = 0.03$; study 2 partial $r = -0.32$, $p = 0.02$). These data suggest that children with greater FM spend less time in PA related to recreational activities than children with lower FM. Therefore, activity time may be more significant in maintaining appropriate body composition in prepubertal children than PA related to EE.

Physical training is used by adults and adolescents to enhance physical performance as well as to achieve and/or maintain body composition. Physical training in children is becoming more common for these same purposes. The response of children to physical training varies just as it does in adolescents and adults.

Barbeau et al.[26] investigated the correlates of body composition changes seen in response to physical training. Seventy-one obese children (22 males and 49 females) with a mean age of 9.7 ± 1.0 years (range 7 to 11 years), and of Caucasian (n = 31) or African-American (n = 40) ethnic origin participated in this study. Body composition including total body mass, fat-free soft tissue, %BF, bone mineral density (BMD), and bone mineral content were measured by DEXA. Testing was conducted at baseline, 4 months, and 8 months. PA was assessed by a 7-day recall interview, and diet by a baseline 1-day food recall with 2-day food recalls at 2 and 4 months of physical training. Children were randomly assigned by sex and ethnicity to one of two groups. Physical training intervention was provided over 8 months with Group 1 receiving training for the first 4 months, and Group 2 receiving training the second 4 months. Physical training sessions were offered 5 days per week (d/wk) with minimum attendance of 3 d/wk. Each session was 40 minutes, with 20 minutes exercising on machines (e.g., treadmill, stationary cycle, and trampoline) and 20 minutes playing games (e.g., basketball, dodge ball, and tag). Heart rate monitoring performed during each session encouraged children to maintain a heart rate of ≥ 150 beats per minute (beats/min).

Barbeau et al.[26] reported mean attendance was 4 d/wk and mean heart rate was 157 ± 7 beats/min per 40-minute session, mean EE was 946 ± 201 Kj per session. Significant increases after 4 months of exercise were seen in total mass, fat-free soft tissue, bone mineral content, and BMD while %BF decreased in the total group. Factors associated with healthier body composition changes with physical training were frequent attendance, male gender, decreased energy intake, and vigorous activity. Older children (≥ 10 years) had greater percent BF decrease, FM at baseline, increases in fat free soft tissue, bone mineral content, and BMD density than younger children. These differences were attributed to normal growth by these authors. They also concluded that frequency and intensity of physical training as well as diet are important correlates of fat loss. Ethnicity did not contribute significantly to body composition changes with physical training.

Sun et al.[27] studied the importance of ethnicity resting energy expenditure (REE) in 98 healthy prepubertal (Tanner[9] Stage I) Caucasian and African-American children. Mean age of Caucasian children (18 females and 21 males) was 8.3 ± 1.4 years (range 5.2 to 10.9 years), and 7.5 ± 1.5 years (range 4.7 to 10.0 years) in African-American children (29 females and 30 males). TEE (by doubly labeled water technique) was measured over 14 days in free-living conditions. REE (indirect calorimetry), body composition (DEXA), Ht (stadiometer), and BW (electronic scale) were also collected. Statistical analysis included two-way (gender and ethnic groups) analysis of covariance with TEE, REE, and activity-related EE as dependent variables while FM and FFM were covariates. Results demonstrated no significant effects of ethnicity on TEE, REE, or activity related EE. Gender did not significantly affect TEE or activity-related EE. However, males did have a significantly higher REE ($P<0.001$) than females. These results do not agree with similar studies conducted[28,29] previously where ethnicity showed a significantly lower REE (> 200 kcal/d) in African-American than Caucasian children.

Goran et al.[30] examined 22 prepubertal children (11 males and 11 females) beginning at a mean age of 5.4 ± 0.9 years. Measurements for TEE, REE, physical activity related EE, reported physical activity, FM, and FFM were obtained three times over a 5-year period. Males and females demonstrated similar increases in BW, FM, and FFM. Significant effects of time and gender on TEE were observed. Females increased EE from year one to year two of the study, but by year five, they had a significant decrease. Reported physical activity in females remained comparable to males until ages 8.5 years and 9.5 years, when there was a significant (50%) decrease. Energy intake did not change during this period. The authors concluded that these results suggest the existence of an energy-conserving mechanism through reduced physical activity prior to puberty in females.

Does reduced EE predispose children to obesity? Goran et al.[31] conducted a longitudinal study in 75 Caucasian children (35 females and 40 males) over a 4-year period to examine this question. The children's mean age was 5.2 ± 0.9 years (range 4 to 7.2 years) at initial testing. Parents of these children were also studied. Parents' mean age at initial testing was 34 ± 5 years in mothers and 37 ± 5 years in fathers. Annual testing was done on the same date as the original visit or within ± 4 weeks. The variables studied were Ht (stadiometer), BW (electronic scale with light clothing), skinfold thicknesses (axilla, chest, subscapular, supra iliac, abdomen, triceps, calf, and thigh), FFM and FM (bioelectric impedance and DEXA), TEE (doubly labeled water), REE (indirect calorimetry), and PA (Minnesota leisure time activity questionnaire). Parents' body composition was determined by underwater weighing, while other variables such as Ht, BW, skinfold thicknesses, and REE were collected in the same manner as the children. Results indicated that the main predictors of change in FM relative to FFM during preadolescence growth are gender (females gained more fat), initial fatness, and parental fatness, but not reduced EE.

B. Type

Exercise is commonly divided into aerobic and anaerobic categories. Basically, aerobic signifies the presence of oxygen while anaerobic signifies absence of oxygen. When these terms are applied to exercise, their definitions expand to include specific metabolic functions. This section will discuss these types of exercise and their implications in childhood.

1. Aerobic

Aerobic fitness depends on the rate of use or uptake of oxygen by muscles during exercise or activity. Increasing fitness levels are expressed by greater capacity or efficiency of this process. $\dot{V}O_{2max}$ is considered a valuable indicator or index of an individual's capacity to perform exercise involving CV, pulmonary, and hematologic systems. $\dot{V}O_{2max}$ is recognized as the single best indicator of aerobic fitness in adults,[32] but not necessarily in children.

Armstrong et al.[33] investigated the practice of using $\dot{V}O_2$ plateau as the standard for establishing $\dot{V}O_{2max}$ during progressive, incremental exercise testing in children. They studied 35 healthy children (18 females and 17 males) with a mean age of 9.9 ± 0.4 years. Three progressively intense treadmill tests to exhaustion were conducted over a 3-week period. Age, gender, Ht, BW, body mass, $\dot{V}O_2$, heart rate, respiratory exchange ratio, blood lactate, minute ventilation, and respiratory frequency were collected at each test. Mean peak $\dot{V}O_2$ values in tests two and three (supra maximal tests) did not significantly differ from values in test one, despite significantly higher indicators (minute ventilation, respiratory frequency, heart rate, respiratory exchange ratio, and blood lactate) of increased anaerobic contribution. There were no significant differences between the children (38.9% female and 35.3% males) who demonstrated a $\dot{V}O_2$ plateau ($\leq 2ml \cdot kg^{-1} \cdot min^{-1}$), and those who did not. $\dot{V}O_{2max}$ in children may not involve a $\dot{V}O_2$ plateau.

Other authors[34,35] agree that $\dot{V}O_{2max}$ may be a less valid indicator of cardiopulmonary function, endurance capacity, and response to training in children and adolescents than in adults. $\dot{V}O_{2max}$ capacity increases at similar rates in males and females up to age 12. It continues to increase in males up to age 18 and plateaus in females around age 14.[35]

McMurray et al.[36] compared the accuracy of two $\dot{V}O_{2max}$ prediction equations [gender-specific physical work capacity (PWC^{GS})[37] and a modified physical work capacity (PWC^{195})[38]] using submaximal cycle ergometry in children. They studied 33 children (18 females and 15 males) with a mean age of 10.0 ± 1.8 years and 10.5 ± 1.2 years for females and males, respectively (age range 7 to 13 years). $\dot{V}O_{2max}$ in all children was measured by a graded treadmill exercise test (GXT). Then each child completed a 9-minute, three-stage, submaximal cycle ergometer test. Their results indicated a significant (p = <0.001) correlation for both prediction equations and the GXT. However, the correlation between the PWC^{195}[38] equation and the GXT (r = 0.807) was higher than the correlation between the PWC^{GS}[37] and the GXT (r = 0.658). These authors conclude the PWC^{195}[38] equation is a more accurate predictor of $\dot{V}O_{2max}$ in children.

2. Anaerobic

The safety and efficacy of resistance or weight training in prepubescent children has been a controversial issue. A 1983 AAP[39] policy statement on weight training and lifting suggested that a minimal benefit was received in prepubescent athletes while maximal benefit of weight training and weight lifting was obtained by postpubertal athletes. The AAP[40] modified this policy statement in 1990 by providing definitions to differentiate weight training, weight lifting, and body building along with recommendations for weight training in pediatric athletes. The AAP[40] supports supervised weight training (by well trained adults), but not maximal competitive weight lifting, power lifting or body building in children prior to Tanner[9] Stage V

An earlier study by Vrijens[41] in 1978 reported no strength gains in prepubescent males aged 10 to 17 years who participated in an 8-week strength training program (1 set, 8–12 repetitions, 3 times/week). Docherty et al.[42] in 1987 reported similar results of no strength gains for 12-year-old hockey and soccer players who trained following their competitive season. Other authors questioned the effectiveness of weight training due to low levels of circulating androgens, lack of motor performance improvements, and potential hazards outweighing risk benefits in prepubescent children.[43-45] However, other studies have shown increased strength in prepubescent children following strength training.[46-48]

Ramsay et al.[49] examined the effects of strength training in 26 prepubertal males (Tanner[9] stage I) aged 9 to 11 years. Thirteen males were assigned to an experimental group receiving progressive resistance training three times per week over 20 weeks. The remaining 13 males served as a control group, and did not receive training. The experimental group utilized circuit training performed under adult supervision. Experimental group training was divided into two 10-week phases. Phase one training consisted of preacher arm curl, double leg extension, leg press, bench press, behind the neck pull down, and sit-up or trunk curl exercises. All exercises were performed at 70% to 75% of one repetition maximum (RM) with 10 to 12 repetitions. Phase two exercises were the same as phase one exercises, but were performed at 80% to 85% of 1 RM with five to seven repetitions.

Data collected from both the experimental and control groups included anthropometry, body composition, measurement of performance, isokinetic and isometric strength, evoked contractile properties, computerized tomography (CAT) scans, and percent motor unit activation of two major muscle groups (elbow flexors and knee extensors). Data collection in both groups coincided with baseline, mid training, and post training of the experimental group. Mid and post training measurements in the experimental group were collected after 2 to 3 days' recovery time from last training session.

Training resulted in significantly increased 1 RM bench press (35%) and leg press (22%), isometric elbow flexion (37%), knee extension strength (25% at 90 degrees and 13% at 120 degrees), isokinetic elbow flexion (26%), knee extension strength (21%), evoked twitch torque of the elbow flexors (30%), and knee extensors (30%) in the experimental group.

III. HEALTH

A. Growth

The term "growth" is defined by the context in which it is used. For purposes of this chapter, growth will be defined as the process by which an individual achieves biological potential. This biological potential is determined by genomic expression of factors such as body composition (Ht and BW) and neurohumoral functions. Additionally, environmental and behavioral factors such as nutritional modulation, mechanical force, and psychosocial experiences combine to influence the final outcome.

1. Genetic and Environmental Factors

a. Physical Growth

Physical growth during the third through fifth years of life is steady at approximately 2.0 kg [4.4 pounds (lbs)] of weight gain, and 6 centimeters (cm) to 8 cm (2.5 inches to 3.5 inches) of height increase per year. Steady growth continues during the early school years with an average of 3 kg to 3.5 kg (6.6 lbs to 7.7 lbs) of weight gain and 6 cm (2.4 inches) in Ht increase. This period of steady growth ends in a preadolescent growth spurt at about age 10 years in females and 12 years in males.[50]

Body composition changes seen during the third through fifth years of life include a loss of lordosis and protuberant abdomen characteristic of late infancy and the toddler years. Baby fat, particularly fat pads covering the arches of the feet, disappear. Neurological development during this period includes refinement of motor skills resulting in the ability to run, skip, jump, and participate in vigorous physical activity.[51]

Body composition changes during the early school years ending in the preadolescent growth spurt include a leaner body configuration with straightening of the spine, and resolution of mild knock knee or flat-footedness that can be seen in early childhood. Neurological maturation results in sophistication of physical activities with refinement of motor and muscular skills.[51]

b. Neurohumoral Factors

Neurohumoral factors associated with the control of growth consist of four stages. In the first or fetal stage, tissue-specific growth factors regulate mitosis, protein synthesis, and differentiation.[52,53] Second, or infancy and early childhood stage, is a period characterized by incremental growth dependent on energy abundance and balance.[54] Third, or childhood through puberty stage, occurs when the brain assumes a central role in stimulating release of growth hormone (GH), thyroid hormones (T3 and T4), and sex steroid (gonadal and adrenal) hormones for the express purpose of facilitating growth.[55-58] Fourth, or late puberty through late adulthood stage, evolves from brain alterations resulting in inhibition of growth in favor of maintenance and repair of lean body tissues.[55,59]

c. Nutritional Modulation

Nutritional status determines the role of neurohumoral growth factors and insulin. Abundance of nutrients and energy increases release of insulin and GH. Insulin expedites cellular uptake of nutrients, stimulates protein and other enzyme synthesis, and inhibits CHO and lipid catabolism. GH functions to stimulate statural and reparative growth.[60,61] Negative nutrient and energy balance have an opposite effect, inhibiting insulin and GH secretion and cellular uptake of CHO, while promoting PRO catabolism.[62,63] Negative energy balance may result from inadequate kilocalorie intake and/or increased EE from PA as well as oxygen shortage and exposure to cold.[64] Psychosocial and behavioral factors influence availability and abundance of nutrient and energy intake as well as PA patterns.

d. Mechanical Force

Mechanical force is a significant stimulus for tissue, cellular, skeletal, and muscle growth. PA produces force by muscle resistance to body parts as they move jointly or in opposition to gravity. Insufficient mechanical force can result in muscle atrophy[65] and bone demineralization.[66,67]

2. Clinical Application

Effects of PA on growth in children have produced conflicting reports. Variability of results occurs due to the wide variety of sports and physical activities available to children. For those children who participate in intensive or competitive PA, the impact of these activities on growth is still uncertain.

More than 30 years ago, Schuck[68] reported decreased growth velocity in young male athletes. Fifteen years later, Buckler and Brodie[69] reported that young male gymnasts had shorter limbs and were smaller than their nongymnast counterparts. However, Astrand et al.[70] in 1963 reported normal growth in 30 female swimmers. More recently, in 1996, Malina et al.[71] reported that 25 male and 13 female athletes were taller and heavier than the reference sample during late childhood. Skeletal age (SA) in active males aged 10 years to 12 years did not differ significantly from chronological age (CA) references until adolescence when SA progressed significantly ($p<0.01$) relative to CA. Active females aged 8 to 18 years had significant ($p<0.05$ and 0.01) differences in Ht, but not BW compared with references. SA in the females was not significantly different from CA references.

Is the type of sport or PA important in determining the impact on growth during childhood? The answer to this question seems to be yes. Studies in children participating in specific sports such as gymnastics (male and female), ballet dancing (female), figure skating (female), and diving (male) have demonstrated shorter stature compared with reference data.[72] One important aspect of this growth issue is skeletal maturation. Both bone accretion and density are important. The relationship between sports activity and growth may be related specifically to the type and intensity of PA. Mechanical loading (ML) and its relationship to BMD may be meaningful.

Grimston et al.[73] studied the effect of significant ML (forces 3 times BW) on BMD in 17 young athletes (MLA) (nine females and eight males). All athletes were healthy, between ages 10 and 16 years, and trained a minimum of 60 minutes three times per week in addition to regular competitive event participation. Athletes who participated in competitive swimming (non MLA) served as controls, and were matched with MLA for age, gender, race, stage of puberty, BW, and average daily training time. BMD measurement of the lumbar spine (L2–L4) and femoral neck (FN) by DEXA, assessment of puberty by Tanner[9] Stage, dietary assessment by 3-day dietary intake records (on two occasions), and assessment of non-weight-bearing hours by PA questionnaire were collected.

The results indicated no significant differences between MLA and non MLA, respectively, in CA (13.2 ± 0.4 years and 12.6 ± 0.4 years), Ht (154.9 ± 2.9 cm and 157.6 ± 3.0 cm), BW (43.6 ± 2.7 kg and 44.5 ± 2.2 kg), years of training (6.4 ± 1.0 years and 5.3 ± 0.7 years), mean times per day of training (2.2 ± 0.2 h/d and 2.1 ± 0.3 h/d), or dietary intake (2392 ± 137 kcal/d and 2443 ± 111 kcal/d). The MLA had significantly ($p<0.05$) greater FN BMD (0.78 ± 0.02 gHA · cm^{-2}) than non MLA (0.72 ± 0.02 gHA · cm^{-2}). Lumbar spine (L2-L4) tended toward greater BMD, but did not reach statistical significance in MLA (0.7 ± 0.03 gHA · cm^{-2}) compared to non MLA (0.66 ± 0.03 gHA · cm^{-2}). When BMD was examined by gender, female MLA were not significantly different from female non MLA, whereas male MLA had significantly greater lumbar spine ($p<0.05$) BMD.

The authors noted that the inability to recruit sedentary control subjects limited the study. The effect of sedentary activity compared with athletes (ML and non ML) would be valuable information. However, the results of this study indicated greater FN BMD in children participating in ML activities than in non-ML activities.

Gunnes and Lehmann[74] confirmed the importance of ML or weight-bearing PA. They prospectively studied forearm trabecular and cortical BMD gain in relation to nutrient intake, ML, and daylight exposure (DE) in 470 healthy children over a 1-year period. Ages of the children at baseline were 8.2 years to 16.5 years. Single photon absorptiometry (SPA) was used to assess BMD. Ht, BW, dietary intake, PA, and DE were collected. The results demonstrated an increased cortical BMD from age 11 years with peaking at age 14.0 ± 0.3 years in females, and 16.0 ± 0.3 years in males. Increase and peak of cortical BMD was delayed by 1 to 2 years in males.

Trabecular BMD was similar between females and males, with adult values being reached at the age of 15 and 16.5 years, respectively. Peak trabecular BMD was observed at a mean of 13 years in females (0.024 g cm^{-2} $year^{-1}$), and 15 years (0.029 g cm^{-2} $year^{-1}$) in males. ML, baseline BMD, Ht and HT gain, BW and BW gain, dietary polyunsaturated fat (PUFA), and sodium chloride (NaCl) were significantly ($p<0.05$) correlated with change in BMD. Using backward stepwise regression analysis, ML was the best predictor of trabecular BMD in children younger than 11 years of age who had a high calcium intake. PUFA intake in females older than 11 years was a significant ($p<0.05$) contributor to trabecular BMD. These authors attributed the role of PUFA intake to possible effects on estrogen metabolism.[75,76] NaCl was negatively associated with trabecular BMD accounting for 10% of the variability in females less than 11 years of age. This negative association may be accounted for by the role NaCl plays in increasing urinary calcium excretion, especially in individuals with marginal calcium intakes.[77]

The authors concluded that ML was the most important environmental predictor of BMD gain in children. A high level of ML activity along with high calcium, and possibly PUFA intakes, while avoiding excessive NaCl intake, may maximize trabecular BMD in this population.

3. Recommendations

The role and impact of PA during childhood continues to be paradoxical. Growth during childhood appears to be controlled by interacting genetic (i.e., neurohumoral growth, anabolic, and sex hormone factors), environmental (i.e., nutrient abundance), and behavioral forces (i.e., PA). The intensity and duration of PA during critical periods of childhood development seem to impact skeletal size and density, although it appears that this effect is sensitive and specific. Negative effects such as delayed or stunted linear Ht or poor skeletal BMD occur when selected activities result in negative energy and nutrient balance. Positive effects include sound mucoskeletal development along with appropriate body composition and overall growth.

All children should be encouraged to participate in PA. Children taking part in selected sports such as gymnastics and ballet, which are associated with growth problems, should be closely monitored with appropriate interventions as required.

Optimal duration and intensity of PA for children is unknown. Many children participating in competitive or high level individual sports train up to 16 hours per week with no apparent problems. Excessive ML can result in epiphyseal growth plate injury and possibly curtail linear Ht growth. PA or sports that involve excessive ML should be avoided.

B. Medical

1. Cardiovascular Status and Benefits

Incidence of mortality from CAD varies greatly among countries around the world. Japan's mortality rate remains much lower than other developed countries despite westernization of its lifestyle.[78] Dwyer et al.[79] explored the hypothesis that differences in childhood lipoprotein concentrations may be responsible.

This study compared data on TC, HDL-C, dietary intake, anthropometry, and activity in 15,948 school-age children from Japan (n = 8542), Australia (n = 3520), and the United States (n = 3886). Data were collected from previously conducted health, fitness, and nutritional surveys.[80-84]

Dwyer et al.[79] demonstrated a significantly ($p<0.001$) higher mean concentration of serum HDL-C (but not TC) in Japanese children than in Australian and U.S. children. The differences in serum HDL-C levels between ages 8 and 10 years and 12 and 15 years were greater ($p<0.001$) for Australian (males-15.2% and females-2.6%) and U.S. (males-9.1% and females-2.7%) children than for their Japanese counterparts (males-4.2% and females-1.9%). Mean serum TC was significantly higher ($p<0.001$) for 8- to 10-year-old children (4.55 mmol/L) than for 12- to 15-year-old children (4.29 mm/L) regardless of nationality. Serum HDL-C to mean TC ratio was higher ($p<0.001$) in Japanese children (0.354) than in Australian (0.321) or U.S. children (0.313) regardless of age. BMI for Australian and Japanese children were similar while U.S. children had higher BMI levels at all ages. Japanese children were more active than Australian children (data not available for U.S. children). Japanese children consumed less total fat from total energy intake (27%) than Australian (37%) or U.S. (36%) children. The authors concluded that childhood differences in food intake and PA may importantly affect later risk of CAD death via a pathway that involves adolescent HDL-C concentration.

PA in adults has been associated with reduced incidence of CAD.[85] Risk factors for CAD appear to begin in childhood.[86,87] PA during childhood is an important factor in potential reduction of CAD risk factors both during childhood and into adulthood.[88,89] Although endurance training in adults has been associated with increased HDL-C, the serum lipoprotein regarded protective against CAD,[90] there are conflicting reports on the same benefit in childhood.

Rowland et al.[91] investigated the influence of a 13-week aerobic training program on serum lipid profiles in 34 healthy sixth-grade students (20 females and 14 males). Mean age of students at the beginning of training was 11.8 ± 0.5 years with a range of 10.9 to 12.9 years. Each child served as his or her own control to minimize genetic effects of trainableness between students.

Serum lipid levels, aerobic fitness ($\dot{V}O_{2max}$, and anthropometric data were collected 13 weeks prior to initiation of training, at initiation of training, and at the end of the 13-week training period. Serum lipid profiles included TC, HDL-C, low density lipoprotein (LDL-C), and triglycerides (Tg). Aerobic fitness was determined by standard cycle ergometer protocol. Anthropometric data included Ht, BW, and skinfold sums.

Training was conducted as part of the usual PE program. Training sessions consisted of 25 minutes of sustained aerobic exercise three times per week. Heart rate monitoring was performed to assess intensity of training [mean heart rate was 175.4 beats per minute (bpm) with a range of 153 bpm to 192 bpm]. Three-day dietary intake records were collected in 11 children (7 females and 4 males) midway through both the 13-week pretraining period, and 13-week training period.

Analysis of 3-day dietary intake records in 11 children showed a small but significant ($p<0.5$) decrease in kilocalorie intake during the training period compared with the pretraining period. Dietary cholesterol (DC) intake during the training period (190 mg ± 64 mg) was significantly ($p<0.5$) lower than the pretraining period (255 mg ± 93 mg). However, when DC was analyzed per 1000 kcals of intake the significance between the training period (100 mg ± 29 mg DC/1000 kcals) and the pretraining period (115 mg ± 34 mg DC/1000 kcals) was lost. Furthermore, there were no significant differences in percent of total caloric intake from CHO, PRO, and fat between the training period (CHO 51.8% ± 6.7%; PRO 14.4% ± 3.0%; fat 33.8% ± 5.1%) and the pretraining period (CHO 54.1% ± 7.9%; PRO 15.9% ± 1.7%; fat 30.0% ± 7.2%).

No significant changes were observed in serum lipid profiles of aerobically trained children. The serum lipid response finding in this study was consistent with similar studies conducted by Linder et al.[92,93] However, a shorter (6-week) study conducted by Gilliam and Burke [94] in 8- to 10-year-old females reported an increase in HDL-C in response to aerobic training.

Another study demonstrating a positive association between aerobic exercise and HDL-C was conducted by Stergioulas et al.[95] Their study consisted of 28 healthy sedentary males aged 10 to 14 years. Eighteen males were randomly assigned to an exercise group, with the remaining ten males serving as controls. Exercise training consisted of aerobic exercise on bicycle ergometer at 75% of physical working capacity during four 60-minute sessions per week over 8 weeks. The control group did not participate in any specific training program. Both groups were instructed not to change their dietary intake or take any medications during the study period. Serum samples for TC, HDL-C, Tg, and prostacyclin (6-keto-PGF1a) were collected. Serum samples were collected before training began, at days 15, 30, and 60 after training was initiated, and 30 days after training ceased. Ht, BW, and physical working capacity were collected at baseline and at the end of the training period with physical working capacity also being collected after 30 days of detraining in both groups.

Stergioulas et al.[95] demonstrated significantly ($p<0.005$) increased mean HDL-C concentration in the exercise group from baseline to post training (1.24 ± 0.07 mmol/L vs. 1.44 ± 0.05 mmol/L, respectively). Change in mean HDL-C concentration in the control group between baseline and post training was not significant. Mean serum 6-keto-PGF1a concentration in the exercise group was also significantly ($p<0.001$) increased from baseline to post training (58.23 ± 2.5 pg/ml vs. 95.4 ± 5.47 pg/ml, respectively). Change in mean serum 6-keto-PGF1a concentration in the control group from baseline to post training was not significant (60.6 ± 3.95 pg/ml vs. 61.7 ± 3.2 pg/ml, respectively). The authors concluded that regular aerobic exercise in young sedentary males can have beneficial effects on serum HDL-C and 6-keto-PGF1a concentrations. These benefits may positively impact CAD prevention.

2. *Anemia*

Nonanemic iron deficiency (NAID), or sports anemia, as it is also known, has been reported in adolescent endurance athletes, particularly long-distance runners.[96-98] NAID has not been reported in childhood athletes. Endurance sports include marathon running, road cycling, triathalons, cross-country skiing, and long-distance running. Other sports that are physically demanding, but do not completely exhaust glycogen stores, including swimming, track, gymnastics, soccer, football, baseball, and dance, are classified as nonendurance sports.[99] Usual childhood athletic activities do not include endurance sports training which is thought to be the etiology of this type of anemia. However, as elite athletes become younger with more-intensive training beginning at younger ages, the probability of seeing this phenomenon in childhood athletes exists.

The prevalence of NAID in high school cross-country runners has been reported as 20%[97,98] to 50%[100] in females and 17% in males.[100] Nickerson et al.[101] investigated 72 high school cross-country runners during the running season for etiological factors associated with NIAD. Iron deficiency (ID) was defined as a normal hemoglobin value (normal value was not defined) with a serum ferritin level of ≤ 12 nanograms (ng) per milliliter (ml) and a transferrin saturation of ≤ 16 %. Iron deficiency anemia (IDA) was defined as a hemoglobin of ≤ 12 milligrams (mg) per deciliter (dl) in females, and ≤ 13 mg/dl in males with serum ferritin level and saturation the same as described above for ID. Runners were 15 to 18 years of age. Runners (females and males) were assigned to one of three groups. Group I (n = 23) received a daily iron supplement (60 mg elemental iron as ferrous sulfate), and was prescribed an iron-rich diet. Group II (n = 21) received a placebo supplement, and was prescribed an iron-rich diet. Group III (n = 22) served as a control, receiving neither an iron supplement nor diet prescription. Diet instructions to increase heme and nonheme iron intake were provided three times during the training season to Groups I and II. Dietary iron records were collected initially and midway through the season in 20 female and 12 male runners.

Nickerson et al.[101] demonstrated that 42% (34% female and 8% male) of the cross-country runners became ID by stated criteria. IDA developed in 14% of the females with ID while none of the males developed IDA. Despite dietary instruction, iron intake did not increase significantly during the study. Iron loss can occur in urine, sweat, and feces. Gastrointestinal (GI) loss has been documented after marathon runs in other studies.[102-104] The effect of possible GI iron loss in these runners was evaluated by heme-compound stool assays. Twenty female runners demonstrated a > 4 mg of hemoglobin per gram of stool in 14 of 90 stool specimens. Only one of the male runners had > 4 mg of hemoglobin per gram of stool in 1 of 5 stool specimens. However, no significant differences in iron loss were seen in 36 prerace and 44 postrace heme-compound stool assays. Iron loss via urine and sweat was not significant.

The authors concluded that low initial iron stores and GI bleeding were associated with NAID. Despite treatment with 60 mg/day of elemental iron supplementation, NAID was not prevented in these runners. However, supplementation of 180 mg/day of elemental iron until indices returned to normal did result in successful treatment of NAID and IDA in these runners.

IV. NUTRITION

The relationship between nutritional intake and exercise performance has been recognized since Greek and Roman times. During the 20th century, understanding of nutrient substrate utilization in energy metabolism has become relatively sophisticated. Consequently, the quest for performance-enhancing energy and nutrient source(s) has intensified for the casual as well as the elite athlete regardless of age. However, this area of research in children is limited.

A. Requirements

Nutritional assessment in children is based on maintaining growth within established parameters. Markers utilized for growth include Ht, BW, Wt/Ht, %BF, and BMI. Monitoring of these markers will reveal imbalance(s) of energy and/or nutrient intake over time. The World Health Organization,[105] publishes nutritional recommendations intended to serve as guidelines for populations of all nations.

1. RDA /DRI

Recommended Dietary Allowances[106] (RDA) are the primary reference values utilized for evaluation and prescription of nutritional intake for healthy individuals in the U.S. The last edition was published in 1989.[106] However, more recently, the Food and Nutrition Board (FNB) has begun to replace the RDAs with a new set of reference values for the U.S. and Canada known as Dietary Recommended Intakes[107] (DRI). The DRIs include values for estimated average requirements, RDA, adequate intakes, and tolerable upper intake levels. The first publication includes values for calcium, phosphorus, magnesium, vitamin D, and fluoride. Use of the DRIs is encouraged, but information is limited to the nutrients listed above. Therefore, until publication of DRIs on all nutrients is available, the RDAs continue to be employed as the primary reference values.

2. *Estimating Energy Needs*

Recommended energy intake for age (Table 3.2) provides one method for estimating energy needs. Adjustments to match individual EE requirements should be accomplished based on monitoring of growth markers over time.[108]

Table 3.2 Recommended Energy and Protein Intakes for Age

	Age (yr)	REE (kcal/kg/d)	Average Energy Needs (kcalAkg $BW^{-1}Ad^{-1}$)	(kcal/d)	Protein (gAkg $BW^{-1}Ad^{-1}$)
Children	1–3	57	102	1300	1.2–1.8
	4–6	48	90	1800	1.2–1.75
	7–10	40	70	2000	1.0–1.5
Males	11–14	32	55	2500	1.0
Females	11–14	28	47	2200	1.0

Adapted from references 106 and 108.

Other modes that estimate energy needs include the REE method,[108] doubly labeled water technique,[109] direct and indirect calorimetry, and heart rate monitoring. The REE method calculates REE/kg of BW as a baseline of EE to which factors such as maintenance, activity, and growth (Table 3.3) are added. Although this method may be subject to wider individual variation, it is readily available and easily utilized in any setting. More-accurate methods, such as doubly labeled water technique, direct and indirect calorimetry, and heart rate monitoring are employed primarily for investigative purposes, and are not readily available outside the research setting.

Table 3.3 REE Method of Estimating Energy Needs

Factors	x REE*/kg Body Weight
Maintenance	0.2
Activity	0.1–0.25
Growth	0.5

Adapted from reference 108
*See Table 3.2

3. *Nutrients — Macro and Micro (Fuel Sources)*

Intensity and duration of PA or exercise determines the source of energy (fuel) utilized by the body. CHO and fat serve as the major sources of energy (fuel) for muscle. PRO provides fuel during prolonged PA or training when CHO and fatty acids (FA) are limited in availability.[110]

PA requiring anaerobic or maximal effort over short periods of time such as sprints, gymnastics, football, figure skating, and ballet primarily utilize adenosine triphosphate (ATP) and phosphocreatine (PCr) as fuel sources. Metabolism of CHO (glucose and glycogen) and FA provide these fuel sources. PA requiring intense effort over longer periods of time or endurance-type activities that involve aerobic mechanisms such as marathon running, basketball, soccer, ice hockey, and wrestling initially utilize CHO as a fuel source. However, over time, FA and PRO provide energy-sustaining fuel sources.[110]

Energy and nutrient intake balanced with expenditure should provide adequate fuel for PA and exercise in children. Rankinen et al.[111] investigated this hypothesis in athletic and non-athletic children. The authors assessed 43 female athletes(FA) (gymnasts, figure skaters, and runners), 49 male (MA) hockey players, 53 non-athletic female controls (FC), and 35 non-athletic male controls (MC). Mean ages of FA and FC were 11.4 ± 0.5 years and 11.5 ± 0.5 years, respectively. Mean ages of MA and MC were 12.5 ± 0.5 years and 12.4 ± 0.5 years, respectively. Four-day dietary intake and activity records, serum trace element status, and anthropometric measures were collected.

Analysis of dietary intake records indicated a significantly higher energy intake in MA than in MC, but not in FA and FC. However, when energy intake was calculated per kilogram BW, FA energy intake was significantly higher than FC. PRO intake was significantly increased in both MA and FA when compared with MC and FC. Dietary micronutrient intakes significantly increased in MA when compared with MC included calcium (Ca), iron (Fe), zinc (Zn), copper (Cu), magnesium (Mg), selenium (Se), vitamins A, D, E, C, thiamin, riboflavin, and niacin. There were no differences in micronutrient intakes between FA and FC, nor were there any significant differences in serum trace element concentration. Serum Zn concentration was significantly higher in MA than MC, but the reverse was true for serum Cu and ferritin. Mean dietary intake of energy, PRO, and micronutrients met or exceeded current RDA/DRI recommendations by MA, but not MC. Mean intakes of Ca, Fe, and Zn were below RDA/DRI-recommended levels in both FA and FC. Serum trace element status for all groups was adequate despite lower than recommended RDA/DRI intakes of some nutrients. The results suggest that additional energy and micronutrient intake beyond RDA/DRI recommendations may not be necessary. However, intense or competitive sports activity may require additional energy and PRO intakes beyond the levels provided by current RDA/DRI recommendations.

Poortmans et al.[112] examined postexercise proteinuria in females (n = 93) and males (n = 77) aged 6 to 18 years. Data collected included urine total protein (TP), albumin, retinol binding protein (RBP), β^2 microglobulin (β^2M), and creatinine. Urine samples were collected prior to and 30 minutes after completion of maximal exercise by the 20-meter shuttle run test.

Results indicated glomerulus permeability and tubular reabsorption increases with age, and excretion rates of all PRO components were related to absolute intensity of exercise ($p<0.001$). Children aged 6 to 9 years demonstrated a gender difference in postexercise proteinuria with enhanced TP, albumin, β^2M, and RBP excretion in males, but not in females. The authors concluded that post-exercise proteinuria is present at maximal exercise in childhood and adolescence, and magnitude of PRO excretion is strictly related to exercise intensity.

4. Fluid

Positive fluid balance is necessary for PA and athletic performance.[113] Inadequate hydration increases body heat storage, decreases blood volume, and results in reduced exercise tolerance.[114] Children have larger body-surface-area to mass ratios than adults, which, in extreme weather conditions of heat or cold result in greater heat loss or heat absorption, respectively. Additionally, thermoregulatory responses are less effective in children than in adults.[115]

Children, similar to adults, do not drink enough fluid to replace losses during PA especially in warm weather.[116] Wilk and Bar-Or[117] demonstrated a 44.5% increase of voluntary fluid intake in non-trained, non-acclimatized children intermittently exercising in a climatic chamber (35°C, 45%–50% relative humidity) by flavoring their water. An additional 45.5% increase in voluntary fluid intake was achieved by adding 6% CHO and 18 mmol/L NaCl to the flavored water. Voluntary fluid replacement prior to and during PA or sports participation may prevent hypo hydration or dehydration altogether.

Rivera-Brown et al.[118] examined the effect of tropical climate (wet bulb globe temperature 30°C ± 1.0°C) on voluntary drinking, drink composition, and fluid balance. Twelve heat-acclimatized male athletes aged 11 to 14 years (mean age 13.4 ± 0.4 years) participated in two 3-hour exercise sessions. Each session consisted of four 20-minute cycling bouts at 60% $\dot{V}O_{2max}$ alternating with 25-minute rest periods. One of two beverages [unflavored water (UFW) or flavored water plus 6% CHO and 18 mmol/L NaCL (FWNaCl)] was offered *ad libitum* during each session. Flavor preferences were predetermined in each athlete. Beverages were then assigned in a random fashion, with each athlete receiving both beverages.

Fluid intake and losses along with serum osmolality, NaCL, hemoglobin, and hematocrit were collected initially and at the end of the study. BW was measured at the beginning and end of each exercise session. Analysis of data demonstrates a 32% higher ($p<0.05$) total intake of FWNaCl beverage than UFW. A pattern of hypohydration (0.94% of initial BW) was observed with UFW whereas euhydration (+0.18% of initial BW) was observed with FWNaCl ($p<0.5$). Despite a 5.5% higher fluid intake than fluid losses with FWNaCl and a negative fluid balance with UFW, no differences were observed in serum volume, osmolality, or electrolyte concentration. These authors concluded that consumption of FWNaCl beverage prevents voluntary dehydration in heat-acclimatized male athletes exercising in a tropical climate.

B. Recommendations

1. Organized Athletics/Physical Activity

The National Institutes for Health[119] recommendation for PA in children (also adults) is to accumulate at least 30 minutes or more of moderate-intensity physical activity on all, or preferably most, days of the week.

The AAP Committee on Sports Medicine and the Committee on School Health[120] have made several recommendations for goals of organized athletics for pre-adolescent children.(Table 3.4) Additionally, they recommend coaches be role models for lifestyle and behavior goals. The coaches' role-modeling goals for childhood athletes should include weight control, fitness, good nutrition, and avoidance of tobacco, alcohol, and drugs.

Table 3.4 Focus of Goals for Organized Athletics in Preadolescent Children

1.	Enjoyment of sports and PA that will be sustained through adulthood
2.	Physical fitness
3.	Basic motor skills
4.	Positive self-image
5.	Balanced perspective on sports in relation to the child's school and community life
6.	Commitment to the values of teamwork, fair play, and sportsmanship

Adapted from reference 120.

The AAP Committee on Sports Medicine[121] has published recommendations on strength training, weight and power lifting, and body building for children and adolescents. These recommendations suggest that strength training programs for prepubescent, pubescent, and postpubescent athletes should be permitted only if conducted by well-trained adults. The adults should be qualified to plan programs appropriate to the athlete's stage of maturation, which should be assessed objectively by medical personnel. Until data demonstrates safety, children and adolescents should avoid the practice of weight lifting, power lifting, and body building, as well as the repetitive use of maximal amounts of weight in strength training programs, until they have reached Tanner[9] Stage V (adult level) of developmental maturity.

2. Energy/Nutrients

RDA/DRI recommended energy and nutrient intakes for age should be utilized for all children including childhood athletes. Energy intake should be adjusted according to individual need to meet energy balance, especially in the very active or very inactive child.

CHO generally provide 55% to 65% of total energy intake in children. There are no studies in children regarding the practice of CHO loading for endurance-type activities or training. Without evidence of beneficial effects in this age group, this practice should be avoided.

PRO usually provides 10% to 15% of total energy intake in children. Table 3.2 provides PRO recommendations based on BW for children. Studies investigating PRO needs in physically active or athletic children are lacking. Data in adult strength and endurance athletes indicates increased PRO need.[122–124] However, without valid clinical data demonstrating beneficial effects of increased PRO intake in physically active or athletic children, current RDA PRO recommendations should be utilized.

The AAP,[125] American Heart Association,[126] and the National Cholesterol Education Program[127] recommend that fat provide 30% of total energy intake, < 10% energy from saturated fat, and < 300 mg cholesterol daily for individuals over 2 years of age. The AAP[125] recommends a minimum level of fat intake that should not be less than 20% of total energy intake.

3. Fluid

Hydration status prior to participating in PA or sports is an important indicator of performance and endurance in adults as well as children. Fluid intake is recommended prior to, during, and at the conclusion of PA.[128] Table 3.5 provides recommendations for fluid intake in physically active children.[128,129] Chilled fluids leave the stomach more rapidly than warm ones and therefore consumption of cold fluids is recommended.[130] Fluid deficits at the conclusion of PA should be replaced based on weight loss. Obtaining body weight at the beginning and at the conclusion of PA is recommended when feasible.

Table 3.5 Recommended Fluid Intake for Physically Active Children

Time	Amount
Prior – 1/2-1 hour	4 oz.–8 oz.
Every 15 min. during	4 oz.
After	16 oz. per pound lost

Adapted from references 128 and 129.

Sport drinks similar to those examined by Wilk and Bar-Or[117] and Rivera-Brown et al.[118] are commercially available. These beverages are beneficial in children who have large fluid losses (sweating) especially in hot, humid weather. They are also beneficial as rehydration solutions when hydration is not adequately maintained during exercise. However, in children who do not have large fluid losses (i.e., exercise < 90 minutes) use of plain water is encouraged.[130]

V. SUMMARY

1. Physically active children and child athletes are more likely to become physically active adults.
2. Aerobic and anaerobic activities are safe, beneficial, and recommended for all children.
3. Physically active children and child athletes grow normally and may have enhanced bone mineralization.
4. Cardiovascular disease risk is positively impacted by physical activity in childhood.

5. Sports anemia is not a risk factor in physically active children or child athletes.
6. Maintaining adequate energy, nutrient, and fluid intakes are essential to good health and enhance physical performance in children.
7. Establishing healthy dietary and physical activity habits in childhood will provide health benefits throughout life.

REFERENCES

1. Rowland, T., Exercise and Children's Health, *Human Kinetics,* Champaign, Illinois, 1990.
2. Sallis, J. F., Simons-Morton, B. G., Stone, E. J., Corbin, C. B., Epstein, L. H., Faucette, N., Iannotti, R. J., Killen, J. D., Klesges, R. C., Petray, C. K., Rowland, T.W., and Taylor, W. C., Determinants of physical activity and interventions in youth, *Med. Sci. Sports Exerc.*, 24, S248, 1992.
3. American Academy of Pediatrics, American Academy of Family Physicians, American Orthopedic Society for Sports Medicine, American Medical Society for Sports Medicine, and the American Osteopathic Academy of Sports Medicine, *Preparticipation Physical Evaluation,* Kansas City, Missouri, American Academy of Family Physicians, 1992.
4. Telama, R. and Yang, X., Physical activity in childhood and adolescence as predictor of physical activity in young adulthood, *Am. J. Prev. Med.,* 13, 317, 1997.
5. Simons-Morton, B. G., McKenzie, T. J., Stone, E., Mitchell, P., Osganian, V., Strikmiller, P. K., Ehlinger, S., Cribb, P., and Nader, P. R., Physical activity in a multiethnic population of third graders in four states, *Am. J. Public Health*, 87, 45, 1997.
6. United States Department of Health and Human Services, *Promoting Health/Preventing Disease: Year 2000 Objectives for the Nation,* Washington, D.C., 1991.
7. Barlow, S. E. and Dietz, W. H., Obesity evaluation and treatment: expert committee recommendations, *Pediatrics*, 102, E29, 1998.
8. Rowland, T., Kline, G., Goff, D., Martel, L., and Ferrone, L., One-mile run performance and cardiovascular fitness in children, *Arch. Pediatr. Adolesc. Med.,* 153, 845, 1999.
9. Tanner, J. M., *Growth at Adolescence,* 2nd ed., Blackwell Scientific, Oxford, 1962.
10. Slaughter, M. H., Lohman, T. G., Boileau, R. A., Horswill, C. A., Stillman R. H., Van Loan, M. D., and Bemben, D. A., Skinfold equations for estimation of body fatness in children and youth, *Hum. Biol.,* 60, 709, 1988.
11. Dennison, B. A., Straus, J. H., Mellits, E. D., and Charney, E., Childhood physical fitness tests: predictor of adult physical activity levels? *Pediatrics*, 82, 324, 1988.
12. President's Council on Youth Fitness, Youth physical fitness, *Government Printing Office,* Washington, D.C., 1961.
13. Flynn, M. A., Nolph, G. B., Baker, A. S., Martin, W. M., Krause, G., Total body potassium in aging humans: a longitudinal study, *Am. J. Clin. Nutr.*, 50, 713, 1989.
14. Depres, J. P., Moorjani, S., Lupien, P. J., Tremblay, A., Nadeau, A., Bouchard, C., Regional distribution of body fat, plasma lipoproteins, and cardiovascular disease, *Arteriosclerosis*, 10, 497, 1990.
15. Pinhas-Hamiel, O., Dolan, L. M., Daniels, S. R., Standiford, D., Khoury, P. R., and Zeitler, P., Increased incidence of non-insulin-dependent diabetes mellitus among adolescents, *J. Pediatr.,* 128, 608, 1996.
16. Tremblay, A., Despres, J. P., Leblanc, C., and Bouchard, C., Sex dimorphism in fat loss in response to exercise training, *J. Obes. Reg.*, 3, 193, 1984.
17. Epstein, L., Wing, R. R., Koeske, R., Ossip, D., and Beck, S. A., A comparison of lifestyle changes and programmed aerobic exercise on weight and fitness changes in obese children, *Behav. Ther.*, 13, 651, 1982.
18. van Dale, D., Saris, W. H. M., Schoffelen, P.F.M., and ten Hoor, F., Does exercise give an additional effect in weight reduction regimes? *Int. J. Obes.,* 11, 367, 1987.
19. van Dale, D., Schoffelen, P. F. M., ten Hoor, F., and Saris, W. H. M., Effects of adding exercise to energy restriction, 24-h energy expenditures, resting metabolic rate, and daily physical activity, *Eur. J. Clin. Nutr.*, 43,441, 1989.
20. Meyer, G. A. L., Janssen, G. M. E., Westerterp, K. R., Verhoeven, F., Saris, W. H. M., and ten Hoor, F., The effect of a 5-month endurance-training program on physical activity: evidence for a sex difference in the metabolic response to exercise, *Eur. J. Appl. Physiol.*, 62, 11, 1991.

21. Blaak, E. E., Westerterp, K. R., Bar-Or, O., Wouters, L.J.M., and Saris, W.H.M., Total energy expenditure and spontaneous activity in relation to training in obese boys, *Am. J. Clin. Nutr.,* 55, 777, 1992.
22. Lohman, T. G., Applicability of body composition techniques and constants for children and youth: advances in pediatric sports science, in: *Human Kinetics*, Boileau, R. A., Ed., Champaign, Illinois, 1984, 29-57.
23. Treuth, M. S., Gigueroa-Colon, G. R., Weinsier, R. L., Butte, N. F., and Goran, M. I., Energy expenditure and physical fitness in overweight versus non-overweight prepubertal girls, *Int. J. Obes.*, 22, 440, 1998.
24. Coward, W. A., Ritz, P., and Cole, T. J., Revision of calculation in the doubly labeled water method for measurement of energy expenditure in humans, *Am. J. Physiol.*, 267, E805, 1994.
25. Goran, M. I., Hunter, T. R., and Johnson, R., Physical activity related energy expenditure and fat mass in young children, *Int. J. Obes.,* 21, 171, 1997.
26. Barbeau, P., Gutin, B., Litaker, M., Owens, S., Riggs, S., and Okuyama, T., Correlates of individual differences in body-composition changes resulting from physical training in obese children, *Am. J. Clin. Nutr.,* 69, 705, 1999.
27. Sun, M., Gower, B. A., Nagy, T. R., Trowbridge, C. A., Dezenberg, C., and Goran, M. I., Total, resting, and activity-related energy expenditures are similar in Caucasian and African-American children, *Am. J. Physiol.,* 274, E232, 1998.
28. Kaplan, A. S., Zemel, B. S., and Stallings, V. A., Differences in resting energy expenditure in prepubertal black children and white children, *J. Pediatr.,* 129, 643, 1996.
29. Morrison, J. A., Alfaro, M. P., Khoury, P., Thornton, B.B., and Daniels, S. R., Determinants of resting energy expenditure in young black girls and young white girls, *J. Pediatr.*, 129,637, 1996.
30. Goran, M. I., Gower, B. A., Nagy, T. R., and Johnson, R. K., Developmental changes in energy expenditure and physical activity in children: evidence for a decline in physical activity in girls before puberty, *Pediatrics,* 101, 887, 1998.
31. Goran, M. I., Shewchuk, R., Gower, B. A., Nagy, T. R., Carpenter, W. H., and Johnson, R. K., Longitudinal changes in fatness in white children: no effect of childhood energy expenditure, *Am. J. Clin. Nutr.,* 67,309, 1998.
32. Astrand, P. O. and Rodahl, K., *Textbook of Work Physiology,* New York, McGraw-Hill, 1986.
33. Armstrong, N., Welsman, J., and Winsley, R., Is peak VO^2 a maximal index of children's aerobic fitness? *Int. J. Sports Med.,* 17, 356, 1996.
34. Rowland, T. W., Oxygen uptake and endurance fitness in children: a developmental perspective, *Ped. Exer. Sci.,* 1, 313, 1989.
35. Bar-Or, O., Metabolic response to acute exercise, in *Pediatric Sports Medicine,* Katz, M. and Carpentier, R. S., Eds., Springer-Verlag, New York, 1983, pp.3-4.
36. McMurray, R. G., Guion, W. K., Ainsworth, B. E., and Harrell, J. S., Predicting aerobic power in children, *J. Sports Med. Phys. Fit.,* 38, 227, 1998.
37. Klissouras, V., Evaluations of physical fitness of schoolchildren: the Eurofit test in youth and fitness, in *Proceedings of the XVth Meeting of International Council for Physical Fitness Research,* Howald, H., Ed., Magglingen, Geneva, 1982, pp.1-12.
38. Mocellin, R., Lindemann, J., Rutenfranz, J., and Sbresny, W., Determination of W170 and maximal oxygen uptake in children by different methods, *Acta. Paediatr. Scand.,* 217, S13, 1971.
39. American Academy of Pediatrics, Policy statement on weight training and weight lifting: information for the pediatrician, *Phys. Sports Med.*, 11, 157, 1983.
40. American Academy of Pediatrics, Strength training, weight and power lifting, and body building by children and adolescents, *Pediatrics,* 86, 801, 1990.
41. Vrijens, J., Muscle strength development in the pre- and postpubescent age, *Med. Sport,* 11, 152, 1978.
42. Docherty, D., Wenger, H. A., Collis, M. L., and Quinney, H.A., The effects of variable speed resistance training on strength development in prepubertal boys, *J. Hum. Mov. Stud.,* 13, 377, 1987.
43. Duda, M., Prepubescent strength training gains support, *Phys. Sportsmed.,* 14, 157, 1986.
44. Jacobson, B. H, and Kulling, F. A., Effect of resistive weight training in prepubescents, *J. Orthop. Sports Phys. Ther.,* 11, 96, 1989.
45. Legwold, G., Does lifting weights harm a prepubescent athlete? *Phys. Sportsmed.,* 10,141, 1982.
46. Ramsay, J. A., Blimkie, C.R.J., Smith, K., Garner, S., MacDougall, J.D., and Sale, D.G., Strength training effects in prepubescent boys, *Med. Sci. Sports Exerc.*, 22, 605, 1990.

47. Pfeiffer, R. D. and Francis, R. S., Effects of strength training on muscle development in prepubescent, pubescent, and postpubescent males, *Phys. Sportsmed.*, 14, 134, 1986.
48. Sewall, L. and Micheli, L., Strength training for children, *J. Ped. Ortho.*, 6, 143, 1986.
49. Ramsay, J. A., Blinkie, J. R., Smith, K., Garner, S., MacDougall, J. D., and Sale, D.G., Strength training effects in prepubescent boys, *Med. Sci. Sports Exerc.*, 22, 605, 1990.
50. Committee on Nutrition, American Academy of Pediatrics, *Pediatric Nutrition Handbook*, 4th ed., Kleinman, R.E., Ed., American Academy of Pediatrics, Elk Grove Village, IL, 1998, 141.
51. Behrman, R. E, and Vaughan, V. C., Developmental pediatrics: growth and development, in *Textbook of Pediatrics,* 13th ed., Nelson, W.E., Ed., W.B. Saunders Company, Philadelphia, 1987, pp.16-17.
52. Heyner, S., Smith R. M., and Schultz, G. A., Temporally regulated expression of insulin and insulin-like growth factors and their receptors in early mammalian development, *Bioessays*, 11, 171, 1989.
53. Hill, D. L. and Han, V. K., Paracrinology of growth regulation, *J. Dev. Physiol.,* 15, 91, 1991.
54. Young, V. R., Steffe, W. P., Pencharz, P. B., Winterer, J. C., and Scrimshaw, N. S., Total human body protein synthesis in relation to protein requirements at various ages, *Nature,* 253, 192, 1975
55. Brook, C. G. D. and Hindmarsh, P. C., The somatotropic axis in puberty, *Endocrinol. Metab. Clin. North Am.,* 21, 767, 1992.
56. Holly, J. M. P., and Wass, J. A. H., Insulin-like growth factors: autocrine, paracrine, or endocrine? New perspectives of the somatomedin hypothesis in the light of recent developments, *J. Endocrinol.,* 122, 611, 1989.
57. Green, H., Morikawa, M., and Nixon, T., A dual effector theory of growth hormone action, *Differentiation,* 29, 195, 1985.
58. Schwartz, H. L., Effect of thyroid hormone on growth and development, in *Molecular Basis of Thyroid Hormone Action,* Oppenheimer, H. and Samuels, H.H., Eds., Academic Press, New York, 1983, pp.413-444.
59. Kennedy, G. C., Interactions between feeding behavior and hormones during growth, *Ann. N. Y. Acad. Sci.,* 157, 1049, 1969.
60. Davidson, M. B., Effect of growth hormone on carbohydrate and lipid metabolism, *Endocrinol. Rev.,* 8, 115, 1987.
61. Hochberg, Z., Hertz, P., Colin, V., Ish-Shalom, S., Yeshurun, D., Youdin, M. B., and Amit, T., The distal axis of growth hormone(GH) in nutritional disorders: GH-binding protein, insulin-like growth factor I (IGF-1), and IGF-1 receptors in obesity and anorexia nervosa, *Metabolism,* 41, 106, 1992.
62. Kelijman, M. and Frohman, L. A., Enhanced growth hormone (GH) responsiveness to GH-releasing hormone after dietary manipulation in obese and non-obese subjects, *J. Clin. Endocrinol. Metabol.,* 66, 489, 1988
63. Mazzeo, R. S., Catecholamine responses to acute and chronic exercise, *Med. Sci. Sports Exerc.,* 23, 839, 1991.
64. Van Helder, W. P., Casey, K., and Radomski, M. W., Regulation of growth hormone during exercise by oxygen demand and availability, *Eur. J. Appl. Physiol.,* 56, 628, 1987.
65. Mc Donough, M.J.N. and Davies, C.T.M., Adaptive response of mammalian skeletal muscle to exercise with high loads, *Eur. J. Appl. Physiol.,* 52, 139, 1984.
66. Aloia, J. F., Cohn, S. H., Ostini, R. H., Cane, R., and Ellis, K., Prevention of involutional bone loss by exercise, *Ann. Int. Med.,* 89, 356, 1978.
67. Morey, E. R. and Baylink, D. J., Inhibition of bone formation during space flight, *Science,* 201, 1138, 1978.
68. Schuck, G. R., Effects of athletic competition on the growth and development of junior high school boys, *Res. Q.,* 33, 288, 1962.
69. Buckler, J. M. and Brodie, D. A., Growth and maturity characteristics of schoolboy gymnasts, *Ann. Hum. Biol.,* 4, 455, 1977.
70. Astrand, P. O., Engstrom, L., Eriksson, B. O., Karlberg, P., Nylander, I., Saltin, B., and Thoren, C., Girl swimmers with special reference to respiratory and circulatory adaptation and gynecological and psychiatric aspects, *Acta. Paediatr,* S147, 1, 1963.
71. Malina, R. M. and Bielicki, T., Retrospective longitudinal growth study of boys and girls active in sport, *Acta. Paediatr.,* 85, 570, 1996.
72. Malina, R. M., Physical growth and biological maturation of young athletes, *Exerc. Sports Sci. Rev.,* 22, 389, 1994.

73. Grimston, S. K., Willows, N. D., and Hanley, D. A., Mechanical loading regime and its relationship to bone mineral density in children, *Med. Sci. Sports Exerci.*, 25, 1203, 1993.
74. Gunnes, M. and Lehmann, E. H., Physical activity and dietary constituents as predictors of forearm cortical and trabecular bone gain in healthy children and adolescents: a prospective study, *Acta. Paediatr., 85, 19, 1996.*
75. Longcope, C., Gorbach, S., Goldin, B., Woods, M., Dwyer, J., Morrill, A., and Warram, J., The effect of a low fat diet on estrogen metabolism, *J. Clin. Endocrin. Metab.*, 64, 1246, 1987.
76. Das, U. N., Can essential fatty acids prevent osteoporosis?, *Med. Sci. Res.*, 22, 163, 1994.
77. Shortt, C., Madden, A., Flynn, A., and Morrissey, P. A., Influence of dietary sodium intake on urinary calcium excretion in selected Irish individuals, *Eur. J. Clin. Nutr.*, 42, 595, 1988.
78. Okayama, A., Ueshima, H., Marmot, M. G., Nakamura, M., Kita, Y., and Yamakawa, M., Changes in total serum cholesterol and other risk factors for cardiovascular disease in Japan, *Int. J. Epidemiol.*, 22, 1038, 1993.
79. Dwyer, T., Iwane, H., Dean, K., Odagiri, Y., Shimomitsu, T., Blizzard, L., Srinivasan, S., Nicklas, T., Wattigney, W., Riley, M., and Berenson, G., Differences in HDL cholesterol concentrations in Japanese, American, and Australian children, *Circulation,* 96, 2830, 1997.
80. Australian Health and Fitness Survey 1985, The fitness, health, and physical performance of Australian school students aged 7-15 years, *ACHPER Publications,* 1985.
81. Department of Community Services and Health, *National dietary survey of schoolchildren (aged 10-15 years): 1985,* Australian Government Publication Service, Canberra, Australia, 1985.
82. Japanese Society of School Health, *Report on a survey of health status of schoolchildren* (in Japanese), 1993.
83. The Japanese Physical Education and School Health Centre, *Promotion of School Feeding Through Cooperation of School, Family, and Community: Report on Dietary Lifestyle Survey* (in Japanese), 1994.
84. Nicklas, T., Webber, L. S., Srinivasan, S. R., and Berenson, G. S., Secular trends in dietary intakes and cardiovascular risk factors of 10-year-old children: the Bogalusa Heart Study (1973-1988), *Am. J. Clin. Nutr.*, 57, 930, 1993.
85. Powell, K. E., Thompson, P. D., Caspersen, C. J., and Kendrick, J. S., Physical activity and the incidence of coronary heart disease, *Annu. Rev. Public Health*, 8, 253, 1987.
86. Williams, C. L., Carter, B. J., and Wynder, E. L., Prevalence of selected cardiovascular and cancer risk factors in a pediatric population: the "Know Your Body" project, New York, *Prev. Med.*, 10, 235, 1981.
87. Szamozi, T., Mihai, K., Peto, J., Makary, A., and Kramer, J., Potential markers of atherosclerotic process in high risk children, *Clin. Biochem.*, 24, 185, 1991.
88. Fletcher, G. F., Balady, G. J., Froelicher, V. F., Hartley, L. H., Haskell, W. L., and Pollock, M. L., Exercise standards: a statement from the American Heart Association, *Circulation,* 91, 580, 1995.
89. Pate, R. R., Pratt, M., Blair, S. N., Haskell, W. L., Macera, C. A., Bouchard, C., Buchner, D., Ettinger, W., Heath, G. W., and King, A. C., Physical activity and public health: a recommendation from the Centers for Disease Control and Prevention and the American College of Sports Medicine, *J. Am. Med. Assoc.*, 273, 402, 1995.
90. Durstine, J. L, and Haskell, W. L., Effects of exercise training on plasma lipids and lipoproteins, *Exerc. Sports Sci. Rev.*, 22, 477, 1994.
91. Rowland, T. W., Martel, L., Vanderburgh, P., Manos, T., and Charkoudian, N., The influence of short-term aerobic training on blood lipids in healthy 10–12-year-old children, *Int. J. Sports Med.,* 17, 487, 1996.
92. Linder, C. W., DuRant, R. H., Gray, R. G., and Harkness, J. W., The effect of exercise on serum lipids in children, *Clin. Res.*, 27, 297, 1979.
93. Linder, C. W., DuRant, R. H., and Mahoney, O. M., The effect of physical conditioning on serum lipids and lipoproteins in white male adolescents, *Med. Sci. Sports Exerc.*, 15, 232, 1983.
94. Gilliam, T. B, and Burke, M., Effects of exercise on serum lipids and lipoproteins in girls 8-10 years, *Artery,* 4, 203, 1978.
95. Stergioulas, A., Tripolitsioti, A., Messinis, D., Bouloukos, A., and Nounopoulos, C., The effects of endurance training on selected coronary risk factors in children, *Acta. Pediatr.*, 87, 401, 1998.

96. Rowland, T. W., Black, S. A., and Kelleher, J. F., Iron deficiency in adolescent endurance athletes, *J. Adolesc. Health Care,* 8, 322, 1987.
97. Nickerson, H. J., Holubets, M C., Tripp, A. D., and Pierce, W. E., Decreased iron stores in high school female runners, *Am. J. Dis. Child.,* 139, 1115, 1985.
98. Nickerson, H. J. and Tripp, A. D., Iron deficiency in adolescent cross country runners, *Phys. Sportsmed.,* 11, 60, 1983.
99. Committee on Nutrition, American Academy of Pediatrics, *Pediatric Nutrition Handbook*, 4th ed., Kleinman, R.E., Ed., American Academy of Pediatrics, Elk Grove Village, IL, 1998, p. 150.
100. Rowland, T. W, and Kelleher, J. F. , Iron deficiency in athletes, *Am. J. Dis. Child.,* 143, 197, 1989.
101. Nickerson, H. J., Holubets, M C., Weiler, B. R., Haas, R. G., Schwartz, S., and Ellefson, M. E., Causes of iron deficiency in adolescent athletes, *J. Pediatr.,* 114, 657, 1989.
102. Halvorsen, F. A., Lyng, J., and Ritland, S., Gastrointestinal bleeding in marathon runners, *Scand. J. Gastroenterol.,* 21, 493, 1986.
103. Porter, A. M. W., Do some marathon runners bleed into the gut?, *Br. Med. J.,* 287, 1427, 1983.
104. Stewart, J. G., Ahlquist, D. A., McGill, D. B., Ilstrup, D. M., Schwartz, S., and Owen, R. A., Gastrointestinal blood loss and anemia in runners, *Ann. Intern. Med.,* 100, 843, 1984.
105. World Health Organization, Food and Agriculture Organization, United Nations University, Energy and protein requirements, *WHO Tech. Rep. Ser., Geneva, Switzerland,* 724, 1985.
106. National Research Council, *Recommended Dietary Allowances,* 10th ed., National Academy of Sciences, Washington, D.C., 1989.
107. Standing Committee on the Scientific Evaluation of Dietary Reference Intakes, *Dietary Reference Intakes,* Food and Nutrition Board, Institute of Medicine, National Academy Press, Washington, D.C., 1997.
108. The Harriet Lane Handbook, *A Manual for Pediatric House Officers,* 15th ed., Siberry, G.K. and Iannone, R., Eds., Mosby, St. Louis, 2000, pg. 484.
109. Schoeller, D. A. and Webb, P., Five-day comparison of the doubly labeled water method with respiratory gas exchange, *Am. J. Clin. Nutr.,* 40, 153, 1984.
110. Hultman, E., Harris, R. C., and Spriet, L. L., Diet in exercise and work performance in *Modern Nutrition in Health and Disease*, Ninth ed., Shils, M. E., Olson, J. A., Shike, M., and Ross, A. C., Eds., Williams and Wilkins, Baltimore, 1999, pp. 761-772.
111. Rankinen, T., Fogelholm, M., Kujala, U., Rauramaa, R., and Uusitupa, M., Dietary intake and nutritional status of athletic and nonathletic children in early puberty, *Int. J. Sport Nutr.,* 5, 136, 1995.
112. Poortmans, J. R., Geudvert, C., Schorokoff, K., and DePlaen, P., Postexercise proteinuria in childhood and adolescence, *Int. J. Sports Med.,* 17, 448, 1996.
113. Committee on Sports Medicine, Climatic heat stress and the exercising child, *Pediatrics,* 69, 808, 1982.
114. Sawaka, M. N. and Pandolf, K. B., Effects of body water loss on physiological function and exercise heat performance, in *Perspectives in Exercise Science and Sports Medicine: Fluid Homeostasis During Exercise,* Gisolfi, C. V. and Lamb, D. R., Eds., Benchmark Press, Indianapolis, IN, 1990, 3, pp. 1-38.
115. Bar-Or, O., Climate and the exercising child, in *Pediatric Sports Medicine,* Katz, M., and Carpentier, R. S., Eds., Springer-Verlag, New York, 1983, pp. 262-264.
116. Bar-Or, O., Dotan, R., Inbar, O., Rothstein, A., and Zonder, H., Voluntary hypohydration in 10- to 12-year-old boys, *J. Appl. Physiol.,* 48,104, 1980.
117. Wilk, B., and Bar-Or, O., Effect of drink flavor and NaCl on voluntary drinking and hydration in boys exercising in the heat, *J. Appl. Physiol.,* 80, 1112, 1996.
118. Rivera-Brown, A. M., Gutierrez, R., Gutierrez, J. C., Frontera, W. R., and Bar-Or, O., Drink composition, voluntary drinking, and fluid balance in exercising, trained, heat-acclimatized boys, *J. Appl. Physiol.*, 86, 78, 1999.
119. National Institutes of Health Consensus Conference, Physical activity and cardiovascular health, *J. Am. Med. Assoc.,* 276, 241, 1996.
120. American Academy of Pediatrics Committee on Sports Medicine and Committee on School Health, *Pediatrics,* 84, 3 583, 1989.
121. American Academy of Pediatrics Committee on Sports Medicine, Strength training, weight and power lifting, and body building by children and adolescents, *Pediatrics,* 86, 801, 1990.
122. Lemon, P. W., Maximizing performance with nutrition: protein and exercise: update 1987, *Med. Sci. Sports Exerc.,* 19, S179, 1987.

123. Burke, L. M. and Read, R. S., Sports nutrition: approaching the nineties, *Sports Med.,* 8, 80,1989.
124. Lemon, P. W., Protein requirements of soccer, *J. Sports Sci.,* 12, S17, 1994.
125. American Academy of Pediatrics Committee on Nutrition, Statement on Cholesterol, *Pediatrics,* 101, 141, 1998.
126. Krauss, R. M., Deckelbaum, R. J., Ernst, N., Fisher, E., Howard, R. M., Knopp, R. H., Kotchen, T., Lichtenstein, A. H., McGill, H. C., Pearson, T. A., Prewitt, T. E., Stone, N. J., Horn, L. V., and Weinberg, R., Dietary guidelines for healthy American adults: a statement for health professionals from the National Committee, American Heart Association, *Circulation,* 94, 1795, 1996.
127. National Cholesterol Education Program, *Report of the Expert Panel on Population Strategies for Blood Cholesterol Education*, National Institutes of Health; National Heart, Lung, and Blood Institute, Bethesda, MD, 90, 140, 1990.
128. Hultman, E., Harris, R. C., and Spriet, L. L., Diet in exercise and work performance in *Modern Nutrition in Health and Disease*, Ninth Edition, Shils, M. E., Olson, J. A., Shike, M., and Ross, A.C., Eds., Williams and Wilkins, Baltimore, 1999, pp. 774-775.
129. Gatorade Fluid Guide, Sport Sciences Institute, Chicago, IL.
130. Timely Statement of The American Dietetic Association: nutrition guidance for child athletes in organized sports, *J. Am. Diet. Assoc.,* 96, 610, 1996.

CHAPTER 4

Nutritional Concerns of Adolescent Athletes

Katherine A. Beals

CONTENTS

I. INTRODUCTION

Adolescence is a time of rapid growth and development. It is estimated that during puberty, adolescents acquire 50% of their adult weight, 20% of their adult height, and 45% of their adult skeletal mass.[1] These rapid growth and developmental rates during adolescence exert a profound effect on energy and nutrient needs. Deficient intakes may delay pubertal development, impede growth and muscle development, and affect cognitive performance.[1,2]

Current reports estimate that more than 50% of children and adolescents in the United States participate in competitive athletics.[3] This includes more that seven million boys and girls involved

0-8493-8199-1/00/$0.00+$.50

in high school sports and an additional 20 million boys and girls between 8 and 16 years of age participating in community-sponsored athletic programs.[4,5] Strenuous physical activity, or sports training, places additional stress on adolescents by augmenting the already existing high nutritional demands of rapid growth.[1] Regular sports training has been shown to increase energy and protein requirements,[6] and may increase the need for certain micronutrients, particularly those important for growth (e.g., folate, iron, zinc, and copper).[7-12] If dietary intake does not meet the exercise-induced increase in nutrient requirements, then sports training has the potential to negatively impact the growth and biological maturation of the adolescent athlete.

Because of the large number of children and adolescents involved in athletics and the potential impact that sports training may have on nutrient requirement, it is critical that the effects of exercise or sport training on the nutritional status of the adolescent athlete be determined. This chapter will summarize the most recent research in the area of sports nutrition as it pertains to adolescent athletes. Particular attention will be given to nutritional status and nutrient requirements of adolescent athletes. In addition, factors that may undermine dietary adequacy (e.g., weight control practices and supplement usage) will be addressed.

II. NUTRITION KNOWLEDGE, ATTITUDES, AND DIETARY PRACTICES

Relatively little research exists describing the nutrition knowledge, attitudes, and dietary practices of adolescent athletes. Nonetheless, the few existing studies are consistent in their findings that, (1) adolescent athletes have only a rudimentary knowledge of general nutritional principles and a poor knowledge of sports nutrition concepts, and (2) increased nutrition knowledge (i.e., through nutrition education) rarely translates into changes or improvements in dietary practices.[5,13-16]

Peron and Endres[15] studied the nutrition knowledge, attitudes, and dietary intakes of 26 female adolescent volleyball players. Forty-six percent of the athletes correctly answered the general nutrition knowledge questions, while 41% correctly answered sports nutrition questions. Athletes were least knowledgeable about the roles of protein and carbohydrate in the diet, carbohydrate loading, and energy expenditure associated with various sports. The athletes demonstrated a positive attitude regarding nutrition, and nutrition knowledge and attitudes were positively correlated, but there was no correlation between knowledge (or attitudes) and dietary intake. For example, 88% of the athletes believed an athlete's diet can affect physical performance, yet most had inadequate intakes of energy, calcium, and iron. Similarly, 42% of the athletes knew that the pre-event meal should be eaten 3–4 hours before an event to avoid gastrointestinal distress, but 80% reported eating their pre-event meal within an hour of the competition.

In one of the largest studies to date on nutritional knowledge in athletes, Schmalz et al[16] examined nutrition beliefs and practices of 381 male and female adolescent athletes. Consistent with the findings of Peron and Endres,[15] the athletes demonstrated some knowledge of diet and health issues, but were basically ignorant with respect to sports nutrition issues. For example, while 95% of the athletes believed that a balanced diet was essential to an athlete's performance, 55% believed that steak and eggs was a good pre-competition meal. Similarly, 52% of the athletes believed that protein supplements were essential for increasing muscle size and strength.

Chapman et al.[13] evaluated the effectiveness of a 6-week sports nutrition education program on the nutrition knowledge and dietary practices of 36 female high school varsity softball players. Despite significant improvements in nutrition knowledge, there were no significant improvements in dietary intake or food choices among the athletes who received nutrition education.

These studies indicate that adolescent athletes are generally uninformed about sound nutritional practices specific to their needs. Moreover, even when adolescent athletes have accurate nutrition knowledge, they rarely put this knowledge into practice by making appropriate dietary choices. This is disturbing, given that many adolescents are at least partly responsible for their food selection and preparation.[15] It is well documented that adolescents routinely choose to consume foods high in fat and simple sugars[16,17] and often skip meals, most notably breakfast.[15,17,18] Adolescent athletes appear to practice similar dietary habits.[15,13-16] Thirteen percent of the athletes in the Schmalz[16] study skipped breakfast altogether, while 26% consumed high-fat, high-sugar breakfast foods (e.g., doughnuts, pastries, etc.). Moreover, only 26% of the athletes reported eating a nutritionally balanced lunch. Similarly, Peron and Endres[15] found that athletes were consuming the largest number of total servings from the "miscellaneous" group of the U.S. Food Guide Pyramid[19] consisting primarily of sodas, sweetened beverages, and concentrated sweets. These substandard dietary practices predispose adolescent athletes to poor nutritional status and place them at an increased risk for nutrient deficiencies.

III. ENERGY INTAKE AND NUTRITIONAL STATUS

Research indicates that, as children grow into their teen years, their average intake of vitamins and minerals on a per calorie basis decreases.[20] This, combined with the fact that nutrient requirements generally increase during adolescence,[21] would suggest that adolescents are at high risk for nutritional deficiencies. This is particularly true for certain nutrients, most notably iron and calcium. According to the 1994–96 Continuing Survey of Food by Individuals, males and females between the ages of 12 and 19, on average, fail to meet the RDA for calcium and iron.[22]

Relatively few studies have examined nutrient intakes of adolescent athletes, and fewer still have assessed multiple measures of nutritional status (i.e., blood levels of multiple micronutrients). The available data indicate that male adolescent athletes tend to consume more calories and higher levels of nutrients than teenage boys who do not participate in athletics.[1,23] The existing data on female adolescent athletes, on the other hand, is currently inconclusive. The limited available research indicates that female athletes have energy and nutrient intakes that fail to meet, meet, or exceed the U.S. Recommended Dietary Allowances (RDAs),[21] and may have either lower, higher, or the same energy and nutrient intakes than their less active counterparts, depending on the sport in which they participate.[8-10,15,23,24] It is important to note that all published studies have relied on self-report diet records, which may not accurately reflect actual nutrient intake.[25-27]

A. Energy Intake

Table 4.1 summarizes the most recent findings from energy intake studies in adolescent athletes. In reviewing the table, it becomes clear that some young athletes report consuming inadequate energy intakes while others report energy intakes well above recommended levels. For example, mean reported energy intakes of male swimmers, football and soccer players, and some female swimmers are adequate.[23,28,29] Conversely, reported energy intakes of female gymnasts, dancers, figure skaters, volleyball players, and male wrestlers appear to be inadequate.[15,24,31-35] Because actual energy requirements of young athletes have not been determined (see following section), and total daily energy expenditure was not measured in these studies, it is not possible to determine whether the energy intakes reported in Table 4.1 are adequate. Moreover, as previously noted, diet records are highly susceptible to inaccuracies, and thus, the seemingly inadequate intakes of some young athletes may be due to underreporting.[25-27] Nonetheless, it is well-recognized that certain groups of athletes, particularly those participating in thin-build or weight dependent sports regularly restrict energy intake in order to meet the body weight and image demands of their sport[3,31,33,36,37] (see following section).

B. Micronutrient Intake and Status

Inadequate energy intakes are generally accompanied by marginal macro- and micronutrient intakes. Indeed, in studies in which athletes reported consuming adequate energy, macro- and

Table 4.1 Self-Reported Energy Intakes of Adolescent Athletes

Reference	Sport	No. of Subjects	Age Range (yr.)	Mean Weight (kg)	Mean Energy Intake (kcal/d)	Mean Energy Intake (kcal/kg/d)
FEMALES:						
Benson et al.1985 (30)	Dance	92	12–17	46.8	1,890	40.8
Rucinski 1989 (33)	Figure Skating	23	13–22	—	1,174	—
Zeigler 1998 (35)	Figure Skating	21	11–16	50.3	1,781	35.4
Benson et al. 1990 (31)	Gymnastics		11–13	12	1,544	39.4
Benardot 1989 (41)	Gymnastics	22	11–14	—	1,706	—
Fogelhom et al. 1995 (167)	Gymnastics Figure Skating	12	16–18	51.7	1,776	—
Loosli and Benson 1986 (168)	Gymnastics	97	11–17	43.2	1,838	42.5
Sundgot–Borgen 1996 (169)	Rhythmic Gymnastics	12	14–20	42	1,703	41
Baer and Tapper 1992* (24)	Running	12	15–17	51.1	1,778	41.5
Benson et al. 1990 (31)	Swimming		11–13	18	1,892	39.5
Berning et al. 1991 (23)	Swimming	10	15–18	58.2	3,573	61.4
Peron and Endres 1985 (15)	Volleyball	26	13–17	—	1,799	—
Beals et. al.1999 (170)	Volleyball	26	14–17	65.2	2,248	34.4
MALES:						
Rucinski 1989 (33)	Figure Skating	17	16–26	—	2,897	—
Hickson et al. 1987 (29)	Football	46	11–14	60.9	2,523	41.4
Hickson et al. 1987 (29)	Football	88	15–18	75.9	3,365	44.3
Rankinen et al. 1995 (1)	Ice Hockey	48	12–13	44.1	2,448	56.7
Schemmel et al. 1988 (34)	Running	14	11–14	—	2,541	66.0
Schemmel et al. 1988 (34)	Running	4	15–18	—	2,736	50.0
Rico–Sanz 1998 (28)	Soccer	119	14–18	67.2	3,785	—
Berning et al. 1991 (23)	Swimming	22	15–18	77.2	5,222	67.6
Hawley and Williams 1991 (43)	Swimming	9	11–14	56.4	3,072	55.0
Van Erp Baart et al. 1989 (171)	Swimming	20	15–18	72.9	3,720	52.6
Horswill et al. 1990 (172)	Wrestling	18	14–17	63.7	—	26.6*
Schemmel et al. 1988 (34)	Wrestling	50	11–14	—	2,459	53.0
Schemmel et al. 1988 (34)	Wrestling	20	15–18	—	2,703	44.0
Roemmich and Sinning 1997 (32)	Wrestiling	9	15.4**	58.0	—	24.7*

* values represent "during season"
** mean age; age range not reported
— value not reported

micronutrient intakes generally met or exceeded recommended levels.[1,23] Conversely, in those studies in which athletes were consuming inadequate energy, macro- and micronutrient intakes typically failed to meet recommendations.[1,8,15,24,30,33,35] For example, Berning et al.[23] examined the energy and nutrient intakes of 22 male (15–18 years) and 21 female (12–17 years) swimmers and found that reported energy intakes of the athletes (5222 kcal/d and 3573 kcal/d for males and females, respectively) far exceeded those reported for the average teenager. In addition, the athletes' average daily intakes of vitamins A and C, thiamin, riboflavin, niacin, calcium, and iron met or exceeded the respective RDA.[23] Similarly, Rankinen et al.[1] compared the dietary intake and nutritional status of 49 adolescent male (12–13 years) hockey players and 43 young adolescent female (11–12 years) gymnasts, figure skaters, and runners to that of 88 male and female, adolescent, nonathletic controls. On average, the male athletes consumed more energy, protein, thiamin, riboflavin, niacin, vitamins C and E, calcium, iron, zinc, copper, and selenium than controls. The female athletes, on the other hand, had similar energy and nutrient intakes to the controls, and in most cases, intakes failed to meet the RDAs. Loosli and Benson[8] found similar inadequate energy and nutrient intakes in 97 competitive female gymnasts 11–17 years of age. Self-reported mean energy intake was only 1838 kcal/d, and 22 gymnasts reported consuming ≤1500 kcal/d, which is considerably less than the RDA for sedentary adolescents.[8] These low energy intakes were accompanied by inadequate micronutrient intakes, with between 41% and 80% of the gymnasts consuming <2/3 of the RDA for calcium, iron, zinc, folate and vitamin B6.[8]

Figure skating, like gymnastics, is a sport in which a low body weight is considered advantageous, and, thus, athletes participating in this sport frequently demonstrate restrictive eating behaviors and subsequent inadequate micronutrient intakes.[33,35,38] For example, Ziegler et al.[35] examined the energy and nutrient intakes of 21 competitive adolescent female figure skaters (11–16 years). Self-reported mean energy intake was only 1781 kcal/d (range 869 kcal/d-2401 kcal/d) and mean calcium and iron intakes were both <2/3 of the RDA. In a similar study of 23 young female figure skaters (13–22 years), Rucinski[33] found mean self-reported energy intake to be only 1174 kcal/d (range 373 kcal/d–2554 kcal/d) and mean micronutrient intakes were consistently ≤50% of the RDA.[33]

Adolescent female runners also frequently report inadequate energy and nutrient intakes. Baer and Taper[24] examined dietary intakes and training status of six amenorrheic and six eumenorrheic adolescent runners. There were no significant differences between the groups in terms of energy or micronutrient intakes and both groups had inadequate intakes of energy, calcium, magnesium, iron, and zinc.

It is interesting to note that, despite the low nutrient intakes frequently reported for adolescent athletes, nutritional status, as measured by blood levels of micronutrients, does not seem to be negatively affected. In the Rankinen et al.[1] study, for example, zinc, copper, and iron status parameters were within normal ranges for the female athletes despite the self-reported inadequate intakes. Similarly, none of the female figure skaters in the Ziegler et al.[35] study presented with iron deficiency anemia even though more than half of the athletes were consuming <2/3 of the RDA for iron. It should be noted, however, that serum ferritin was not measured in the Ziegler et al[35] study; thus, some of the athletes may have been iron depleted.

The lack of an association between micronutrient intakes and status measures could be viewed as further evidence for under-reporting among female adolescent athletes. However, it should be noted that very few of the aforementioned studies monitored weight changes (to ascertain weight stability) and none provided an indication of the length of time that the athletes had been following their particular eating patterns. Adolescents are notorious for inconsistent and erratic eating patterns such that what they consume (or fail to consume) might vary greatly from week to week. Thus, the intakes reported in the aforementioned studies may very well be accurate. It also should be emphasized that clinical nutrient deficiencies can take several months or even years to develop, which may further explain why the inadequate nutrient intakes seen in these short-term studies did not correspond to clinical nutritional deficiencies. More studies assessing nutritional status as well as longitudinal studies to assess changes in nutritional status with training are desperately needed.

Failure to meet energy and nutrient requirements will impair athletic performance and negatively impact health. Some health consequences of inadequate energy and nutrient intakes include short stature and delayed puberty,[39,40] electrolyte imbalances and dehydration,[41-43] increased susceptibility to athletic injuries,[44] menstrual dysfunction,[24,45,46] decreased bone mineral density, and increased risk of stress fractures and premature osteoporosis.[47–49] Thus, it is crucial that adolescents (and their parents) make every effort to meet the energy and nutrient requirements that accompany participation in sport. The following sections will outline what is currently known with respect to the energy and nutrient needs of adolescent athletes.

IV. ENERGY AND MACRONUTRIENT REQUIREMENTS

A. Energy Requirements

Because there are so few well-designed studies on energy balance in adolescent athletes, it is difficult to state with confidence the energy requirements of this group.[50] Nonetheless, it is generally accepted that regular exercise, particularly of an intense nature, will increase an adolescent's energy requirements.[50] It is well recognized that adult athletes have greater energy needs than their sedentary counterparts.[50] It has been recommended that adult athletes consume 40–50 $kcal/kg^{-1}$ or (1.8–2.2 times basal metabolic rate (BMR))[50] Extrapolating from studies done on adult athletes, one can theorize that energy and macronutrient needs increase with exercise training in the adolescent athlete. Adolescent athletes not only need to meet demands of daily living and support growth and development, but they also need energy to support physical training, speed recovery from intense training, prevent injury, and maintain normal menstrual function.[50]

Only two studies have examined the effects of exercise training on energy balance in previously sedentary boys and girls and both used doubly labeled water to measure total daily energy expenditure. Blaak et al.[51] reported a 12% increase in total daily energy expenditure in obese boys cycling 5 days/wk for 45 min. at 55–67% Vo_{2max}. Similarly, Eliekim et al.[52] reported that total daily energy expenditure of formally sedentary girls was 15% higher than a sedentary control group (34.5 $kcal/kg^{-1}$ vs. 32.2 $kcal/kg^{-1}$, respectively) after 5 weeks of endurance-type training performed 5 days/wk. These training studies indicate that just 1 hour of moderate-intensity, endurance-type exercise performed 5 days/wk can significantly increase energy expenditure and, thus, energy requirements. Because most adolescent athletes easily exceed the duration, intensity, and frequency of the exercise bouts described in the above training studies, it is safe to assume that energy needs of adolescent athletes are substantially greater; exactly how much greater remains unknown. What is known is that energy requirements will be influenced by the energy demands of the specific sport, the athlete's age and gender, and potential changes in energy intake and spontaneous physical activity associated with exercise training.[50]

It has been estimated that energy needs of moderately active adolescents may be 1.5–2.0 times greater than that for sedentary or "normally" active adolescents.[8] However, this estimate was not based on actual measures of energy balance in active adolescents. The RDAs for "normally" active adolescent males and females are listed in Table 4.2. A recently published method for estimating increased energy needs in competitive sports uses the RDAs for energy with additional calories to reflect increased energy demands of athletes in training.[53] For example, using this method, a weight-stable 11–14-year-old female athlete training rigorously would require an additional 5 kcal per lb (2.3 kcal/kg), while a 15–18-year-old female athlete would require an additional 4 kcal per lb (1.8 kcal/kg).

Table 4.2 The Recommended Dietary Allowances for Energy and Protein for Adolescents

Gender	Age (yr)	Energy Intake (kcal/kg/d)	Protein Intake (kcal/kg/d)
Males	11–14	55	1.0
	15–18	45	0.9
Females	11–14	47	1.0
	15–18	40	0.8

* Adapted from Reference 21

B. Macronutrient Requirements

Because carbohydrate is the predominant fuel used during high intensity exercise and because the body's glycogen stores are limited, most of the increased energy intake associated with exercise should come from carbohydrate. Specific carbohydrate recommendations for adult athletes have not been determined. Nonetheless, it is generally recommended that adolescent athletes (especially endurance athletes) consume 55–60% of their total daily energy intake from carbohydrate.[54,55] It is important to note, however, that this may not be sufficient if energy intake is inadequate. For this reason, it may be more accurate to express carbohydrate intake relative to body weight for example, 7–10 g/kg/d.[6] These same recommendations would most likely be appropriate for adolescent athletes, as well.

There are currently no published studies documenting the protein needs of adolescent athletes; thus, specific protein intake recommendations for this group cannot be made. However, it is well documented that adult athletes have greater protein needs than their sedentary counterparts, often as high as twice the current RDA for protein.[56,57] Moreover, relative protein requirements (per kg of body weight) of sedentary or "normally active" adolescent males (11–18 years) and young adolescent females (11–14 years) are greater than those of sedentary adults.[21] Thus, one can assume that, to support the increased demands of physical training, the protein needs of adolescent athletes are greater than those of their more sedentary counterparts. As a general rule, protein intake should be sufficient for the adolescent athlete if it represents 12–15% of total energy intake.[6] Assuming energy intake is adequate, this would provide 1.2–2.0 g/kg/d (120–250%) of the RDA, depending on the age of the adolescent.[6]

While consuming adequate fat is generally not problematic for the typical teenager, fat avoidance has been identified in some adolescent females and young athletes involved in thin-build and weight-dependent sports.[8,39,58] Thus, adolescent athletes, particularly females, should be educated as to the importance of adequate dietary fat. It is recommended that fat intake compose 25–30% of the adolescent's daily energy intake. As with adults, the emphasis should be placed on limiting saturated fat and emphasizing mono- and polyunsaturated fats.

V. FLUID AND ELECTROLYTE REQUIREMENTS

It is generally accepted that the thermoregulatory response of adolescents is less efficient than that of adults, although these differences diminish as the adolescent reaches late puberty.[59,60] Adolescents have a lower sweat rate, higher ratio of surface area to body mass (which leads to greater heat exchange with the environment), and increased metabolic heat production than adults.[59,61,62] Bar-Or et al.[61] showed that young adolescents experience a significantly greater rise in body core temperature than adults for the same level of dehydration. Thus, the margin for detrimental fluid loss before thermoregulation is compromised may be less in adolescents than in adults. Furthermore, research indicates that young athletes do not instinctively drink enough to replenish losses and maintain euhydration during prolonged exercise, and may not recognize when to stop exercise despite marked heat strain.[63,64] These findings emphasize the importance of carefully monitoring the adolescent's fluid intake prior to, during, and following exercise. The primary strategy is to enhance thirst and convince athletes to drink frequently, even when they are not thirsty. Coaches (and parents) should make sure the athlete begins practice fully hydrated by consuming 500 ml of fluid (17 fl oz.) 10–20 minutes prior to practice.[65] Athletes should be encouraged to drink 150–300 ml (5–10 fl oz.) of fluid every 15–20 minutes during practice and fully rehydrate after practice by consuming 50% over and above the volume of fluid ingested to restore pre-exercise body weight (approximately 24 fl oz. for every lb. or 300 ml. For every kg of body weight lost).[65-67] Weighing the athlete before and after practice can provide an estimate of fluid losses and, thus, replenishment requirements. Serial weighing can also identify the athlete who is becoming chronically dehydrated during several training sessions, as well as predict how much fluid the athlete needs for subsequent workouts.[54]

Plain water is the most economical source of fluid and is appropriate for low- to moderate-intensity exercise lasting <60 minutes. However, carbohydrate-replacement beverages (sports drinks) have been shown to delay fatigue and enhance performance in moderate- to high-intensity exercise lasting >60 minutes (e.g., running, cycling, soccer) and high-intensity, interval-type sports (e.g., field and ice hockey, rugby, tennis, basketball), sports in which adolescents frequently participate.[66,68-70] Moreover, it has been recently shown that children's thirst and fluid intake can be enhanced during exercise by flavoring the beverage and adding NaCl and carbohydrate in amounts typically found in sports drinks (e.g., 18 mmol/L NaCl and 6–8% carbohydrate solution).[71,72] Thus, sports drinks as well as water should be made readily available to adolescents before, during, and after exercise, to encourage fluid consumption and prevent voluntary dehydration.

VI. MICRONUTRIENT REQUIREMENTS

A. Iron

One area of particular concern in adolescent athletes is low body iron stores. Iron deficiency will not only impair athletic performance but can interfere with normal growth and maturation of the adolescent and negatively impact gastrointestinal, neurological, and immune function.[12,73] Low levels of storage iron are common during periods of rapid growth, and, during puberty, the iron requirements are significantly increased due to increases in body mass, blood volume, and hemoglobin concentrations, accentuating the need for adequate iron stores.[12,74] These same parameters may also increase as a result of exercise, further exaggerating the need for iron during growth.[12,73]

A number of studies have evaluated iron status in young athletes.[75-79] In general, iron deficiency without anemia is more common than iron deficiency anemia and both are more common in female than male athletes, except for boys 11–14 years old.[80]. Female adolescent athletes are particularly susceptible to depleted body iron stores due to menstrual losses and poor dietary intake. It has been estimated that 35–45% of female adolescent athletes suffer from hypoferritinemia.[81] It remains controversial, however, whether adolescent athletes are at a greater risk for iron deficiency than nonathletes, because few studies have included a non-athletic control group. Nonetheless, studies that have followed young athletes through their competitive season indicate that exercise, particularly that of a high-impact nature (e.g., running), may promote iron depletion. Rowland et al.[79] followed serum ferritin levels, hemoglobin, and red cell indices in 30 male and 20 female high school cross-country runners during a competitive season. Initial findings indicated that 40% of girls and 3% of boys suffered from iron depletion (serum ferritin <12 ng/mL). At the end of the season, the prevalence had increased to 45% of girls and 17% of boys. Similarly, Nickerson et al.[75] found that 14 of 41 of female high school runners (34%) became iron deficient during the course of the competitive season. However, Rowland and Kelleher[78] found no significant changes in serum ferritin levels in female high school swimmers from the beginning to the end of the competitive season. Thus, the impact of exercise on iron status may be "sport-specific."

Inadequate dietary intake coupled with increased requirements is undoubtedly the primary cause of iron deficiency in adolescent athletes. Assuming that the typical diet contains 6 mg of iron per 1000 kcal, the adolescent athlete would have to consume 2500 kcal/d to meet iron requirements. While such an energy intake is relatively common among male adolescent athletes, as previously described, many female athletes consume <2000 kcal/d. The bioavailability of dietary iron must also be considered. Limited evidence suggests that female and young male adolescent athletes consume sources of iron that are less bioavailable (i.e., more non-heme and less heme iron).[12] In addition to low intake of bioavailable iron, iron deficiency in adolescent athletes may be caused by iron losses in sweat, gastrointestinal bleeding from gut ischemia, hematuria, and intravascular hemolysis caused by mechanical trauma to the foot.[81] Willows et al.[12] found that iron deficient adolescent female runners were more likely to suffer from gastrointestinal blood losses than runners who weren't iron deficient. Similarly, among 20 female high school runners studied by Nickerson et al.,[76] nine had iron losses via gastrointestinal bleeding and seven of those nine had iron deficiency.

Because of the high prevalence of iron deficiency, iron status should be assessed in all adolescent athletes prior to and during the competitive season. It is well recognized that iron deficiency anemia will impair athletic performance and, thus, should be treated promptly with oral iron supplementation under a doctor's supervision. It remains controversial, however, whether iron deficiency without anemia will negatively impact athletic performance.[81] Animal studies indicate that non-anemic iron deficiency impairs endurance exercise capacity,[82,83] but most studies have failed to support this conclusion in humans.[84,85] Nonetheless, performance issues aside, attention to those with iron depletion is important for at least two reasons, (1) iron depletion predisposes athletes to iron deficiency anemia, and (2) iron depletion may have a broader negative impact on health, including impaired intellectual performance and attention span, increased susceptibility to infection, and gastrointestinal diseases.[9] Thus, adolescent athletes, particularly females, should be encouraged to eat an iron-rich diet and taught how to increase the bioavailability of the iron they do consume. In cases where the female athlete is unable or unwilling to consume adequate iron from food sources, it may be prudent for her to take a daily multivitamin/mineral supplement containing the RDA for iron.

B. Calcium

Adolescence is a critical time for the development of bone mass and is considered the most crucial period in terms of the influence of calcium on bone status[86,87] Although peak bone mass is not achieved until the second or third decade of life, the majority of bone mineral deposition occurs during adolescence, with approximately 40% of bone mass acquired during the pubertal growth spurt.[88,89]

The maximal amount of bone mass attained by young adulthood is dependent upon genetic, hormonal, and lifestyle factors. Although genetic factors are the primary determinants of peak bone mass, lifestyle factors such as exercise and diet are considered important contributors largely because they can be modified.[90,91] While a variety of dietary factors are necessary for the development of optimal bone mass, by far the most studied nutrient for its role in bone health is calcium.[48,92] A large body of literature including epidemiological evidence, randomized clinical trials, and metabolic balance studies indicates that dietary calcium is a key determinant of bone mass accretion.[89,93-103] Epidemiological studies suggest that variations in calcium intake early in life may account for a 5–10% difference in adult peak bone mass.[89,100,104] Randomized clinical trials in children and adolescents all show greater increments in bone mass and bone mineral density with calcium supplementation, whether in the form of supplements, fortified foods, or dairy products.[92,94,95,99] For example, in a 12-month longitudinal study of 48 girls 9–13 years of age, Chan et al.[95] found that increasing calcium intake from 728 mg/d to at least 1200 mg/d (mean intake 1437 mg/d) with diary products produced significantly greater increases in lumbar bone density and total body bone mineral content. Similarly, Lloyd et al.[99] found that girls who consumed approximately 1300 mg/d of calcium gained 1.3% more bone mass than those consuming only 960 mg/d. The age of the individual or stage of the growth period during which calcium is consumed may be as important, if not more so, than the amount consumed in terms of maximizing gains in bone mineral density. In a recent double-blind, placebo-controlled study, 45 pairs of identical twins ages 6–14 were randomly assigned to consume either 908 mg/d (baseline calcium consumption) or 1612 mg/d of calcium (via supplementation with calcium carbonate malate). After 3 years, the prepubertal twin from each pair who had consumed the higher calcium level had a greater rate of increase in bone mineral density at the radius and lumbar spine. Among the twin pairs who were postpubertal, or who had gone through puberty during the course of the study, the calcium-supplemented twin received no benefit.[92] It should be noted, however, that the skeletal advantage seen with calcium supplementation is not maintained, (at least not significantly) if calcium supplementation is ceased. For example, in a follow-up to the Johnston et al.[92] twin study, Slemeda et al.[105] reported that the observed differences in bone density in the twins were no longer statistically significant following 1 year of cessation of calcium supplementation. This suggests that high calcium intakes must be maintained throughout adolescence to achieve increased bone mass.

Dietary survey data indicate that adolescents, particularly females, are not consuming adequate calcium, and, thus, are at high risk for poor bone health.[22,106-111] Albertson et al.[111] collected 14-day food records from 4000 girls ages 11–18 years at 2-year intervals (from 1980–1992). The percentage of girls consuming <2/3 of the RDA for calcium increased with advancing age. In fact, more than 75% of 15–18 year-olds were consuming <2/3 of the RDA for calcium during the 1990–92 interval. According to the most recent U.S. Department of Agriculture's Continuing Survey of Food Intakes by Individuals (CSFII 1994–1996), calcium consumption for 12–19-year-old males and females was, on average 1145 mg/d and 771 mg/d, respectively.[22]

To date, no similar large-scale studies have been conducted to ascertain average calcium intakes in adolescent athletes. Nonetheless, combined data from the existing studies on nutrient intakes in adolescent athletes indicate that most male athletes are consuming adequate calcium, wherea most female athletes, particularly those participating in sports that emphasize leanness (e.g., gymnastics, figure skating, running) fall far short of the requirement (see previous section on nutritional status).[8,24,33,35]

Numerous studies have observed a greater bone density in athletes compared with nonathletes. Unilateral control studies consistently report a significantly greater bone mineral density in the dominant arms of Little League baseball players, elite female tennis players, and elite female squash players.[112-114] Retrospective and cross-sectional studies tend to demonstrate a positive relationship between regular weight-bearing exercise and bone density.[90,115,116] Prospective studies also support the bone-mass-enhancing effects of exercise.[89,117,118] For example, Matkovic et al.[89] followed 260 teenagers for 11 years and found that regular exercise was associated with greater hip and spine bone density in men and higher hipbone density in women.

It should be noted, however, that even though weight-bearing exercise promotes higher bone density, it cannot compensate for the effects of a poor diet, particularly low calcium intake, on bone. Indeed, increasing physical activity without providing adequate nutriture to support bone formation could actually result in bone mineral loss.[48,90,119] Additionally, intense exercise combined with inadequate energy intake in female adolescent athletes may lead to menstrual dysfunction, which can result in significantly decreased bone density (see subsequent section on the Female Athlete Triad).[87,120-122] Bachrach et al.[47] found that despite high levels of physical activity, young anorexic women had significantly lower bone mineral densities. Calcium and physical activity may also interact on a different level. Physical activity of sufficient intensity and duration to cause excessive sweating may produce increased calcium losses, thereby increasing the need for calcium.[90] Calcium losses in sweat were generally thought to be small and have little impact on calcium requirements. However, a study in male collegiate basketball players indicated that calcium losses in sweat were substantial and, if not balanced by increased calcium intakes, could lead to calcium deficiency and potentially decreased bone mineral density.[123]

In summary, appropriate exercise and adequate nutrition during the growing years are clearly essential if the adolescent athlete hopes to attain genetically predetermined peak bone mass. The current Adequate Intake for 11–18-year-olds is 1300 mg/d.[124] This intake appears adequate to support maximal calcium retention and corresponds reasonably well to the threshold of 1480 mg/d identified for this age group by Matkovic and Heanney.[125]

VII. WEIGHT CONTROL AND DISORDERED EATING

A. Dieting and Weight Loss Practices

Adolescence is characterized by a heightened awareness of physical appearance and a concomitant preoccupation with body weight and shape. Studies conducted over the past 2 decades have described increasingly widespread body weight dissatisfaction and body image disturbances among adolescents, particularly adolescent females. A 1972 survey of teenagers found that only 6% were concerned about their weight,[126] while a similar survey conducted 10 years later indicated that 31% of teenagers worried that they weighed too much.[127] Eisele et al.[128] found that while 81% of 12–14-year-old girls sampled were within or below the normal range of weight for height, 78% would prefer to weigh less and only 14% reported being satisfied with their current weight. Similarly, in a study of 326 high school girls, Moses et al.[129] found that 51% of the underweight girls described themselves as extremely fearful of becoming fat and 36% reported weight preoccupation. Body weight dissatisfaction frequently leads to dieting and the use of unhealthy weight control methods. Casper et al.[130] found that 61% of adolescent girls surveyed reported dieting during the previous year. Moreover, many of those surveyed reported using unhealthy weight control methods including fasting (51%), diet pills (16%), and vomiting (12%).[130] Similarly, Moore[131] found that of 1728 10th-graders, 11% had vomited, 7% had used laxatives, and 4% had used diuretics for weight loss.

Although no similar large-scale studies of dieting behaviors have been conducted with adolescent athletes, results from several smaller studies have indicated that dieting and the use of unhealthy weight loss methods occur with a frequency similar to that seen in nonathletes.[31,132-135] For example, Dummer et al.[135] examined the prevalence of dieting and the use of pathogenic weight control methods among 487 female and 468 male adolescent swimmers (9–18 years). Fifteen percent of the girls and 3.6% of the boys reported using pathogenic weight control methods including vomiting (12.7% of girls and 2.7% of boys), diet pills (10.7% of girls and 6.8% of boys), laxatives (2.5% of girls, and 4.1% of boys), and diuretics (1.5% of girls and 2.8% of boys).

Researchers have long speculated that excessive weight preoccupation and chronic dieting may be predisposing factors to the more serious clinical eating disorders anorexia and bulimia nervosa.[136-138] Indeed, many individuals with eating disorders report that the onset of disorder was preceded by a period of strict dieting.[136] Because dieting is common among adolescents regardless of participation in sport, the risk of developing eating disorders in this age group is high.

Whether adolescent athletes are at a greater risk for developing eating disorders than their more sedentary counterparts remains controversial. Research in this area is limited by small sample sizes, lack of control samples, and the use of nonvalidated questionnaires. Moreover, the guilt associated with eating disorders combined with the fear of losing his/her position on the team may make athletes reluctant to respond truthfully to questionnaires.[139,140] It has been hypothesized that the stress of competition, pressure of competing in sports that emphasize a low body weight, and personality characteristics (i.e., perfectionist, goal-oriented), may predispose some athletes to developing eating disorders. Studies investigating eating disorders in *college-aged* populations have consistently demonstrated an increased risk among female athletes, particularly those competing in sports that emphasize leanness.[37,141-143] The comparative lack of research on eating disorders among *adolescent* athletes is unfortunate, given that adolescence is considered the most vulnerable period for the development of eating disorders.[136] Moreover, many college-aged athletes report that their eating disorders and pathogenic weight control behaviors began during their teen years.[36,132,135] Nonetheless, the limited existing research suggests an increased risk of eating disorders among adolescent athletes relative to nonathletic adolescent controls. For example, Brooks-Gunn et al.[132] compared the prevalence of eating disorder symptoms among groups of adolescent ballet dancers (n = 64), figure skaters (n = 25), and swimmers (n = 72) with nonathletes (n = 424). They found that the athletes exhibited more eating disorder symptoms and restrained eating than the nonathletes, with the dancers and swimmers demonstrating the highest prevalence. Similarly, Mallick et al.[133] found that the prevalence of self-reported eating disorders, dieting, and the use of pathogenic weight control behaviors were significantly greater in female high school athletes (n = 87) participating in track, swimming, gymnastics, and ballet than non-athletic controls (n = 120).

It should be noted, however, that not all studies have found an increased prevalence of eating disorders among athletes. Traub and Blinde[134] compared 100 adolescent female athletes (softball, basketball, volleyball, and track/cross country athletes) and 110 nonathletes in terms of behavioral and psychological traits associated with eating disorders and use of pathogenic weight control behaviors. Sport-by-sport comparisons were also investigated to determine if athletes in specific sports were at an increased risk. Athletes were more perfectionistic and more likely to exhibit bulimic tendencies than nonathletes; however, both groups reported a similar prevalence of dieting. In addition, there were no significant differences between the athletic groups with respect to weight control behaviors. It is noteworthy, however, that almost 25% of athletes reported fasting, 15% reported using diet pills, and 10% reported using laxatives for weight control. Similarly, Benson et al.[31] investigated the prevalence of disordered eating behaviors in two groups of Swiss adolescent athletes (12 gymnasts and 18 swimmers) and 34 non-athletic adolescent controls. The gymnasts were chosen to represent a sport that emphasized leanness, while the swimmers were supposed to represent a sport that does not emphasize leanness. All three groups reported a similar prevalence of body weight preoccupation and drive for thinness; however, the swimmers reported a significantly greater degree of body dissatisfaction than the gymnasts and controls. The authors maintained that the study provided evidence that disordered eating behaviors are equally pervasive in athletes and nonathletes and are not more prevalent in sports that emphasize leanness. However, many researchers would argue that swimming, due to the revealing attire, is a sport that emphasizes leanness, and, in more recent studies, it has been classified as such.[36,37,58,144]

Severe energy restriction and the use of pathogenic weight control methods not only have profound short-term effects on adolescent athletes including chronic fatigue, hypoglycemia, and an increased risk of illness and injury, but also pose significant long-term health risks that include growth retardation, nutritional deficiencies, cardiovascular abnormalities, electrolyte imbalances, menstrual dysfunction and the resulting osteopenia and premature osteoporosis.[145,146] Due to the pervasiveness among female athletes and the significant health threat, these final two complications—menstrual dysfunction and osteoporosis—combined with disordered eating have collectively been recognized as the Female Athlete Triad.[147]

B. The Female Athlete Triad

While any one of the disorders of the triad can, and do, occur in isolation, they often follow a typical developmental pattern. The female athlete who feels pressured to achieve or maintain a low body weight may develop disordered eating. The resulting energy restriction and pathogenic weight control behaviors predispose her to menstrual dysfunction, subsequent decreased bone mineral density, and premature osteoporosis.[147] It is currently not known how many young female athletes are affected by the triad of disorders. It is estimated that between 15–62% of young female athletes suffer from some form of disordered eating.[140,147] Amenorrhea occurs with alarming frequency in female athletes, with prevalence estimates ranging from 3.5–66%, depending upon the sport being studied.[147] The prevalence of premature osteoporosis in the young female athlete is currently unknown, largely due to the lengthy time course of the development of the disease and the relatively recent identification of the disease in female athletes.[147] Nonetheless, several studies have documented significantly decreased bone mineral density in young amenorrheic athletes, thus placing them at a greater risk for osteoporosis in the future. For example, Drinkwater et al.[122] found that amenorrheic runners with a chronological age of 24.9 years had a bone mineral density equivalent to that of women 51.2 years of age. Moreover, in a 4-year follow-up study, Drinkwater et al.[148] reported that while bone mineral density increased in the athletes with resumption of menses, it still remained well below the average for their age group, indicating that bone lost as a result of amenorrhea can never be fully regained. The increased risk of scoliosis[149] and stress fractures in athletes with delayed menarche or amenorrhea is a serious consequence of decreased bone density.[149-151] Interestingly, the increased incidence of stress fractures is associated with aberrant eating patterns and concomitant nutritional deficiencies even before changes in bone mineral density are observed.[152]

The *adolescent* female athlete is perhaps at the greatest risk for developing the disorders of the triad. Psychological and societal pressures as well as biological factors render adolescence a particularly "time-sensitive" period.[153] Additionally, skeletal integrity is vulnerable during this time as the most rapid growth and development of the skeleton occurs during adolescence.[153] Because of the significant risk of developing one or more of the disorders of the triad, all adolescent female athletes should be screened. The pre-participation physical exam provides the best opportunity for screening for disorders of the triad. Questions should address menstrual history, age of menarche, weight history, and unusual diets or methods of weight loss as well as other signs and symptoms of eating disorders. The presence of any one of the disorders of the triad should warrant immediate attention and further evaluation.[147]

C. Disordered Eating in Male Athletes — The Special Case of "Making Weight"

Population studies and clinical samples consistently report a lower prevalence of eating disorders among men than women. This, combined with the fact that few sports demand that men meet specific body weight or size requirements would indicate that eating disorders should be relatively uncommon among male athletes. And, in fact, studies of eating disorders and pathogenic weight control behaviors among male athletes have confirmed this presumption.[140,153] The sport of wrestling appears to be an exception, as data from this sport indicates that dieting, pathogenic weight control behaviors, and eating disorders are pervasive.[155-158] It is common practice for wrestlers to restrict food and fluid intake throughout the competitive season in order to compete at one to three weight classes below their normal weight[156] in the belief that they will gain a competitive advantage over smaller opponents. In ever-desperate attempts to make weight, many wrestlers resort to pathogenic weight control methods. For example, Nelson-Steen and Brownell[156] examined weight loss practices among 368 high school wrestlers and found that 13% used a sauna once a week, 26% fasted once a week, and 31% restricted fluids at least once a week. Laxatives, diuretics, and vomiting were used by 2% of athletes once a week and 6% once a month. Forty-three percent of the athletes reported being "preoccupied with food and weight" and 20% reported feeling "often" or "always" out of control when eating. Similarly, in a study of 125 high school wrestlers, Weissinger et al.[158] found that pathogenic weight control behaviors were disturbingly prevalent with 51% reporting fasting, 15% vomiting, 14% using diet pills, 10% using diuretics, and 8% using laxatives. Lakin et al.[155] found that almost 3% of the 716 high school wrestlers studied met the diagnostic criteria for bulimia nervosa. Similarly, Oppliger et al.[157] found that 1.7% of 713 high school wrestlers demonstrated behaviors consistent with bulimia nervosa.

From a performance standpoint, the food and fluid restriction commonly used to "make weight" can lead to liver and muscle glycogen depletion, dehydration, reduced muscular strength, and decreased time to fatigue.[159] The risks associated with pathogenic weight control methods were described in the previous section. One additional risk that has been suggested is a decrease in resting metabolic rate, theoretically from the repeated cycles of weight loss and regain. Nelson-Steen et al.[160] reported that wrestlers who experienced repeated cycles of weight loss and regain had a 14% lower resting metabolic rate than those who did not engage in weight cycling. This could make future weight loss attempts more difficult, leading to more-drastic pathogenic weight control methods and perhaps the development of clinical eating disorders.

Despite medical warnings, as well as national and state rules regulating weight loss, rapid and dangerous weight loss methods continue to dominate the sport of wrestling.[161] Thus, coaches and parents must understand the consequences of rapid and extreme weight loss methods and be educated as to healthy alternatives for achieving a suitable competitive weight.[54]

VIII. SUPPLEMENT USE

Athletes searching for the competitive edge frequently turn to nutritional supplements, and adolescent athletes are no exception. While the prevalence of supplement use among all adolescents (20–25%) is estimated to be somewhat less than in adults (35–40%),[162] research suggests that adolescent athletes may be more frequent consumers of supplements than their non-athletic counterparts.[14,163] In addition, adolescents participating in contact sports, where size and strength are essential, are more apt to consume supplements.[162,163] For example, Massad et al.[163] found that the prevalence of supplement use was highest among football players, wrestlers, and boxers. Similarly, Sobal and Marquart[162] found that athletes participating in wrestling and ice hockey reported the highest usage of nutritional supplements.

When queried, the majority of athletes believe that supplements will improve performance and, in fact, performance enhancement is one of the most frequently cited reasons for using supplements.[162,163] Other frequently reported reasons for supplement usage include to increase energy, make up for a "poor" diet, enhance the immune system, or treat an illness. It's not surprising that the most frequently consumed supplements include multivitamin/mineral preparations, vitamin C, protein supplements, and carbohydrate/electrolyte beverages.[162-164]

Unfortunately, many well-meaning but misinformed parents and coaches advise adolescent athletes to take supplements with the idea that they will promote early athletic development, improve performance, or provide "health insurance."[55] Although vitamin and mineral supplementation may improve the nutritional status and, perhaps, performance of adolescents with inadequate dietary intakes or overt deficiencies, there is not scientific evidence to support the indiscriminant use of supplements to hasten or improve athletic development.[165,166] Indeed, the unsupervised and indiscriminate use of supplements can be costly and, when used in place of a sound nutrition program, can compromise performance as well as health. Large doses of certain vitamins and minerals may be toxic and the risk of consuming toxic amounts is far greater with supplements than with food. Moreover, the efficacy and safety of most of today's popular supplements have yet to be established. Providing young athletes with supplements can also give them a false sense of security and encourage faulty eating habits. Young athletes may come to erroneously attribute any improvement in performance to whatever supplement they are taking as opposed to training and a balanced diet. This type of false reinforcement may subsequently encourage experimentation with other more potent and dangerous ergogenic aids such as steroids.[55]

Because adolescent athletes consider parents, coaches, and athletic trainers to be important sources of nutrition information, they play a key role in dispelling nutrition myths and misconceptions and emphasizing that regular food can promote muscle growth and development. Adolescent athletes must be taught that their nutritional needs can be readily met by consuming a balanced and varied diet that contains sufficient energy to support their increased energy expenditure.

IX. SUMMARY AND CONCLUSIONS

Adolescence is frequently considered a nutritionally vulnerable period because of the characteristic rapid physical and psychological changes. High levels of physical activity can add to that vulnerability by increasing the adolescent's already high nutritional demands. Currently, there is relatively little scientific data documenting energy and nutrient needs of adolescent athletes; thus, it is difficult to make recommendations with certainty. Nonetheless, despite the lack of research, it is safe to assume that adolescent athletes have greater energy, macronutrient, and fluid requirements than their more sedentary counterparts. Unfortunately, with a few exceptions, research suggests that many adolescent athletes are not meeting those elevated requirements. Of particular concern are adolescent female athletes participating in sports that emphasize leanness, who, because of their inadequate intake, are placing themselves at risk for micronutrient deficiencies and a myriad of health consequences, most notably amenorrhea and premature osteoporosis. Thus, the challenge for health professionals is to help the athlete establish good eating habits at an early age. To this end, educational efforts should be aimed at the athlete, the athlete's parents and coach. Information regarding basic nutritional concepts as well as sport-specific requirements should be provided so as to promote optimal health and performance of the adolescent athlete.

REFERENCES

1. Rankinen, T., Fogelholm, M., Kujala, U., Rauramaa, R., and Uusitupa, M. Dietary intake and nutritional status of athletic and nonathletic children in early puberty. *Int. J. Sport Nutr.* 5:136-150, 1995.
2. Southon, S., Wright, A.J.A., Finglas, P.M., Bailey, A.L., and Belstein, J.L. Micronutrient intake and psychological performance of school children. Consideration of the value of calculated nutrient intakes for the assessment of micronutrient status in children. *Proc. Nutr. Society.* 51:315-324, 1992.
3. McKeag, D. Adolescents and exercise. *J. Adolesc. Health Care.* 7:1215-1305, 1986.
4. Squire, D. Heat illness: Fluid and electrolyte issues for pediatric and adolescent athletes. *Sports Med.* 37:1085-1097, 1990.
5. Lipp, E.J. and Trimble, N. Health behaviors of adolescent male football players. *Pediatric Nursing.* 19;395-399, 1993.
6. Lemon, P.W.R. Nutrition for muscular development of young athletes. In: *Perspectives in Exercise Science. vol. 2. Youth, Exercise, and Sport.* C.V. Gisolfi and D.R. Lamb (Eds). Indianapolis: Benchmark Press, 1989, pp. 369-396.
7. King, J. Does poor zinc nutriture retard skeletal growth and mineralization in adolescents? *Am. J. Clin. Nutr.* 64:375-376, 1996.
8. Loosli, A.R. and Benson, J. Nutritional intake in adolescent athletes. *Ped. Clin. N. Am.* 37(5):1143-1152, 1990.
9. Rowland, T.W. Iron deficiency in the young athlete. *Ped. Clin. N. Am.* 37(5): 1153-1163, 1990.
10. Rowland, T.W., Stagg, L., and Kelleher, J.F. Iron deficiency in adolescent girls. Are athletes at an increased risk? *J. Adolesc. Health.* 12:22-31, 1991.
11. Tsui, J.C. and Nordstrom, J.S. Folate status of adolescents: Effects of folic acid supplementation. *J. Am. Diet. Assoc.* 90:1551-1556, 1990.
12. Willows, N.D., Grimston, S.K., Roberts, S., Smith, D.J., and Hanley, D.A. Iron and hematologic status in young athletes relative to puberty: A cross-sectional study. *Pediatr. Exer. Sci.* 5:367-376, 1993.
13. Chapman, P., Ramses, B., Toma, R.V., and Jacob, M. Nutrition knowledge among adolescent high school female athletes. *Adolescence.* 32:437-446, 1997.
14. Douglas, P.D. and Douglas, J.G. Nutrition knowledge and food practices of high school athletes. *J. Am. Diet. Assoc.* 84:1198-1202, 1984.
15. Perron, M. and Endres, J. Knowledge, attitudes, and dietary practices of female athletes. *J. Am. Diet. Assoc.* 85:573-576, 1985.
16. Schmalz, K. Nutritional beliefs and practices of adolescent athletes. *J. School Nursing.* 9:18-22, 1993.
17. Thakur, N. and D'Amico, R. Relationship of nutrition knowledge and obesity in adolescence. *Family Med.* 31:122-127, 1999.
18. Munoz, K.A., Kreps-Smith, S.M., Ballard-Barbash, R., and Cleveland, L.E. Food intakes of U.S. children and adolescents compared with recommendations. *Pediatrics.* 100:323-329, 1997.
19. United States Department of Agriculture Human Nutrition Information Service. *The Food Guide Pyramid.* Hyattsville, MD, USDA Human Nutrition Information Service, 1992.
20. Nicklas, T. Dietary Studies of children: the Bogalusa Heart Study experience. *J. Am. Diet. Assoc.* 95:1127-1133, 1995.

21. Food and Nutrition Board, Commission on Life Sciences, National Research Council. *Recommended Dietary Allowances*. 10th Edition. Committee on Dietary Allowances 1. Washington, D.C., National Academy Press, 1989.
22. United States Department of Agriculture, Agricultural Research Service. *Food and Nutrient Intake by Individuals in the United States, 1-day. 1994-1996: Continuing Survey of Food Intakes by Individuals, 1994-1996*. Washington, D.C., U.S. Department of Agriculture, Agricultural Research Service. 1999.
23. Berning, J., Troup, J.P., Yanhandel, P.J., Daniels, J. and Daniels, N. The nutritional habits of young adolescent swimmers. *Int. J. Sport Nutr.* 1:240-248, 1991.
24. Baer, J.T. and Taper, J.L. Amenorrheic and eumenorrheic adolescent runners: Dietary intake and exercise training status. *J. Am. Diet. Assoc.* 92:89-91, 1992.
25. Bandini, L.G., Schoeller, D.A., Cyr, H.N., and Dietz, W.H. Validity of reported energy intake in obese and non-obese adolescents. *Am. J. Clin. Nutr.* 52:421-425, 1990.
26. Black, A.E., Prentice, A.M., Goldberg, G.R., Jebb, S.A., Bingham, S.A., Livingston, M.B.E., and Coward, W.A. Measurements of total energy expenditure provide insights into the validity of dietary measurements of energy intake. *J. Am. Diet. Assoc.* 93:572-579, 1993.
27. Schoeleer, D.A. Limitations in the assessment of dietary energy intake by self-report. *Metabolism.* 44:18-22, 1995.
28. Rico-Sanz, J. Body composition and Nutritional Assessment in Soccer. *Int. J. Sport Nutr.* 8:113-123, 1998.
29. Hickson, J.F., Duke, M.A., Risser, W.L., Johnson, C.W., Palmer, R. and Stockton, J.E. Nutritional intake from food sources of high school football athletes. *J. Am. Diet. Assoc.* 87:926-927, 1987.
30. Benson, J., Guillino, D., and Loosli, A. Inadequate nutrition and chronic caloric restriction in adolescent ballerinas. *Phys. Sportsmed.* 13:79-90, 1985.
31. Benson, J.E., Allemann, Y., Theintz, G.E., and Howald, H. Eating problems and calorie intake levels in Swiss adolescent athletes. *Int. J. Sportsmed.* 11:249-252, 1990.
32. Roemmich, J.N. and Sinning, W.E. Weight loss and wrestling training: Effects on nutrition, growth, maturation, body composition, and strength. *J. Appl. Physiol.* 82:1751-1759, 1997.
33. Rucinski, A. Relationship of body image and dietary intake of competitive ice skaters. *J. Am. Diet. Assoc.* 89:98-100, 1989.
34. Schemmel, R.A., Ryder, E., Moeggenberg, J.A., and Conn, C.A. Comparison of nutrient intakes between elite wrestlers and runners. In: *Competitive Sports for Children and Youth*. Brown, E.W. and Branta, C.R. (Eds). Champaign, Ill.: Human Kinetics, 1988, pp. 27-38.
35. Zeigler, P., Hensley, S., Roepke, J.B., Whitaker, S.H., Craig, B.W., and Drewnowski, A. Eating attitudes and energy intakes of female skaters. *Med. Sci. Sports Exer.* 30;583-586, 1998.
36. Beals, K., and Manore, M. Behavioral, physiological, and psychological characteristics of female athletes with subclinical eating disorders. *Int. J. Sport Nutr.* In press.
37. Sundgot-Borgen, J. Prevalence of eating disorders in elite female athlete. *Int. J. Sport Nutr.* 3;29-40, 1993.
38. Delistraty, D.A., Reisman, E.J., and Snipes, M. A physiological and nutritional profile of young female figure skaters. *J. Sports Med. Phys. Fitness.* 32:149-155, 1992.
39. Pugliese, M.T., Lifshitz, F., Grad, G., Fort, P., and Marks-Katz, M. Fear of obesity: A cause of short stature and delayed puberty. *N. Engl. J. Med.* 309:513-518, 1983.
40. Smith, W.J., Underwood, L.E., and Clemmons, D.R. Effects of caloric or protein restriction on insulin-like growth factor-1 (IGF-1) and IGF-binding proteins in children and adults. *J. Clin. Endocrin.Metabol.* 80:443-449, 1995.
41. Benardot, D., Schwarz, M., and Heller, D.W. Nutrient intake in young, highly competitive gymnasts. *J. Am. Diet. Assoc.* 89:401-403, 1989.
42. Esroy, G. Dietary status and anthropometric assessment of child gymnasts. *J. Sportsmed. Phys. Fitness.* 31:577-580, 1991.
43. Hawley, J.A. and Williams, M.M. Dietary intake of age group swimmers. *Br. J. Sports Med.* 25:154-158, 1991.
44. Marcus, R., Cann, C., Madvig, P., Minkoff, J., Goddard, M., Bayer, M., Martin, M., Goudiani, L., Haskell, W., and Genan, H. Menstrual function and bone mass in elite women distance runners: Edocrine and metabolic features. *Ann. Int. Med.* 102:158-163, 1985.

45. Meyerson, M., Guitin, B., Warrne, M.P., May, M.T., Contento, T., Lee, M., Pi-Sunyer, F.X., Pierson, R.N., and Brooks-Gunn, J. Resting metabolic rate and energy balance in amenorrheic and eumenorrheic runners. *Med. Sci. Sports Exer.* 23:15-22, 1991.
46. Williams, N.I., Young, J.C., McAurthur, J.W., Bullen, B., Skinnar, G.S., and Turnbull, B. Strenuous exercise with caloric restriction. Effect on LH secretion. *Med. Sci. Sports Exer.* 27:1390-1398, 1995.
47. Bachrach, L.K., Guido, D., Katzman, D., Lift, I.F., and Marcus, R. Decreased bone mineral density in adolescent girls with anorexia nervosa. *Pediatrics*. 86:440-447, 1990.
48. Weaver, C.M., Peacock, M., and Johnston, C. Adolescent nutrition in the prevention of postmenopausal osteoporosis. *J. Clin. Endocrinol. Metabol.* 84;1839-1843, 1999.
49. Wolman, R.L., Clark, P., McNally, E., Harries, M.G., and Reeve, J. Dietary calcium as a statistical determinant of spinal trabecular bone density in amenorrheic and oestrogen replete athletes. *Bone Min. Res.* 17;415-423, 1992.
50. Thompson, J.L. Energy balance in young athletes. *Int. J. Sport Nutr.* 8:160-174, 1998.
51. Blaak, E.E., Westerter, K.R., Bar-Or, O., Wouters, L.J.M., and Saris, W.H.M. Total energy expenditure and spontaneous physical activity in relation to training in obese boys. *Am. J. Clin. Nutr.* 55:777-782, 1992.
52. Eliekim, A., Barstow, T.J., Brasel, J.A., Ajie, H., Lee, W-N.P., Renslo, R., Berman, N., and Cooper, D.M. Effect of exercise training on energy expenditure, muscle volume and max O_2 uptake in female adolescents. *J. Pediatr* 129:537-543, 1996.
53. Nevin-Folino, N.L. Sports nutrition for children and adolescents. In: *Handbook of Pediatric Nutrition*. Queen, P.M. and Lang, C.E. (Eds.). Gaithersburg, MD: Aspen Publishers, Inc. 1993, pp. 187-205.
54. Nelson-Steen, S. Nutrition for the school-aged child. In: *The Child and Adolescent Athlete*. Bar-Or, O. (Ed). Oxford, London. Blackwell Science. 1996a, pp. 260-273.
55. Nelson-Steen, S. Timely statement of the ADA: Nutritional guidance for adolescent athletes in organized sports. *J. Am. Diet. Assoc.* 96:611-612, 1996b.
56. Lemon, P.W.R. Effect of exercise on dietary protein requirements. *Int. J. Sport Nutr.* 8:426-447, 1998.
57. Tarnopolsky , M.A., Atkinson, S.A., MacDougall, J.D., Chesley, A., Phillips, S., and Schwarcz, H.P. Evaluation of protein requirements for trained strength athletes. *J. Appl. Physiol.* 73:1986-1995, 1992.
58. Sundgot-Borgen, J. Nutrient intakes of elite athletes suffering from eating disorders. *Int. J. Sport Nutr.* 3:431-442, 1993.
59. Bar-Or, O. The young athlete: Some physiological considerations. *J. Sports Sci.* 13;S31-S33, 1995.
60. Falk, B. Bar-Or, O., and MacDougall, J.D. Thermoregulatory responses of pre-, mid-, and late-pubertal boys to exercise in dry heat. *Med. Sci. Sports Exer.* 24:688-694, 1992.
61. Bar-Or, O. Temperature regulation during exercise in children and adolescents. In: *Perspectives in Exercise. Science. Vol. 2. Youth, Exercise, and Sport*. C.V. Gisolfi and D.R. Lamb (Eds.) Indianapolis: Benchmark Press. 1989, pp. 335-367.
62. Meyer, R., Bar-Or, O. MacDougall, D., and Heigenhauser, G.J.F. Sweat electrolyte loss during exercise in the heat: Effects of gender and maturation. *Med. Sci. Sports Exer.* 24:776-781, 1992.
63. Bar-Or, O., Dotan, R., Inbar, O., Rthstein, A., and Zonder, H. Voluntary hypohydration in 10–12-year-old boys. *J. Applied Physio*. 48:104-108, 1980.
64. Iuliano, S., Naughton, G., Collier, G., and Carlson, J. Examination of the self-selected fluid intake practices by junior athletes during a simulated duathlon event. *Int. J. Sport Nutr.* 8;10-23, 1998.
65. American College of Sports Medicine. Position Stand. Exercise and fluid replacement. *Med. Sci. Sports Exer.* 28:I-vii, 1996.
66. Horswill, C.A. Effective fluid replacement. *Int. J. Sport Nutr.* 8:175-195, 1998.
67. Shirreffs, S.M., Taylor, A.J., Leiper, J.B., and Maughan, R.J. Post-exercise rehydration in man: Effects of volume consumed and drink sodium content. *Med. Sci. Sports Exer.* 28:1260-1271, 1996.
68. Burke, L.M. and Hawley, J.A. Fluid balance in team sports: Guidelines for optimal practices. *Sports Med.* 24:38-54, 1997.
69. Davis, J.M., Jackson, D.A., Broadwell, M.S., Queary, J.L., and Lambert, C.L. Carbohydrate drinks delay fatigue during intermittent high-intensity cycling in active men and women. *Int. J. Sport Nutr.* 7:230-235, 1997.
70. Welsh, R.S., Byam, S., Bartoli, W., Burke, J.M., Williams, H., and Davis, J.M. Influence of carbohydrate ingestion on physical and mental function during intermittent high-intensity exercise to fatigue. *Med. Sci. Sports Exer..* 31; S123, 1999.

71. Rivera-Brown, A.M., Gutierrez, R., Gutierrez, J.C., Frontera, W.R., and Bar-Or, O. Drink composition, voluntary drinking, and fluid balance in exercising, trained, heat-acclimatized boys. *J. Appl. Physiol.* 86:76-84, 1999.
72. Wilk, B. and Bar-Or, O. Effect of drink flavor and NaCl on voluntary drinking and rehydration in boys exercising in the heat. *J. Appl. Physiol.* 80: 1112-1117, 1996.
73. Schmidt, W., Maasen, N., Trsot, F., and Boening, D. Training-induced effects on blood volume, erythrocyte turnover, and hemoglobin oxygen properties. *Eur. J. Appl. Physiol.* 57:490-498, 1988.
74. Raunikar, R.A. and Sabio, H. Anemia in the adolescent athlete. *Am. J. Dis. Child.* 146:1201-1205, 1992.
75. Nickerson, H.J., Holubets, M.C., Weiler, B.R., Haas, R.G., Schwartz, S., and Ellefson, M.E. Causes of iron deficiency in adolescent athletes. *J. Pediat.* 114:657-663, 1989.
76. Nickerson, H.J., Holubets, M., Tripp, A.D., and Pierce, W.G. Decreased iron stores in high school runners. *Am. J. Dis. Child.* 139:1115-1119, 1985.
77. Risser, W.L., Lee, E.J., Poindexter, H.B.W., West, M.S., Pivarnick, J.M., Risser, J.M.H., and Hickson, J.F. Iron deficiency in female athletes: its prevalence and impact on performance. *Med. Sci. Sports Exer.* 20:116-121, 1988.
78. Rowland, T.W., and Kelleher, J.F. Iron deficiency in athletes. Insights from high school swimmers. *Am. J. Dis Child.* 143:197-200, 1989.
79. Rowland, T.W., Black, S.A., and Kelleher, J.F. Iron deficiency in adolescent endurance athletes. *J. Adolesc. Health Care.* 8:322-328, 1987.
80. Risser, W.L. and Risser, M.H. Iron deficiency in adolescents and young adults. *Phys. Sportsmed.* 18(12):87-101, 1990.
81. Rowland, T.W. Iron deficiency in the adolescent athlete. In:*The Child and Adolescent Athlete.* Bar-Or, O. (ed). Oxford, London. Blackwell Science. 1996, pp.274-286.
82. Finch, C.A., Miller, L.R., Inamidar, A.R., Person, R., Seiler, K., and Mackler, B. Iron deficiency in the rat: Physiological and biochemical studies of muscle dysfunction. *J. Clin. Invest.* 447-453, 1976.
83. Willis, W.T., Gohil, K., Brooks, G.A., and Dallman, P.R. Iron deficiency: improved exercise performance within 15 hours of iron treatment in rats. *J. Nutr.* 120:909-916, 1990.
84. Celsing, F., Ekblom, B., Sylven, C., Everett, J., and Astrand, P.O. Effect of chronic iron deficiency anemia on myoglobin content, enzyme activity, and capillary density in the human skeletal muscle. *Acata Med. Scand.* 223:451-457, 1988.
85. Newhouse, I.J., Clement, D.B., Tauton, J.E., and McKenzie, D.C. The effects of prelatent/latent iron deficiency on physical work capacity. *Med. Sci. Sports Exer.* 21:263-268, 1989.
86. Bailey, D.A. The role of physical activity in the regulation of bone mass during growth. In: *The Child and Adolescent Athlete.* Bar-Or, O. (ed). Oxford: Blackwell Science. 1996a, pp.138-152.
87. Orr, S.M. Bone density in adolescents. *N. Engl. J. Med.* 325:1646-1648, 1991.
88. Matkovic, V. Calcium and peak bone mass. *J. Int. Med.* 231:151-156, 1992.
89. Matkovic, V., Jelic, T., Wardlow, G.M., Illich, J.Z., Goel, P.K., Wright, J.K., Andon, M.B., Smith, K.T., and Heany, R.P. Timing of peak bone mass in Caucasian females and its implications for the prevention of osteoporosis. *J. Clin. Inves.* 93:799-808, 1994.
90. Barr, S. and McKay, H.A. Nutrition, exercise, and bone status in youth. *Int. J. Sport Nutr.* 8;124-142, 1998.
91. Krall, E.A. and Dawson-Hughes, B. Heritable and life-style determinants of bone mineral density. *J. Bone Min. Res.* 8:1-9,1993.
92. Heaney, R.P. Protein intake and the calcium economy. *J. Am. Diet. Assoc.* 93;1259-1260, 1993.
93. Andon, M.B., Lloyd, T., and Matkovic, V. Supplementation trials with calcium citrate malate: Evidence in favor of increasing the calcium RDA during childhood and adolescence. *J. Nutr.* 124;1412S-1417S, 1994.
94. Cadogan, J., Eastell, R., Jones, N., and Barker, M.E. Milk intake and bone mineral acquisition in adolescent girls: randomized, controlled intervention trial. *Br. Med. J.* 315:1255-1260, 1997.
95. Chan, G.M., Hoffman, K., and McMurray, M. Effects of dairy products on bone and body composition in pubertal girls. *J. Pediatr.* 126;551-556, 1995.
96. Halioua, L. and Anderson, J.J.B. Lifetime calcium intake and physical activity habits: independent and combined effects on the radial bone of healthy premenopausal Caucasian women. *Am. J. Clin. Nutr.* 49;534-541, 1989.

97. Johnston, C.C., Miller, J.Z., Slemenda, C.W., Reister, T.K., Hui, S., Christian, J.C., and Peacock, M. Calcium supplementation and increases in bone mineral density in children. *N. Engl. J. Med.* 327;82-87, 1992.
98. Lee, W.T.K., Leung, S.S.F., Wang, S.H., Xu, Y.C., Zeng, W.P., Lau, J., Oppenheimer, S.J., and Cheng, J.C.Y. Double-blind controlled calcium supplementation and bone mineral accretion in children accustomed to a low-calcium diet. *Am. J. Clin. Nutr.* 60;774-750, 1994.
99. Lloyd, T., Andon, M.B., Rollings, N., Martel, J.K., Landis, R., Demers, L.M., Eggli, D.F., Kieselhorst, K., and Kulin, H.E. Calcium supplementation and bone mineral density in adolescent girls. *J. Am. Med. Assoc.*. 270;841-844, 1993
100. Matkovic, V., Kostial, K., Simonovic, I., Buzina, R., Brodarec, A., and Nordin, C. Bone status and fracture rates in two regions of Yugoslavia. *Am. J. Clin. Nutr.* 32:540-549, 1979.
101. Matkovic, V., Fontana, D., Tominac, C., Goel, P., and Chesnut, C.H. Factors that influence peak bone mass formation: a study of calcium balance and the inheritance of bone mass in adolescent females. *Am. J. Clin. Nutr.* 52;878-888, 1990.
102. Nieves, J.W., Golden, A.L., Siris, E., Kelsey, J.L., and Lindsay, R. Teenage and current calcium intake are related to bone mineral density of the hip and forearm in women aged 30–39 years. *Am. J. Epidemiology.* 141;342-351, 1995.
103. Soroko, S., Holbrook, T.L., Edelstein, S., and Barret-Conner, E. Lifetime milk consumption and bone mineral density in older women. *Am. J. Pub. Health.* 84;1319-1322, 1994.
104. Sandler, R.B., Slemenda, C.W., LaPorte, R.E., Cauley, J.A., Schramm, M.M., Barresi, M.L., and Kriska, A.M. Postmenopausal bone density and milk consumption in childhood and adolescence. *Am. J. Clin. Nutr.*. 42;270-274,1985.
105. Slemenda, C.W., Reister, T.K., Peacock, M., and Johnston, C.C. Bone growth in children following the cessation of calcium supplementation. *J. Bone Min. Res.* 8(suppl 1):S145, 1993.
106. Abrams, S.A., and Stuff, J.E. Calcium metabolism in girls: current dietary intakes lead to low rates of calcium absorption and retention during puberty. *Am. J. Clin. Nutr.* 60;739-743, 1994.
107. Eck, L.H., and Hackett-Renner, C. Calcium intake in youth: sex, age, and racial differences in NHANES II. *Preventive Med.* 21;473-482, 1992.
108. Harel, Z., Riggs, S., Vaz, R., White, L., and Menzies, G. Adolescents and calcium: what they do and do not know and how much they consume. *J. Adolesc. Health.* 22;225-228, 1998.
109. Frank, C.C., Webber, L.S., Nicklas, T.A., and Berenson, G.S. Sodium, postassium, calcium, magnesium, and phosphorus intakes of infants and children: Bogalusa Heart Study. *J. Am. Diet. Assoc.* 88;801-807, 1988.
110. Fleming, K.H. and Heimbach, J.T. Consumption of calcium in the U.S.: Food sources and intake levels. *J. Nutr.* 124;1426S-1430S, 1994.
111. Albertson, A.M., Tobelmann, R.C., and Marquart, L. Estimated dietary calcium intake and food sources for adolescent females 1980-1992. *J. Adol. Health.* 20;20-26, 1997.
112. Haapasalo, H., Kannus, P., Sievnen, H., Heinonen, A., Oja, A., and Vuori, I. Long-term unilateral loading and bone mineral density and content in female squash players. *Calcif. Tissue Int.* 54:249-255, 1994.
113. Haapasalo, H., Sievanen, H., Kontulainene, S., Kannus, P., Jarvinen, M., and Vuori, I. High bone mineral content in male tennis players playing arm is due to big bone size not density. *Med. Sci. Sports Exer.* 31:S137, 1999.
114. Watson, R. Bone growth and physical activity in young males. In: *International Conference on Bone Mineral Measurements.* Mazess, R. (Ed.) Washington, DC:DHEW Publication. NIH 75-683. 1974, pp.380-385.
115. Bailey, D.A., Faulkner, R.A., and McKay, H.A. Growth, physical activity, and bone mineral acquisition. In: *Exercise and Sport Sciences Reviews* (vol. 24). J.O. Holloszy (Ed.) Baltimore, MD. Williams and Wilkins, 1996b, pp. 233-266.
116. Snow, C.M. Exercise and bone mass in young and premenopausal women. *Bone.* 18;51S-55S, 1996.
117. Gunnes, M. and Lehman, E. Physical activity and dietary constituents as predictors of forearm cortical and trabecular bone gain in healthy children and adolescents: a prospective study. *Acata Paedriatrica.* 85:19-25, 1996.

118. Morris, F.L., Naughton, G.A., Gibbs, J.L., Carlson, J.S., and Wark, J.D. Prospective 10-month exercise intervention in pre-menarcheal girls: positive effects on bone and lean mass. *J. Bone Min. Res.* 12:1453-1462, 1997.
119. Lennkh, C., Zwaan, M., Bailer, U., Strnad, A., Nagy, C., El-Giamal, N., Wiesnagrotzki, S., Vytiska, E., Huber, J., and Kasper, S. Osteopenia in anorexia nervosa: specific mechanisms of bone loss. *J. Pysch. Res.* 33:349-356, 1999.
120. Cann, C.E., Martin, M.C., Genant, H.K., and Jaffe, R.B. Decreased spinal mineral content in amenorrheic women. *J. Am. Med. Assoc.* 251:626-629, 1984
121. Drinkwater, B.L., Bruemmer, B., and Chestnut III, C.H. Menstrual history as a determinant of current bone density in young athletes. *J. Am. Med. Assoc.* 263:545-548, 1990.
122. Drinkwater, B.L., Nilson, K., Chestnut III, C.H., Bremmer, W.J., Shainholtz, S., and Southworth, M.B. Bone mineral content of amenorrheic and eumenorrheic athletes. *N. Engl. J. Med.* 311:277-281, 1984.
123. Klesges, R.C., Ward, K.D., Shelton, M.L., Applegate, W.B., Cantler, E.D., Palmieri, G.M., Harmon, K., and Davis, J. Changes in bone mineral content in male athletes: Mechanisms of action and intervention effects. *J. Am. Med. Assoc.* 276:226-230, 1996.
124. National Academy of Sciences. Washington, D.C. *Dietary Reference Intakes: Calcium, Phosphorous, Magnesium, Vitamin D, and Fluoride.* Food and Nutrition Board. Institute of Medicine. Washington, D.C.: National Academy of Sciences Press. 1997.
125. Matkovic, V. and Heanney, R.P. Calcium balance during human growth: Evidence for threshold behavior. *Am. J. Clin. Nutr.* 55:992-996, 1992.
126. Sternleib, J.J. and Munson, L.A. A survey of health problems, practices, and needs of youth. *Pediatrics.* 49:117-180, 1972.
127. Feldman, W., Hadgson, C., Corber, S., and Quinn, A. Health concerns and health-related behaviors of adolescents. *J. Can. Med. Assoc.* 134:489-496, 1983.
128. Eisele, J., Hersgaard, D., and Light, H.K. Factors related to eating disorders in young adolescent girls. *Adolescence.* 21:283-301, 1986.
129. Moses, N., Banilivy, M.M., and Lifshitz, F. Fear of obesity among adolescent girls. *Pediatrics.* 83:393-398, 1989.
130. Casper, R.C. and Offer, D. Weight and dieting concerns in adolescents. Fashion or symptom? *Pediatrics.* 86:384-390, 1990.
131. Moore, D.C. Body image and eating behavior in adolescent girls. *Am. J. Dis. Child.* 144:475-481, 1990.
132. Brooks-Gunn, J., Burrow, C., Warren, M.P. Attitudes toward eating and body weight in different groups of female adolescent athletes. *Int. J.Eating Disorders.* 7:749-757, 1988.
133. Mallick, M.J., Whipple, T.W., and Huerta, E. Behavioral and psychological traits of weight-conscious teenagers: A comparison of eating disordered patients and high- and low-risk groups. *Adolescence.* 85:157-168, 1987.
134. Traub, D.E. and Blinde, E.M. Eating disorders among adolescent female athletes: Influence of athletic participation and sport team membership. *Adolescence.* 27:833-48, 1992.
135. Dummer, G.M., Rosen, L.W., Heusner, W.W., Roberts, P.J., and Counsilman, J.E. Pathogenic weight control behaviors of young competitive swimmers. *Phys. Sportsmed.* 15:75-84, 1987.
136. Garner, D.M., Rosen, L.W., and Barry, D. Eating disorders among athletes. *Child Adolesc. Psych. Clin. N. Am.* 7:839-857, 1998.
137. Streigel-Moore, R., Silberstein, L.R., and Rodin, J. Toward an understanding of the risk factors for bulimia. *Am. Psych.* 41:246-263, 1986.
138. Yates, A. Current perspectives on eating disorders 1: History, psychological and biological aspects. *J. Am. Acad. Child Adolesc. Psych.* 28:813-828, 1989.
139. O'Conner, P.J., Lewis, R.D., and Kirchner, E.M. Eating disorder symptoms in female college gymnasts. *Med. Sci. Sports Exer.* 27:550-555, 1995.
140. Wilmore, J.H. Eating disorders in the young athlete. In:*The Child and Adolescent Athlete*. Bar-Or, O. (Ed). Oxford, London. Blackwell Science. 1996, pp.287-303.
141. Davis, C. and Cowles, M. A comparison of weight and diet concerns and personality factors among female athletes and nonathletes. *J. Psychosom. Res.* 33:527-536, 1989.
142. Stoutjesdyk, D. and Jevne, R. Eating disorders among high performance athletes. *J,.Youth Adolesc.* 22:271-282, 1993.

143. Sundgot-Borgen, J. and Corbin, C. Eating disorders among female athletes. *Phys. Sportsmed.* 15(2):89-95, 1987.
144. Beals, K.A. and Manore, M.M. Nutritional status of female athletes with subclinical eating disorders. *J. Am. Diet. Assoc.* 98:419-425,1998
145. Benson, J.E., Engelbert-Fenton, K.A., and Eisenman, P. Nutritional aspects of amenorrhea in the female athlete triad. *Int. J. Sport Nutr.* 6:134-145, 1996.
146. Palla, B. and Lilt, I.F. Medical complications of eating disorders in adolescence. Pediatrics. 81:613-620, 1988.
147. American College of Sports Medicine. Position Stand. The female athlete triad. *Med. Sci. Sports Exer.* 29:I-ix, 1997.
148. Drinkwater, B.L., Nilson, K., Ott, S., and Chestnut III, C.H. Bone mineral density after resumption of menses in amenorrheic athletes. *J. Am. Med. Assoc.* 256:380-382, 1986.
149. Warren, M.P., Brooks-Gunn, J., Hamilton, L.F., Warren, L.F., and Hamilton, W.G. Scoliosis and fractures in young ballet dancers: Relation to delayed menarche and secondary amenorrhea. *N. Engl. J. Med.* 314:1348-1353, 1986.
150. Chan, G.M., Hess, M., Hollis, J., and Book, L.S. Bone mineral status in childhood accidental fractures. *Am. J. Dis. Child.* 139:569-570, 1984.
151. Warren, M.P., Brooks-Gunn, J., Fox, R.P., Lancelot, C., Newman, D., and Hamilton, W.G. Lack of bone accretion and amenorrhea: Evidence for a relative osteopenia in weight-bearing bones. *J. Clin. Endocrinol. Metabol.* 72:847-853, 1991.
152. Frusztajer, N.T., Dhuper, S., Warren, M.P., Brooks-Gunn, J., and Fox, R.P. Nutrition and the incidence of stress fractures in ballet dancers. *Am. J. Clin. Nutr.* 51:779-783, 1990.
153. Yeager, K.K., Agostini, R., Nattiv, A., Drinkwater, B.L. The female athlete triad: disordered eating , amenorrhea, osteoporosis [commentary]. *Med. Sci. Sports Exer.* 25:775-777, 1993.
154. Petrie, T.A. Differences between male and female college lean sport athletes, nonlean sport athletes, and nonathletes on behavioral and psychological indices of eating disorders. *J. Appl. Sport Psychol.* 8:218-230, 1996.
155. Lankin, J.A., Steen, S.N., and Oppliger, R.A. Eating behaviors, weight loss methods, and nutrition practices among high school wrestlers. *J. Community Health Nur.* 7:223-234, 1990.
156. Nelson-Steen, S. and Brownell, K.D. Patterns of weight loss and regain in wrestlers; has the tradition changed? *Med. Sci. Sports Exer.* 22:762-768, 1990.
157. Oppliger, R.A., Landry, G.L., Foster, S.W., and Lambrecht, A.C. Bulimic behaviors among interscholastic wrestlers: A statewide survey. *Pediatrics.* 91:826-831, 1993.
158. Weissinger, E., Housh, T.J., Johnson, G.O. Weight loss behaviors in high school wrestling: Wrestler and parent perceptions. *Pediat. Exer. Sci.* 3:64-73, 1991.
159. Brownelll, K.D., Steen, S.N., and Wilmore, J.H. Weight regulation practices in athletes; analysis of metabolic and health effects. *Med. Sci. Sports Exer.* 19:546-556, 1987.
160. Nelson-Steen, S., Oppliger, R.A., and Brownell, K.D. Metabolic effects of repeated weight loss and regain in adolescent wrestlers. *J. Am. Med. Assoc.* 260:47-50, 1988.
161. American College of Sports Medicine: Position Stand. Weight loss in Wrestlers. *Med. Sci. Sports Exer.* 28:ix-xii, 1996.
162. Sobal, J. and Marquart, L.F., Vitamin/mineral supplement use among high school athletes. *Adolescence.* 29:835-843, 1994.
163. Massad, S.J., Shier, N.W., Koceja, D.M., and, N.T., High school athletes and nutritional supplements: A study of knowledge and use. *Int. J. Sport Nutr.* 5:232-245, 1995.
164. Krowchuk, D.P., Agnlin, T.M., Goodfellow, D.B., Stancin, T., Williams, P., and Zimet, G.D. High school athletes and the use of ergogenic aids. *Am. J. Dis. Child.* 143:486-489, 1989.
165. Haymes, E.M. Vitamin and mineral supplementation in athletes. *J. Sports Nutr.* 1:146-149, 1991.
166. Singh, A., Maoses, F.M., and Deuster, P.A. Chronic multivitamin/mineral supplement does not enhance physical performance. *Med. Sci. Sports Exer.* 24:726-732, 1992.
167. Fogelholm, G.M., Kukkonen-Harjula, T.K., Taipale, S.A., Sievanen, H.T., Oja, P., and Vuori, I.M. Resting metabolic rate and energy intakes in female gymnasts, figure skaters, and soccer players. *Int. J. Sports Med.* 16;551-556, 1995.
168. Loosli, A., Benson, J., Gillian, D. Nutrition habits and knowledge in competitive female gymnasts. *Phys. Sportsmed.* 14:8-15, 1986.

169. Sundgot-Borgen, J. Eating disorders, energy intake, training volume, and menstrual function in high-level modern rhythmic gymnasts. *Int. J. Sport Nutr.* 6:100-109, 1996.
170. Beals, K.A., Woolf, K, and Corte, C.Nutritional and menstrual status of elite adolescent volleyball players. *J. Am. Diet. Assoc.* 99:A-39, 1999.
171. Van Erp Baart A.M.J., Saris, W.H.M., Brinkhorst, R.A. and Elvers, J.W.H. Nationwide Survey on nutritional habits in elite athletes. Part I. Energy, Carbohydrate, Protein and Fat Intake. *Int. J. Sports Med.* 10:S3-S10,1989.
172. Horswill, C.A., Park, S.H., and Roemich, J.N. Changes in protein nutritional status of adolescent wrestlers. *Med. Sci. Sports Exer.* 25:599-604, 1990.

CHAPTER 5

Nutritional Concerns of Elderly Athletes

Melissa D. Ripley, Paul N. Taylor, Ira Wolinsky, and Dorothy Klimis-Zacas

CONTENTS

I. INTRODUCTION

Many older Americans do not engage in regular physical activity.[1-3] Among men and women aged 50–59 years, 18% of the men and 30% of the women do not.[2] These proportions slowly increase with increasing age, reaching 40% among men and 62% among women aged 80 years and over.[2] The lower proportion of women engaging in physical activity, compared with men of the same age range, may be due to socialization, which has fostered negative attitudes among women toward exercise.[4,5] Unfortunately, the gender difference in physical activity participation is reflected in measures of muscle strength and aerobic capacity, which are lower among women than among men. Both measures decline with increasing age, at a greater rate in women than in men.[1,2] Encouraging women to exercise may lessen this "gender gap." In addition to the

0-8493-8199-1/00/$0.00+$.50

general benefits of exercise for older women,[6] female exercisers may be more satisfied with their body image than nonexercising women, and this satisfaction may increase with age among the exercisers.[7]

In 1998, there were approximately 34 million people age 65 and older.[8] By 2030, this number is projected to reach 69 million, approximately 20% of the U.S. population.[9] This age group is expected to grow modestly until 2010, then more dramatically as the "baby-boom" generation (people born between 1946 and 1964) begins to enter the group.[10] The baby boomers, unlike previous generations, are not comfortable with the physical decline usually associated with aging, and are more devoted to fitness and wellness.[1,11]

The "very old" agc group (85+ years) is especially fast-growing, projected to increase from 1.4% of the population to 2.4% by 2030, then to 4.6% by 2050.[12] In 1997, life expectancy at birth reached 76.5 years.[13] Continuing increases in longevity are attributed to decreasing mortality from chronic diseases, whereas earlier increases in life expectancy were attributed to decreases in infant and child mortality.[14] Today, people aged 65 years can expect to live until the age of 82.5.[15] Considering that the risk for many chronic diseases and physical disabilities increases with age, we must now ask what will be the overall quality of these added years for these individuals. At least one-third of the elderly population have self-reported limitations due to chronic conditions, while more than 50% report having at least one disability.[14,16] At least some of the physiological changes that are associated with aging are also related to inactivity.[17] The overall health benefits attributed to regular physical activity for the elderly athlete include better functional capacity, less physical and musculoskeletal disability, less need of medical care, lower body weight, and better cardiovascular fitness (Figure 5.1).[18,50]

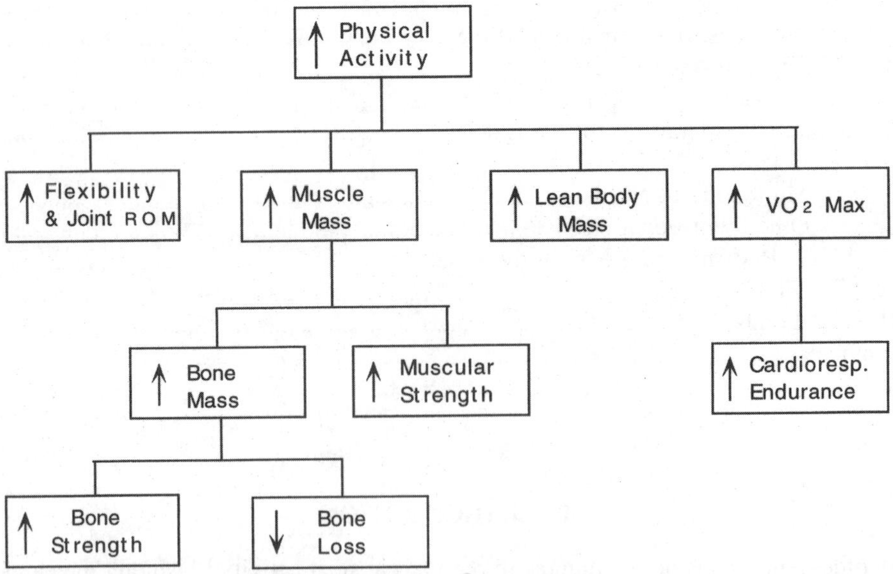

Figure 5.1 The influence of increased physical activity among older adults. (Adapted from Seto, J. L., et al., *Clin. Sports Med.*, 10:401-429, 1991. With permission.)

Unfortunately, there is scant information available to elderly athletes concerning how their nutritional needs may differ from those of younger athletes. The information that does exist is based on younger populations or on older populations that are less functionally capable than the typical elderly athlete.[1] The need for this information is great and will continue to increase, not only in respect to the growing elderly population, but also in regard to the increasing number of these individuals involving themselves in some form of physical activity or sport.

II. OVERLYING CHARACTERISTICS OF THE ELDERLY

A. Physiological Aspects

1. Body Composition and Muscular Strength

Aging brings about many changes in physical condition. Among these changes, body fat increases,[19] at the expense of muscle and bone, both of which decrease.[17] Most of the body fat increase accumulates in the abdominal area.[19] With a decrease in muscle (or lean body mass), which is more metabolically active tissue, the body uses fewer calories to function and thus the basal metabolic rate of the elderly is lower.[20] The decline in resting metabolic rate is also attributed to other factors including Na-K pump activity, increasing fat mass, lower maximal aerobic power, and menopausal status.[21] Total energy needs also decrease concomitant with a decline in energy expenditure due to decreased physical activity. If caloric intake is not reduced, weight gain may occur.

As one ages, total body composition changes due to the decrease in fat-free mass and increasing body fat.[20] Sedentary elders have a higher body fat percentage than their active peers,[22] and there is some evidence that those with a high percent body fat have high levels of disability.[23] While total body weight may not change with aging, loss of muscle is usually great. An increase in body fat tends to equal the weight that is lost from a decrease in muscle mass.

By controlling energy intake and exercising, the elderly can maintain the same body fat levels as much younger individuals.[24] Regular aerobic or endurance exercise produces fat loss in this population;[25] however, the amount lost is not enough to completely balance aging-associated body composition changes. A dual-component program of aerobic and strength training is needed to preserve lean body mass[25,26] and to increase the metabolism of endogenous fat stores.[27] Fat oxidation, in general, is lower in the elderly than in younger adults,[27,28] but can be increased after endurance training with no significant changes in lipolysis or free fatty acid availability during exercise.[27]

Positive benefits are associated with exercise for the elderly[29] and include increased muscle strength. A decrease in muscle strength, as occurs with aging, is one of the major causes of disability.[20] For example, decreases in walking and chair-rising speeds are associated with a decrease in strength.[30] Even small increases in muscle strength in the elderly can slow functional decline and provide a better quality of life.[31] The decrease in mobility and physical performance as one ages is directly linked to loss of muscle mass.[32-34] This is attributed to the combined loss from both types of muscle fibers, but especially from type II fibers.[30,35] Reduced muscle fiber size also occurs with aging. A decline in muscle mass begins after age 30, becoming more exaggerated after the age of 50.[36-38] Muscle strength, however, usually does not differ dramatically until approximately age 70, when reduced contractile strength of muscle becomes evident.[36,39,40]

Resistance training helps to lessen the normal muscle loss and loss of muscle strength that are associated with aging.[41-43] With strength training, it is possible to substantially increase both upper- and lower-body strength while also increasing total fat-free mass and decreasing total fat mass by the same amount.[44]

Dietary supplements are often prescribed for elderly and/or rehabilitation patients in need of weight gain. When combined with a program of strength training, the supplements might influence increases in lean and adipose tissues without affecting strength gain,[45] but by themselves, multi-nutrient supplements are not effective in counteracting muscle weakness and frailty among the very elderly.[46] Likewise, neither chromium picolinate nor creatine monohydrate, both popular supplements among athletes, enhances muscle size or power development,[47] muscle strength or lean body mass accretion,[47,48] or endurance[48] in older men participating in resistance training.

At or around age 65, muscle mass is about 80% of what it was at age 20, with the loss occurring in the lower extremities more quickly than in the upper extremities.[49] As well, muscle strength begins to decline rapidly after approximately age 50.[50] However, the elderly are able to regain strength as easily as younger people,[51] and regular exercise may also ameliorate age-related diseases.[52] The strength gain comes, not from changes in muscle mass, but from an increased ability to recruit more muscle units and fibers as well as a possible increase in neural activation.[53,54] Aging-associated body composition changes are also very similar to those that occur with certain diseases: exercise, nutrition, vascular and neurologic abnormalities, and hormones all have effects similar to those of aging on body composition changes.[55]

Age-specific formulae and tables should be used when determining body composition of older adults.[56] Because stature decreases with increasing age, height should be measured rather than taken from self-reports.[1] In elderly women, there are several differences among health-related factors based on the level of physical activity, including body weight and body mass index, flexibility of the hip and spine, and endurance.[57]

Obesity is common among the elderly[58,59] until the age of approximately 75 years, after which it occurs less often.[60] Many diseases, including myocardial infarction, stroke, hypertension, hyperlipidemia, and diabetes, as well as overall mortality, are associated with obesity.[61-63] Obese elderly should be encouraged to make dietary and lifestyle changes, to include reducing total fat intake (i.e., balancing the dietary energy profile), avoiding micronutrient deficiencies, and increasing intake of dietary fiber.[60] Energy balance is more likely among women and fat loss is less significant.[64]

2. Cardiovascular Functions

Heart disease is the number one cause of death for those aged 65 years and over.[65] Age-related changes in the healthy heart include cellular hypertrophy and increased impedance to left ventricular ejection,[66] decreased maximal heart rate due to reduced contractility of the myocardium,[52,67] and increased systolic blood pressure.[68] Arterial function and structure also change with age, showing increasing vascular stiffness and accumulations of lipids, collagen, and minerals.[69] Finally, the ability of the muscles to use oxygen declines 8–10% per decade, and most of this decrease is due to inactivity.[17] Fortunately, regular exercise may reduce the rate of this decline.[29,31,70-72]

There is enough evidence to support an inverse correlation between physical activity and heart disease to influence public health policy regarding lifelong physical activity and physical fitness.[18,29,73-76] Atherosclerosis, too, is influenced by exercise-induced metabolic changes,[77-81] as is hypertension.[82-86] Whereas earlier reports of the benefits of regular exercise in preventing heart disease rarely included women or non-white individuals, several recent papers have extended our understanding,[87-89] although more studies are needed, especially concerning racial and ethnic differences.[87,90,91]

3. Bone Health

Dietary calcium and vitamin D are important to bone fracture risk, especially among women, who may have poor mineral and vitamin intakes, and to the elderly, who may suffer decreased mineral and vitamin absorption.[92] A decline in calcium absorption is a normal consequence of aging,[93] beginning at approximately age 60 for women and age 70 for men.[94] This decrease in absorption is associated with low calcium intake, hypercalciuria, and decreased blood levels of 1,25-dihydroxy vitamin D,[93] and can eventually lead to osteoporosis and bone fractures. There are also seasonal differences in vitamin D levels and bone mineral density in northern-latitude-dwelling elderly women,[95] and overt vitamin D deficiency has been implicated as a contributing factor of syndrome X (in which degenerative vascular disease increases with glucose intolerance and diabetes).[96]

Gender, hormonal status, heredity, and calcium and vitamin D intake influence bone mass, which declines 5–10% per decade after age 40;[93] up to 6% per year after menopause.[97] More than 30% of women over age 65 will develop spinal fractures due to age-related loss of bone density, and the number of total fractures among Americans is expected to rise substantially in the next 50 years.[17] An awareness of adequate dietary calcium and its role in the prevention of osteoporosis has received continuing emphasis in the literature of nutrition.[98-101]

Physical activity is important in the prevention of hip fractures,[102] whereas physical inactivity has been noted as a significant risk factor for the occurrence of hip fractures and possibly osteoporosis.[101,103] High-intensity strength training for postmenopausal women has a protective effect on bone density and improves muscle mass and strength.[98,102,104-106] Continued resistance exercise increases bone mass and reverses the loss of skeletal calcium in the elderly,[92,106-108] and aerobic exercise may similarly affect bone density.[109] Elderly athletes would do well to exercise in moderation, however, using a well-planned regimen after consulting with a physician, for there is some evidence to indicate that endurance athletes may suffer an uncoupling of bone cell metabolism and consequent loss of bone density.[110,111]

Falls occur with increasing frequency as aging progresses, in both men[112,113] and women.[114-116] Regular exercise, by increasing strength and balance, may reduce the risk of falling.[92,100,102,108]

Lifelong regular exercise has become part of the prescription for reducing age-related loss of bone mass.[29,117,118] Even patients with osteoarthritis, which is often associated with obesity, can exercise if they focus on lower intensity, longer duration activities that place less impact on the joints.[119] These may be simple, job-related activities[120] or more leisurely pursuits.[29,105]

4. *Gastrointestinal and Alimentary Functions*

By itself, aging has no significant adverse effects on caloric intake and nutritional status of healthy elderly individuals.[121] Although many physiological factors can affect these two parameters, overall gastrointestinal function remains largely unchanged by aging.[122] However, specific gastrointestinal parameters may show age-related changes in some elderly individuals, such as a slowing of gastric emptying time,[123] an increase in esophageal (e.g., reflux disease)[124] and colonic (diarrhea, irritable bowel syndrome, constipation, etc.) disorders,[124,125] changes in intestinal absorption,[122,126-130] decreased insulin production and sensitivity,[131-133] and, perhaps most important, a loss of reserve capacity, which may compromise gastrointestinal function during periods of stress.[134] Some of these can be partially overcome or prevented by exercise.[52]

Several other age-related physical and physiological changes have the potential to compromise nutrition in some individuals. Many will lose some or all of their natural teeth as they age, conditions that may be associated with lower than recommended intakes for some important nutrients.[135,136] Difficulty chewing food is a logical consequence of tooth loss, occurring even if the missing teeth are replaced with dentures, and may lead to patterns of food avoidance and dietary inadequacies.[137]

The sense of smell seems to decrease with age, but there is limited information addressing the mechanisms of this aging-related sensory loss. Most researchers agree, however, that perceived aging-related loss of taste is actually a function of olfactory ability.[138-142] Sensory-specific satiety, i.e., a decrease in the perceived pleasantness of a food as it is consumed, may change with age and may be entirely absent in people over the age of 65.[143,144] More research is needed to determine whether, as one ages, observed declines in olfactory ability, appetite, and hunger, together with perceived decline in tasting ability, are linked to inactivity and/or other physical or psychosocial variables.[121]

Research concerning the effects of exercise on gastrointestinal function is relatively recent, although infrequent observations have been made since William Beaumont's landmark studies over 100 years ago.[145] What seems clear is that the gastrointestinal tract functions optimally at rest, that both upper and lower gastrointestinal disorders can occur with even moderate exercise, and that female exercisers seem to be more affected by digestive maladies than male exercisers.[146-151] Wise athletes of any age would do well to develop an individualized regimen to minimize or eliminate their specific gastrointestinal discomfort(s) when exercising.

B. Physical Aspects

The risk of injury resulting from exercise, physical activity, or sports is a concern for all age groups. Older runners report rates of musculoskeletal injuries similar to those of younger runners with the same running distance,[152,153] and there seem to be few differences in the kinds of injuries suffered by athletes over 60 years of age compared to athletes aged 21–25 years, although the older athletes' injuries are more likely due to overuse.[154] In the older athlete, the ability of body systems to adapt to high levels of loading is diminished, and the safety margin of an exercise dose declines with aging.[155] Muscle is the most common acutely injured tissue among active elderly athletes, with the lower extremities the most susceptible to injury.[154,155] More degenerative and inflammatory injuries, as opposed to fractures, dislocations, sprains, and contusions, are seen in the older athlete.[18]

C. Psychological Aspects

Physical mobility, mental alertness, and cognitive function influence the independence, self-esteem, and quality of life of the elderly.[156] Regular exercise positively influences spontaneous activity in the elderly,[64] and may also help to preserve cognitive function[29,157-166] and to alleviate the symptoms and behaviors of depression.[29,165,167] Staying physically fit through regular exercise also seems to help individuals with daily activities, improves overall quality of life, and lessens feelings of loneliness and social isolation.[161,168,169]

III. NUTRITIONAL CONSIDERATIONS FOR THE ELDERLY

As individuals age, energy needs decrease, so less energy intake is needed to maintain weight.[19,30,170-172] As the energy requirements change, food intake adjusts such that older individuals eat less.[123,173] In some, the risk for malnutrition of certain nutrients, especially calcium and vitamins B_{12} and D, increases,[19,172] while in others, overweight is a concern, as mentioned above.[58-64]

By being more physically active, older adults can control or maintain weight while taking in more calories than their non-exercising peers, thus increasing the likelihood of having nutritionally balanced diets. If weight loss is a goal, then maintenance energy intake must be reduced by roughly 3,500 kcal per week to result in a weight loss of about 1 pound (2.2 kg) per week.[174] The obese elderly can safely lose up to 1% of body weight per week, but must permanently modify behavior and food choices.[175]

To maintain acceptable weight, energy intake and energy expenditure must be balanced. The Harris-Benedict equations are commonly used to measure basal metabolic rate (BMR, in kilocalories/day), taking into account body weight (W, in kilograms), height (L, in centimeters), and age (A, in years).[174,176]

$$\text{Women: BMR} = 655.1 + 9.56W + 1.85L - 4.7A$$

$$\text{Men: BMR} = 66.5 + 13.7W + 5L - 6.8A$$

These equations can be used by individuals of any age to estimate energy needs for weight maintenance. However, these formulas tend to overestimate the needs of inactive women[1] and obese individuals,[174] and to underestimate the needs of active women and elderly men.[1]

Exercise may increase energy requirements from 20 to >70% of the BMR, depending on its frequency, intensity, duration, and type.[174,177] Energy needs as determined by total energy expenditure (TEE) and resting energy expenditure (REE) [or resting metabolic rate (RMR)] and by body composition may be higher in elderly men than are recommended by the National Research

Council.[178,179] In assessing conflicting experimental evidence, some scientists have speculated that higher energy needs for older athletes are due to an increase in thermic responses to eating among those elders who are more physically active than in those who are not exercising, and also suggest that large variations in TEE are due mainly to differences in total physical activity.[21,180] Their equations[21,181-184] for predicting the TEE and RMR of older individuals may be more accurate than the Harris-Benedict equations[174,176] for this age group, keeping in mind that RMR measurements are less precisely defined than BMR measurements.[174] More research to determine the energy needs of the elderly athlete, as well as to verify the validity of the age-specific TEE and RMR equations, is warranted.

A. Macronutrient Needs

Current broad dietary guidelines for those aged 51+ years are presently the same as for adults aged <51 years. Carbohydrates should compose 50–60% of the diet, protein 10–20%, and fat should contribute 30% or less of total energy.[179,185-187] Although recent research indicates that the metabolism of carbohydrates and fats changes with age,[27,188] there is presently no reason to change the broad guidelines for most of the elderly population.[172] There are subpopulations, however, for whom fat intake should be slightly more than 30% of total energy.[172,189]

Reference protein (eggs, meats, milk, fish) requirements for the elderly might be higher than recommended (currently 0.75g/kg/d),[190] although there is considerable controversy. Campbell et al.[191] suggested 1.0–1.25 g/kg of high quality protein for elderly adults, based on a short-term nitrogen balance study, although they also noted that the efficiency of nitrogen retention and protein use during resistance training is higher in older adults who consumed 0.8 g protein/kg/day (essentially, the RDA) rather than 1.62 g protein/kg/day.[192] A review of six nitrogen balance studies[193] led to the conclusion that protein recommendations were probably too low for the elderly, but that further research was needed before making revisions. More-recent research[194] and a review[195] show that revising the current RDA for reference protein in the elderly remains controversial.

B. Micronutrient Needs

Recommended dietary allowances (RDAs) and dietary reference intakes (DRIs)for those aged 51 and over are presently the same as for those aged < 50 years (except that calcium, vitamin D, vitamin B_6 and magnesium RDIs are highter for both sexes, and the RDA for iron is lower for females after the age of 51 years).[277] The requirements for some other minerals and vitamins, e.g., vitamins A, and B_{12}, and folic acid, may change with increasing age.[172,196,197] Some older individuals do not consume the recommended amounts of vitamins and minerals due to alcohol abuse, low energy intake, socioeconomic factors, or some combination of these factors.[171,198] Older adults may also be more susceptible to exercise-induced oxidative damage, requiring greater amounts of antioxidants to compensate for this damage.[199]

The recommendation for adequate calcium intake was recently raised from 800 mg/d to 1.2–1.4 g/d.[200] The best ways to increase calcium in the diet include drinking more milk and choosing other low-fat dairy products. For those who will not consume dairy products for reasons of lactose intolerance, lactose-free dairy products are available and many manufacturers offer calcium-fortified orange juice. In some cases (e.g., aversion to dairy products), calcium supplements may have to be taken. It is important to remember that vitamin D status must also be adequate to maximize the nutritional value of calcium,[93] and that protein, fiber, and sodium are also important cofactors.[201]

The recommendation for adequate vitamin D intake was recently raised from 200 to 600 IU.[200] Older adults are at risk for inadequate vitamin D due to less effective endogenous production as a consequence of aging[202] or as a consequence of limited sun exposure.[95] Vitamin D-fortified foods (e.g., milk) or vitamin D supplements may need to be emphasized for the elderly.[172]

When the dietary recommendations for vitamins B_6, B_{12} and riboflavin were recently revised, the recommendation for vitamin B_6 intake was reduced (from 2.0 mg/d to 1.7 mg/d, and from 1.6 mg/d to 1.5 mg/d, for men and women aged 51+ years, respectively), the recommendation for vitamin B_{12} intake was increased from 2.0 mg/d to 2.4 mg/d for both sexes aged 51+ years, and the recommendation for riboflavin intake was decreased (from 1.4 mg/d to 1.3 mg/d, and from 1.2 mg/d to 1.1 mg/d, for men and women aged 51+ years, respectively).[203,204] The requirements for these three nutrients, however, might be greater for subpopulations of older adults, based on recent research.[196,205-207] Because many elderly people do not adequately absorb vitamin B_{12}, fortified food products or supplements may be indicated.[172,204]

Other micronutrients, such as vitamins C and E, may be necessary for older adults in amounts greater than those recommended for younger populations.[198,208] Higher intakes of vitamins C and and E have been recommended and might be preventive for specific pathologies such as cataracts[198,209–211] and cancer.[212-219] Kanter[220] linked the healthful act of exercise with increased free-radical production due to increased metabolism. Experiments in which supplements of vitamin E (800 mg) were given to a group of healthy elderly show that serum vitamin E levels are increased without any adverse side effects[221] and support the hypothesis that vitamin E is protective against oxidative injury associated with exercise.[222] In the long term, 4 months of vitamin E supplement use improved clinically relevant indexes of cell-mediated immunity in healthy elderly adults.[223] The Food and Nutrition Board of the Institute of Medicine reviewed the 1989 (and subsequent)[218,224,225] and proposed[217,226] recommendations for dietary intakes of vitamins C and E (and other antioxidant nutrients), and issued a report in 1999.[204] Subsequently, the recommendations for vitamins C and E were increased (vitamin C from 60 mg/d for men and women aged 51+ years to 90 mg/d and 75 mg/d, respectively; vitamin E from 10 mg/d for men and 8 mg/d for women aged 51+ years to 15mg/d for men and women), and the recommendations for selenium were decreased for men aged 51+ years (from 70 μg/d to 55 μg/d; the recommendation for women aged 51+ years is unchanged, 55 μg/d).[277]

Iron, which maintains the oxygen-carrying capacity of blood, should be a concern of all athletes,[227-231] including the elderly. Iron insufficiency, with or without anemia, is an important contributor to "restless legs syndrome," which is common in many older adults.[232] The iron requirements for male endurance athletes and postmenopausal female runners may be as much as 8 mg/day higher than the current RDA (10 mg/day)[233] to avoid signs and symptoms of anemia.[234] However, greater levels of iron intake may also have adverse effects such as an increased risk for cardiovascular disease and cancer.[235,236] Most nutrition scientists recommend choosing foods rich in heme iron as opposed to iron supplements,[227,228,237] unless clinical evidence, e.g., measures of serum ferritin, indicate a need for supplements on an individual basis.[238]

Requirements for other micronutrients are presently under review.[204] Because excessive intakes of several vitamins and minerals can be toxic, multi-vitamin/mineral supplements, if used, should not exceed current recommended levels.[1] "Complete" liquid supplements or modular macronutrient supplements are not needed for physically active older individuals.[239]

C. Other Nutritional Needs

Water is an essential nutrient for people of all ages.[240,241] Thirst diminishes with aging,[242-246] possibly leading to dehydration.[240–242,247] Adequate water intake is important for temperature regulation, especially during exercise.[241] Reduced renal responsiveness, heat tolerance, skin blood flow, and possibly sweating capabilities among the elderly increase the likelihood for dehydration.[244,248–250] Malabsorption, diuretic use, liver disease, and alcohol use may also contribute to dehydration.[94,172,240,241]

Dietary fiber is important in diets for the elderly,[172] many of whom suffer constipation and other intestinal disorders.[17,172,251] Increasing the amount of fiber in the diet may alleviate these problems. Recommendations for dietary fiber intake for adults are within the range of 20–35 g/d,[252] but most older (age 70 years and over) adults consume only 14–16 g/d.[172] Other benefits to be enjoyed from increasing dietary fiber include lower blood cholesterol levels and lower incidences of cancers and cardiovascular diseases.[172,253,254]

IV. NUTRITIONAL RECOMMENDATIONS FOR THE ELDERLY

There are significant differences in nutrient intakes between active older persons and their sedentary peers. For example, active women have higher intakes of iodine and calcium than inactive women, and active men have higher intakes of energy, carbohydrate, carotene, vitamin E, vitamin C, and calcium,[255] but whether these differences affect overall nutritional status of either group is unknown. Other researchers report that elderly sportsmen have nutrient intakes more compatible with RDAs than do non-exercising elderly men, yet some were deficient in certain vitamins and minerals.[256] Clearly, nutrition and exercise recommendations should be made on an individual basis, considering individual lifestyles and preferences. Both aerobic and strength training exercises are beneficial for elderly athletes.[31] Endurance exercise benefits include improvements in VO_{2max} and cardiovascular capacity, and metabolic changes that slow glucose clearance.[30] Strength (resistance) training increases both muscle strength and mass, in even the frail elderly.[24]

The elderly population is heterogeneous, including individuals with varying functional capacities, fitness levels, and health status, and spanning a large range of age. A physician should complete the initial assessment of an extremely sedentary elderly person about to begin an exercise program. There are at least two caveats to consider when assessing the elderly for an exercise program: 1) older adults have a reduced maximum exercise capacity, and 2) older adults have an increased prevalence of diseases that may alter exercise tolerance.[257] A health history and a survey of risk factors relating to disease must be taken, and usual exercise habits noted. Blood pressure, pulse rate, body weight, and blood lipids should be assessed before prescribing an exercise regimen.[257]

Nutritional recommendations for the elderly athlete should follow current dietary recommendations for relatively healthy, active, older adults. A modification of the recommendations within the Food Guide Pyramid,[187] proposed for people aged 70 years and over, should optimize nutrient intakes consistent with the changing nutrient and energy needs of aging people.[172] This Modified Food Pyramid for 70+ Adults (Figure 5.2) reflects the needs for fewer servings of more nutrient-dense foods, for more high-fiber foods, for supplements of calcium and vitamins B_{12} and D, and for water.[172]

A. Fluids

Older athletes should drink at least eight glasses of water every day to meet resting metabolic needs. The RDA for water for adults at rest under average conditions of environmental exposure is currently 1 ml/kcal of energy expenditure,[258] about 2.2 l/d for women and 2.9 l/d for men.[259] Individual differences in physical activity, medication use, renal function, and ambient temperature will affect the total amount of fluid needed,[172] and the RDA can be increased to 1.5 ml/kcal without risking water intoxication.[258] A variety of fluid sources, except alcohol, coffee, and tea (because of their diuretic effects), can be used in calculating fluid intake.[172,241] For most older recreational athletes, water is sufficient as a rehydration beverage, and if exercise lasts for up to an hour, then 100 to 150 ml every 10 to 15 min of cool (15–22°C) water is enough.[260] For exercise sessions lasting more than an hour, an effort should be made to hyperhydrate up to 2 hours before beginning exercise by drinking 100 to 200 ml of fluid every 10 to 15 min, increasing to 400 to 500 ml 10 to 15 min before commencing exercise.[261] To facilitate hyperhydrating, a fluid containing 50 to 100 g/l carbohydrate and 10 to 30 m*M*/l NaCl can be substituted for plain water.[241,261]

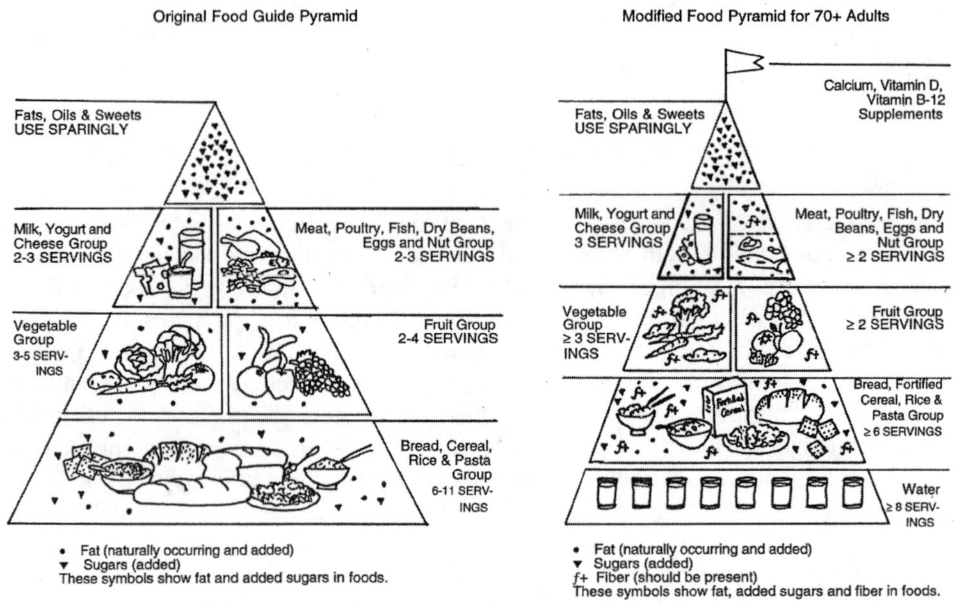

Figure 5.2 The modified food guide pyramid for people over seventy years of age. (Adapted from Russell, R. M., et al., *J. Nutr.* 129:751-753, 1999. With permission.)

B. Foods

The older athlete should consume a varied diet that includes six or more servings of bread, fortified cereals, rice, and pastas, focusing on whole-grain and enriched foods. These food choices make important contributions of dietary fiber and folic acid. Foods fortified with folate may help the elderly to lower blood homocysteine levels, possibly reducing the risk of cardiovascular disease.[172]

Three or more servings of deeply colored (green, orange, yellow) vegetables should be eaten daily to provide vitamin C, folic acid, vitamin A, and fiber. Cruciferous vegetables (beets, broccoli, cabbage, kale), which contain antioxidant phytochemicals, are recommended for their potential to prevent cancer.[172]

Two or more servings of fruit are recommended every day. To contribute dietary fiber, eating whole fruit rather than fruit juice is recommended.[172]

Three servings of dairy products (milk, yogurt, cheese) should be eaten daily, making an effort to choose low-fat products. These foods are important sources of protein, calcium, riboflavin, and vitamin D (fortified milk and yogurt).[172]

Meats, poultry, fish, dry beans, eggs, and nuts should provide two or more servings per day, with food choices made based on variety, preference, availability, cost, ease of preparation, and tenderness.[172] Lean cuts of red meats should be chosen no more than twice per week, with portion sizes limited to about 3 oz. (~85 g). Fish, a good source of omega-3 fatty acids, may lower the risk of cardiovascular disease if consumed at least once every week. Dry-bean dishes provide dietary fiber and protein. Eggs are an excellent source of reference protein,[190] and nuts may be cardioprotective if eaten weekly in modest amounts of about 5 oz. (~142 g), by virtue of their omega-3 fatty acids and mostly unsaturated fats.[262]

Fats, oils, and sweets should be used sparingly, especially in the older adult, whose energy needs have declined. The general guidelines for the U.S. population, that total fat intake should be ≤ 30% of energy, with saturated fat limited to 8–10% of energy, and cholesterol ≤ 300 mg/d,[186] should be applicable to the older adult populations.[172,263] Most would agree that trans fatty acids, found mostly in products containing hydrogenated fats, should be limited because of adverse effects similar to, or greater than, those of saturated fats,[172,263-267] while others believe that more convincing evidence is needed.[268-270]

Many older adults may not be receiving maximum nutritional benefits from calcium and vitamins B_{12} and D, for reasons mentioned above, and may therefore need to take dietary supplements of one or more of these nutrients.[172] Several research reports[99,271,272] and reviews[273-276] contain recommendations regarding indications, contraindications, and doses.

V. SUMMARY

In the next 30 years, the proportion of the U.S. population aged 65 years and over is expected to increase to 20%. The process of aging is characterized by tendencies toward involution and functional impairment, and most people can expect an increased proportion of abdominal fat, reduced lean body mass, and reduced bone mineral density to accompany aging.

Regular physical exercise, consisting of a balanced aerobic and resistance-training exercise regimen, can modify many of the aging-related physiological and metabolic changes and improve quality-of-life factors for the older adult. Even the frail elderly and the very-old elderly groups can participate in well-planned, low-risk, life-improving exercise programs.

Group heterogeneity, lower energy requirements, greater likelihood of morbidity and use of pharmaceuticals will dictate individual exercise and nutrition prescriptions. Choices of foods with greater nutrient density, dietary fiber, and disease-preventing nutrients should be emphasized. Adequate hydration and the need for a deliberate rehydration plan are especially important for physically active elders.[241] Supplements of calcium, vitamin D and vitamin B_{12}, nutrients that for many of the elderly may be inadequately ingested, absorbed or metabolized, should be considered. Finally, we cannot overemphasize the importance of seeking qualified, continuing medical and dietary advice to individualize the exercise and nutrition program for optimum health and longevity.

REFERENCES

1. Rock, C. L., Nutrition and the older athlete, in *Nutrition in Exercise and Sport*, 3rd ed., Driskell, J. and Wolinsky, I., Eds., CRC Press, Boca Raton, FL, 1998, pp. 481-494.
2. Crespo, C. J., Keteyian, S. J., Heath, G. W., and Sempos, G. T., Leisure-time physical activity among U.S. adults. Results from the third national health and nutrition examination survey, *Arch. Intern. Med.*, 156, 93, 1996.
3. Yusuf, H. R., Croft, J. B., Giles, W. H., Anda, R. F., Casper, M. L., Caspersen, C. J., and Jones, D.A., Leisure-time physical activity among older adults. 1990, *Arch. Intern. Med.*, 156, 1321, 1996.
4. Wilcox, S. and Storandt, M., Relations among age, exercise, and psychological variables in a community sample of women, *Health Psychol.*, 15, 110, 1996.
5. Lee, C., Factors related to the adoption of exercise among older women, *J. Behav. Med.*, 16, 323, 1993.
6. O'Brien, S. J. and Vertinsky, P. A., Unfit survivors: exercise as a resource for aging women, *Gerontologist*, 31, 347, 1991.
7. Wilcox, S., Age and gender in relation to body attitudes. Is there a double standard of aging?, *Psychol. Women Quart.*, 21, 549, 1997.
8. Hobbs, F. B. and Damon, B. L., U.S. Bureau of the Census, Current Population Reports, Special Studies, P23-190, *65+ in the United States*, U.S. Government Printing Office, Washington, D.C., 1996, p. 8-3.
9. Day, J. C., U.S. Bureau of the Census, Current Population Reports, P25-1130, *Population Projections of the United States by Age, Sex, Race, and Hispanic Origin: 1995 to 2050*, U.S. Government Printing Office, Washington, D.C., 1996, p. 9.

11. Hobbs, F. B. and Damon, B. L., U.S. Bureau of the Census, Current Population Reports, Special Studies, P23-190, *65+ in the United States*, U.S. Government Printing Office, Washington, D.C., 1996, p. 1-1.
10. Chernoff, R., Baby boomers come of age: nutrition in the 21st century, *J. Am. Diet. Assoc.*, 95, 650, 1995.
12. U.S. Bureau of the Census, Current Population Reports, Special Studies, P23-193, *How We're Changing. Demographic State of the Nation: 1997*, U.S. Government Printing Office, Washington, D.C., 1997, p. 1.
13. Ventura, S. J., Anderson, R. N., Martin, J. A., and Smith, B. L., Births and deaths: preliminary data for 1997, *Nat. Vital Stat. Rep.*, 47, 5, 1998.
14. Pamuk, E., Makuc, D., Heck, K., Reuben, C., and Lochner, K., Socioeconomic status and health chartbook. Health, United States, 1998, National Center for Health Statistics, Hyattsville, MD, 1998, 88.
15. Peters, K. D., Kochanek, K. D., and Murphy, S. L., Deaths: final data for 1996, *Nat. Vital Stat. Rep.*, 47, 21, 1996.
16. McNeil, J. M., Americans With Disabilities: 1994-95, U.S. Bureau of the Census, Current Population Reports, Household Economic Studies No. P70-61, U.S. Government Printing Office, Washington, D.C., 1997, p. 2.
17. Nieman, D. C., Physical activity and aging, in *Fitness and Sports Medicine, an Introduction*, Bull Publishing, Palo Alto, CA, 1990, pp. 359-385.
18. Hunter, S. C., The ageless athlete, *J. Med. Assoc. Ga.*, 81, 283, 1992.
19. Ausman, L. M. and Russell, R. M., Nutrition in the elderly, in *Modern Nutrition in Health and Disease*, 8th ed., Shils, M. E., Olson, J. A., and Shike, M., Eds., Lea and Febiger, Philadelphia, 1994, pp. 770-780.
20. Evans, W. J., Effects of aging and exercise on nutrition needs of the elderly, *Nutr. Rev.*, 54, S35, 1996.
21. Poehlman, E. T., Arciero, P. J., and Goran M. I., Endurance exercise in aging humans: effects on energy metabolism, *Exerc. Sport Sci. Rev.*, 22, 251, 1994.
22. Voorrips, L. E., van Staveren, W. A., and Hautvast, J. G., Are physically active elderly women in a better nutritional condition than their sedentary peers? *Eur. J. Clin. Nutr.*, 45, 545, 1991.
23. Visser, M., Harris, T. B., Langlois, J., Hannan, M. T., Roubenoff, R., Felson, D. T., Wilson, P. W., and Kiel, D. P., Body fat and skeletal muscle mass in relation to physical disability in very old men and women of the Framingham Heart Study, *J. Gerontol. A. Biol. Sci. Med. Sci.*, 53, M214, 1998.
24. Fielding, R. A., The role of progressive resistance training and nutrition in the preservation of lean body mass in the elderly, *J. Am. Coll. Nutr.,* 14, 587, 1995.
25. Evans, W. J. and Cyr-Campbell, D., Nutrition, exercise, and healthy aging, *J. Am. Diet. Assoc.*, 97, 632, 1997.
26. Evans, W. J. and Campbell, W. W., Sarcopenia and age-related changes in body composition and functional capacity, *J. Nutr.*, 123, 465, 1993.
27. Sial, S., Coggan, A. R., Hickner, R. C., and Klein, S., Training-induced alterations in fat and carbohydrate metabolism during exercise in elderly subjects, *Am. J. Physiol.*, 274, E785, 1998.
28. Calles-Escandon, J. and Poehlman, E. T., Aging, fat oxidation, and exercise, *Aging (Milano)*, 9, 57, 1997.
29. American College of Sports Medicine Position Stand. Exercise and physical activity for older adults, *Med. Sci. Sports Exerc.*, 30, 992, 1998.
30. Evans, W. J., Exercise, nutrition, and aging, *Clin. Geriatr. Med.*, 11, 725, 1995.
31. Chandler, J. M. and Hadley, E. C., Exercise to improve physiologic and functional performance in old age, *Clin. Geriatr. Med.*, 12, 761, 1996.
32. Whipple, R. H., Wolfson, L. I., and Amerman, P. M., The relationship of knee and ankle weakness to falls in nursing home residents, *J. Am. Geriatr. Soc.*, 35, 13, 1987.
33. Blair, S. N., Physical activity, physical fitness, and health, *Res. Q. Exerc. Sport*, 64, 365, 1993.
34. McArdle, W. D., Katch, F. I., and Katch, V. L., Physical activity, health, and aging, in *Exercise Physiology: Energy, Nutrition, and Human Performance*, 4th ed., Williams and Wilkins, Baltimore, 1996, pp. 634-668.
35. Sipila, S., Viitsalo, J., Era, P., and Suominen, H., Muscle strength in male athletes aged 70-81 years and a population sample, *Eur. J. Appl. Physiol.*, 63, 399, 1991.

36. Brooks, S. V. and Faulkner, J. A., Skeletal muscle weakness in old age: underlying mechanisms, *Med. Sci. Sports Exerc.*, 26, 432, 1994.
37. Grimby, G., Muscle performance and structure in the elderly as studied cross-sectionally and longitudinally, *J. Gerontol. A Biol. Sci. Med. Sci.*, 50, 17, 1995.
38. Monemi, M., Eriksson, P. O., Eriksson, A., and Thornell, L. E., Adverse changes in fibre-type composition of the human masseter versus biceps brachii muscle during aging, *J. Neurol. Sci.*, 154, 35, 1998.
39. Doherty, T. J., Vandervoort, A. A., Taylor, A. W., and Brown, W. F., Effects of motor unit losses on strength in older men and women, *J. Appl. Physiol.*, 74, 868, 1993.
40. Booth F. W., Weeden, S. H., and Tseng, B. S., Effect of aging on human skeletal muscle and motor function, *Med. Sci. Sports Exerc.*, 26, 556, 1994.
41. Brown, A. B., McCartney, N., and Sale, D. G., Positive adaptations to weight-lifting training in the elderly, *J. Appl. Physiol.*, 69, 1725, 1990.
42. Aniansson, A., Grimby, G., and Hedberg, M., Compensatory muscle fiber hypertrophy in elderly men, *J. Appl. Physiol.*, 73, 812, 1992.
43. Roman, W. J., Fleckenstein, J., Stray-Gundersen, J., Alway, S. E., Peshock, R., and Gonyea, W. J., Adaptations in the elbow flexors of elderly males after heavy-resistance training, *J. Appl. Physiol.,* 74, 750, 1993.
44. Treuth, M. S., Ryan, A. S., Pratley, R. E., Rubin, M. A., Miller, J. P., Nicklas, B. J., Sorkin, J., Harman, S. M., Goldberg, A. P., and Hurley, B. F., Effects of strength training on total and regional body composition in older men, *J. Appl. Physiol.*, 77, 614, 1994.
45. Meredith, C. N., Frontera, W. R., and Evans, W. J., Body composition in elderly men: effect of dietary modification during strength training, *J. Am. Geriatr. Soc.*, 40, 155, 1992.
46. Fiatarone, M. A., O'Neill, E. F., Ryan, N. D., Clements, K. M., Solares, G. R., Nelson, M. E., Roberts, S. B., Kehayias, J. J., Lipsitz, L. A., and Evans, W. J., Exercise training and nutritional supplementation for physical frailty in very elderly people, *New Engl. J. Med.*, 330, 1769, 1994.
47. Campbell, W. W., Joseph, L. J., Davey, S. L., Cyr-Campbell, D., Anderson, R. A., and Evans, W. J., Effects of resistance training and chromium picolinate on body composition and skeletal muscle in older men, *J. Appl. Physiol.*, 86, 29, 1999.
48. Bermon, S., Venembre, P., Sachet, C., Valour, S., and Dolisi, C., Effects of creatine monohydrate ingestion in sedentary and weight-trained older individuals, *Acta Physiol. Scand.*, 164, 147, 1998.
49. Brown, M., Special considerations during rehabilitation of the aged athlete, *Clin. Sports Med.*, 8, 893, 1989.
50. Seto, J. L. and Brewster, C. E., Musculoskeletal conditioning of the older athlete, *Clin. Sports Med.*, 10, 401, 1991.
51. Aniansson, A. and Gustafsson, E., Physical training in elderly men with special reference to quadriceps muscle strength and morphology, *Clin. Physiol.*, 1, 87, 1981.
52. Lowenthal, D. T., Kirschner, D. A., Scarpace, N. T., Pollock, M., and Graves, J., Effects of exercise on age and disease, *South. Med. J.*, 87, S5, 1994.
53. Frontera, W. R., Meredith, C. N., O'Reilly, K. P., Knuttgen, H. G., and Evans, W. J., Strength conditioning in older men: skeletal muscle hypertrophy and improved function, *J. Appl. Physiol.*, 64, 1038, 1988.
54. Stamford, B. A., Exercise and the elderly, *Exerc. Sport Sci. Rev.*, 16, 341, 1988.
55. Lowenthal, D. T., Kendrick, Z. V., and Powers, S., The effects of exercise training on skeletal muscle in humans and aging Fischer 344 rats, in *Musculoskeletal Soft-Tissue Aging: Impact on Mobility*, Buckwalter, J. A., Goldberg, V. M., and Woo, S. L.-Y., Eds., American Academy of Orthopaedic Surgeons, Rosemont, IL, 1993, 201.
56. Durnin, J. V. and Wormersley, J., Body fat assessed from total body density and its estimation from skinfold thickness: measurements of 481 men and women aged from 16 to 72 years, *Br. J. Nutr.*, 32, 77, 1974.
57. Voorrips, L. E., Lemmink, K. A., van Heuvelen, M. J., Bult, P., and van Staveren, W. A., The physical condition of elderly women differing in habitual physical activity, *Med. Sci. Sports Exerc.*, 25, 1152, 1993.
58. Schlienger, J. L., Pradignac, A., and Grunenberger, F., Nutrition of the elderly: a challenge between facts and needs, *Horm. Res.*, 43, 46, 1995.

59. Seim, H. C. and Holtmeier, K. B., Treatment of obesity in the elderly, *Am. Fam. Physician*, 47, 1183, 1993.
60. Ortega, R. M. and Andres, P., Is obesity worth treating in the elderly? *Drugs and Aging*, 12, 97, 1998.
61. Bidlack, W. R., Interrelationships of food, nutrition, diet and health: the National Association of State Universities and Land Grant Colleges White Paper, *J. Am. Coll. Nutr.*, 15, 422, 1996.
62. Carek, P. J., Sherer, J. T., and Carson, D. S., Management of obesity: medical treatment options, *Am. Fam. Physician*, 55, 551, 1997.
63. Ortega, R. M., Fernandez-Azuela, M., Encinas-Sotillos, A., Andres, P., and Lopez-Sobaler, A. M., Differences in diet and food habits between patients with gallstones and controls, *J. Am. Coll. Nutr.*, 16, 88, 1997.
64. Westerterp, K. R., Alterations in energy balance with exercise, *Am. J. Clin. Nutr.*, 68, 970S, 1998.
65. Hoyert, D. L., Kochanek, K. D., and Murphy, S. L., Deaths: final data for 1997, *Nat. Vital Stats. Rep.*, 47, 8, 1999.
66. Weisfeldt, M., Aging, changes in the cardiovascular system, and responses to stress, *Am. J. Hypertens.*, 11, 41S, 1998.
67. Salmasi, A. M. and Dore, C., Variation of aortic blood velocity with age at rest and during exercise in normal subjects, *Clin. Auton. Res.*, 5, 19, 1995.
68. Lindeman, R. D., Tobin, J., and Shock, N. W., Longitudinal studies on the rate of decline in renal function with age, *J. Am. Geriatr. Soc.*, 33, 278, 1985.
69. Marin, J., Age-related changes in vascular responses: a review, *Mech. Aging Dev.*, 79, 71, 1995.
70. Pickering, G. P., Fellmann, N., Morio, B., Ritz, P., Amonchot, A., Vermorel, M., and Coudert, J., Effects of endurance training on the cardiovascular system and water compartments in elderly subjects, *J. Appl. Physiol.*, 83, 1300, 1997.
71. Siscovick, D. S., Fried, L., Mittelmark, M., Rutan, G., Bild, D., and O'Leary, D. H., Exercise intensity and subclinical cardiovascular disease in the elderly. The Cardiovascular Health Study, *Am. J. Epidemiol.*, 145, 977, 1997.
72. Yataco, A. R., Fleisher, L. A., and Katzel, L. I., Heart rate variability and cardiovascular fitness in senior athletes, *Am. J. Cardiol.*, 80, 1389, 1997.
73. Public health focus: physical activity and the prevention of coronary heart disease, *Morb. Mortal. Wkly. Rep.*, 42, 669, 1993.
74. Blair, S. N., Physical activity, fitness, and coronary heart disease, in *Physical Activity, Fitness, and Health. International Proceedings and Consensus Statement*, Bouchard, C., Shephard, R. J., and Stephens, T., Eds., Human Kinetics Publishers, Champaign, IL, 1994, pp. 579-590.
75. Whaley, M. H. and Blair, S. N., Epidemiology of physical activity, physical fitness and coronary heart disease, *J. Cardiovasc. Risk*, 2, 289, 1995.
76. Leon, A. S., Myers, M. J., and Connett, J., Leisure time physical activity and the 16-year risks of mortality from coronary heart disease and all causes in the Multiple Risk Factor Intervention Trial (MRFIT), *Int. J. Sports Med.*, 18, S208, 1997.
77. De Backer, G., Physical activity and psychosocial variables in atherosclerosis, *Acta Cardiol. Suppl.*, 29, 107, 1988.
78. Moore, S., Physical activity, fitness, and atherosclerosis, in *Physical Activity, Fitness, and Health. International Proceedings and Consensus Statement*, Bouchard, C., Shephard, R. J., and Stephens, T., Eds., Human Kinetics Publishers, Champaign, IL, 1994, pp. 570-578.
79. Bernadet, P., Benefits of physical activity in the prevention of cardiovascular diseases, *J. Cardiovasc. Pharmacol.*, 25, S3, 1995.
80. Fletcher, G. F., The antiatherosclerotic effect of exercise and development of an exercise prescription, *Cardiol. Clin.*, 14, 85, 1996.
81. Niebauer, J. and Cooke, J. P., Cardiovascular effects of exercise: role of endothelial shear stress, *J. Am. Coll. Cardiol.*, 28, 1652, 1996.
82. American College of Sports Medicine. Position Stand. Physical activity, physical fitness, and hypertension, *Med. Sci. Sports Exerc.*, 25, i, 1993.
83. Fagard, R. H. and Tipton, C. M., Physical activity, fitness, and hypertension, in *Physical Activity, Fitness, and Health. International Proceedings and Consensus Statement*, Bouchard, C., Shephard, R. J., and Stephens, T., Eds., Human Kinetics Publishers, Champaign, IL, 1994, pp. 633-655.

84. Miller, N. H., Physical activity: one approach to the primary prevention of hypertension, *Am. Assoc. Occupat. Health Nurs. J.,* 43, 319, 1995.
85. Borhani, N. O., Significance of physical activity for prevention and control of hypertension, *J. Hum. Hypertens.,* 10, S7, 1996.
86. Yang, Y. C., Huang, S. C., Wu, J. S., and Chang, C. J., Community-based study on the relationship between physical activity and hypertension, *J. Formos. Med. Assoc.*, 95, 110, 1996.
87. Folsom, A. R., Arnett, D. K., Hutchinson, R. G., Liao, F., Clegg, L. X., and Cooper, L. S., Physical activity and incidence of coronary heart disease in middle-aged women and men, *Med. Sci. Sports Exerc.*, 29, 901, 1997.
88. Garber, C. E., The benefits of physical activity on coronary heart disease and coronary heart disease risk factors in women, *Women's Health Issues*, 7, 17, 1997.
89. Haapanen, N., Miilunpalo, S., Vuori, I., Oja, P., and Pasanen, M., Association of leisure time physical activity with the risk of coronary heart disease, hypertension and diabetes in middle-aged men and women, *Int. J. Epidemiol.*, 26, 739, 1997.
90. Lip, G. Y., Luscombe, C., McCarry, M., Malik, I., and Beevers, G., Ethnic differences in public health awareness, health perceptions and physical exercise: implications for heart disease prevention, *Ethn. Health.*, 1, 47, 1996.
91. Pereira, M. A., Folsom, A. R., McGovern, P. G., Carpenter, M., Arnett, D. K., Liao, D., Szklo, M., and Hutchinson, R. G., Physical activity and incident hypertension in black and white adults: the Atherosclerosis Risk in Communities Study, *Prev. Med.*, 28, 304, 1999.
92. Lewis, R. D. and Modlesky, C. M., Nutrition, physical activity, and bone health in women, *Int. J. Sports Nutr.*, 8, 250, 1998.
93. Wolinsky, I., Taylor, P. N., Klimis-Tavantzis, D. J., and Arnaud, S. B., Calcium nutrition in the elderly, in *Handbook of Nutrition in the Aged*, 2nd ed., Watson, R. R., Ed., CRC Press, Boca Raton, FL, 1994, pp. 355-362.
94. Fahey, P. J., Boltri, J. M., and Monk, J. S., Key issues in nutrition. Supplementation through adulthood and old age, *Postgrad. Med.*, 81, 123, 1987.
95. Rosen, C. J., Morrison, A., Zhou, H., Storm, D., Hunter, S. J., Musgrave, K., Chen, T., Wei, W., and Holick, M. F., Elderly women in northern New England exhibit seasonal changes in bone mineral density and calciotropic hormones, *Bone Miner.*, 25, 83, 1994.
96. Boucher, B. J., Inadequate vitamin D status: does it contribute to the disorders composing syndrome 'X'?, *Br. J. Nutr.*, 79, 315, 1998.
97. Mosekilde, L., Minisymposium, osteoporosis, and calcium, *J. Intern. Med.*, 231, 145, 1992.
98. Singh, M. A., Combined exercise and dietary intervention to optimize body composition in aging, *Ann. N. Y. Acad. Sci.*, 854, 378, 1998.
99. Storm, D., Eslin, R., Porter, E. S., Musgrave, K., Vereault, D., Patton, C., Kessenich, C., Mohan, S., Chen, T., Holick, M. F., and Rosen, C. J., Calcium supplementation prevents seasonal bone loss and changes in biochemical markers of bone turnover in elderly New England women: a randomized placebo-controlled trial, *J. Clin. Endocrinol. Metab.*, 83, 3817, 1998.
100. Lane, J. M. and Nydick, M., Osteoporosis: current modes of prevention and treatment, *J. Am. Acad. Orthop. Surg.*, 7, 19, 1999.
101. O'Connell, M. B., Prevention and treatment of osteoporosis in the elderly, *Pharmacotherapy*, 19, 7S, 1999.
102. Butler, R. N., Davis, R., Lewis, C. B., Nelson, M. E., and Strauss, E., Physical fitness: benefits of exercise for the older patient. 2, *Geriatrics*, 53, 46, 1998.
103. Burckhardt, P., Are hip fractures preventable with nutrition measures and exercise in the elderly?, *Osteoporosis Int.*, 3, S56, 1996.
104. Nelson, M. E., Fiatarone, M. A., Morganti, C. M., Trice, I., Greenberg, R. A., and Evans, W. J., Effects of high-intensity strength training on multiple risk factors for osteoporotic fractures, *J. Am. Med. Assoc.*, 272, 1909, 1994.
105. Iwamoto, J., Takeda, T., Otani, T., and Yabe, Y., Effect of increased physical activity on bone mineral density in postmenopausal osteoporotic women, *Keio J. Med.*, 47, 157, 1998.
106. Layne, J. E. and Nelson, M. E., The effects of progressive resistance training on bone density: a review, *Med. Sci. Sports Exerc.*, 31, 25, 1999.

107. Bassey, E. J., Rothwell, M. C., Littlewood, J. J., and Pye, D. W., Pre- and postmenopausal women have different bone mineral density responses to the same high-impact exercise, *J. Bone Miner. Res.*, 13, 1805, 1998.
108. Bemben, D. A., Exercise interventions for osteoporosis prevention in postmenopausal women, *J. Okla. State Med. Assoc.*, 92, 66, 1999.
109. Kelley, G. A., Aerobic exercise and bone density at the hip in postmenopausal women: a meta-analysis, *Prev. Med.*, 27, 798, 1998.
110. Voss, L. A., Fadale, P. D., and Hulstyn, M. J., Exercise-induced loss of bone density in athletes, *J. Am. Acad. Orthop. Surg.*, 6, 349, 1998.
111. Crespo, R., Revilla, M., Villa, L. F., Usabiaga, J., Leibar, X., and Rico, H., Transient dissociation of bone metabolism induced by high performance exercise: a study in elite marathon runners, *Calcif. Tissue Int.*, 64, 287, 1999.
112. Grisso, J. A., Kelsey, J. L., O'Brien, L. A., Miles, C. G., Sidney, S., Maislin, G., LaPann, K., Moritz, D., and Peters, B., Risk factors for hip fracture in men. Hip Fracture Study Group, *Am. J. Epidemiol.*, 145, 786, 1997.
113. Schwartz, A. V., Kelsey, J. L., Sidney, S., and Grisso, J. A., Characteristics of falls and risk of hip fracture in elderly men, *Osteoporos. Int.*, 8, 240, 1998.
114. Slemenda, C., Prevention of hip fractures: risk factor modification, *Am. J. Med.*, 103, 65S, 1997.
115. Dargent-Molina, P., Risk factors and prevention of fractures in the elderly, *Curr. Opin. Rheumatol.*, 10, 357, 1998.
116. Hill, K., Schwarz, J., Flicker, L., and Carroll, S., Falls among healthy, community-dwelling, older women: a prospective study of frequency, circumstances, consequences and prediction accuracy, *Aust. N. Z. J. Pub. Hlth.*, 23, 41, 1999.
117. Joakimsen, R. M., Magnus, J. H., and Fnneb, V., Physical activity and predisposition for hip fractures: a review, *Osteoporos. Int.*, 7, 503, 1997.
118. Henderson, N. K., White, C. P., and Eisman, J. A., The roles of exercise and fall risk reduction in the prevention of osteoporosis, *Endocrinol. Metab. Clin. North Am.*, 27, 369, 1998.
119. Kovar, P. A., Allegrante, J. P., MacKenzie, C. R., Peterson, M. G., Gutin, B., and Charlson, M. E., Supervised fitness walking in patients with osteoarthritis of the knee: a randomized controlled trial, *Ann. Intern. Med.*, 116, 529, 1992.
120. Sinaki, M., Fitzpatrick, L. A., Ritchie, C. K., Montesano, A., and Wahner, H. W., Site-specificity of bone mineral density and muscle strength in women: job-related physical activity, *Am. J. Phys. Med. Rehabil.*, 77, 470, 1998.
121. Casper, R. C., Nutrition and its relationship to aging, *Exp. Gerontol.*, 30, 299, 1995.
122. Saltzman, J. R. and Russell, R. M., The aging gut. Nutritional issues, *Gastroenterol. Clin. North Am.*, 27, 309, 1998.
123. Clarkston, W. K., Pantano, M. M., Morley, J. E., Horowitz, M., Littlefield, J. M., and Burton, F. R., Evidence for the anorexia of aging: gastrointestinal transit and hunger in healthy elderly vs. young adults, *Am. J. Physiol.*, 272, R243, 1997.
124. Kay, L. and Avlund, K., Abdominal syndromes and functional ability in the elderly, *Aging (Milano)*, 6, 420, 1994.
125. O'Keefe, E. A., Talley, N. J., Zinsmeister, A. R., and Jacobsen, S. J., Bowel disorders impair functional status and quality of life in the elderly: a population-based study, *J. Gerontol. A Biol. Sci. Med. Sci.*, 50, M184, 1995.
126. Webster, S. G. P. and Leeming, J. T., Assessment of small-bowel function in the elderly using a modified xylose tolerance test, *Gut*, 16, 109, 1975.
127. Castleden, C. M., Volans, C. N., and Raymond, K., The effect of aging on drug absorption from the gut, *Age Aging*, 6, 138, 1977.
128. Webster, S. G., Wilkinson, E. M., and Gowland, E., A comparison of fat absorption in young and old subjects, *Age Aging*, 6, 113, 1977.
129. Montgomery, R. D., Heaney, M. R., Ross, I. N., Sammons, H. G., Barford, A. V., Balakrishnan, S., Mayer, P. P., Culank, L. S., Field, J., and Gosling, P., The aging gut: a study of intestinal absorption in relation to nutrition in the elderly, *Q. J. Med.*, 47, 197, 1978.

130. Wallis, J. L., Lipski, P. S., Mathers, J. C., James, O. F., and Hirst, B. H., Duodenal brush-border mucosal glucose transport and enzyme activities in aging man and effect of bacterial contamination of the small intestine, *Dig. Dis. Sci.*, 38, 403, 1993.
131. Davidson, M. B., The effect of aging on carbohydrate metabolism: a review of the English literature and a practical approach to the diagnosis of diabetes mellitus in the elderly, *Metab. Clin. Exp.*, 28, 687, 1979.
132. Gudat, U., Berger, M. and Lefèbvre, Physical activity, fitness, and non-insulin-dependent (Type II) diabetes mellitus, in *Physical Activity, Fitness, and Health. International Proceedings and Consensus Statement*, Bouchard, C., Shephard, R. J., and Stephens, T., Eds., Human Kinetics Publishers, Champaign, IL, 1994, pp. 669-683.
133. Ahren, B. and Pacini, G., Age-related reduction in glucose elimination is accompanied by reduced glucose effectiveness and increased hepatic insulin extraction in man, *J. Clin. Endocrinol. Metab.*, 83, 3350, 1998.
134. Evers, B. M., Townsend, C. M., Jr., and Thompson, J. C., Organ physiology of aging, *Surg. Clin. North Am.*, 74, 23, 1994.
135. Appollonio, I., Carabellese, C., Frattola, A., and Trabucchi, M., Influence of dental status on dietary intake and survival in community-dwelling elderly subjects, *Age Aging*, 26, 445, 1997.
136. Papas, A. S., Palmer, C. A., Rounds, M. C., and Russell, R. M., The effects of denture status on nutrition, *Spec. Care Dentist*, 18, 17, 1998.
137. Hildebrandt, G. H., Dominguez, B. L., Schork, M. A., and Loesche, W. J., Functional units, chewing, swallowing, and food avoidance among the elderly, *J. Prosthet. Dent.*, 77, 588, 1997.
138. Cain, W. S., Reid, F., and Stevens, J. C., Missing ingredients: aging and the discrimination of flavor, *J. Nutr. Elder.*, 9, 3, 1990.
139. Weiffenbach, J. M. and Bartoshuk, L. M., Taste and smell, *Clin. Geriatr. Med.*, 8, 543, 1992.
140. Murphy, C., Nutrition and chemosensory perception in the elderly, *Crit. Rev. Food Sci. Nutr.*, 33, 3, 1993.
141. Kaye, J. A., Oken, B. S., Howieson, D. B., Howieson, J., Holm, L. A., and Dennison, K., Neurologic evaluation of the optimally healthy oldest old, *Arch. Neurol.*, 51, 1205, 1994.
142. Nordin, S. and Murphy, C., Odor memory in normal aging and Alzheimer's disease, *Ann. N. Y. Acad. Sci.*, 855, 686, 1998.
143. Rolls, B. J. and McDermott, T. M., Effects of age on sensory-specific satiety, *Am. J. Clin. Nutr.*, 54, 988, 1991.
144. Rolls, B. J., Appetite, hunger, and satiety in the elderly, *Crit. Rev. Food Sci. Nutr.*, 33, 39, 1993.
145. Moses, F. M., Physical activity and digestive processes, in *Physical Activity, Fitness, and Health. International Proceedings and Consensus Statement*, Bouchard, C., Shephard, R. J., and Stephens, T., Eds., Human Kinetics Publishers, Champaign, IL, 1994, pp. 383-400.
146. Moses, F. M., The effect of exercise on the gastrointestinal tract, *Sports Med.*, 9, 159, 1990.
147. Green, G. A., Gastrointestinal disorders in the athlete, *Clin. Sports Med.*, 11, 453, 1992.
148. Brouns, F. and Beckers, E., Is the gut an athletic organ? Digestion, absorption and exercise, *Sports Med.*, 15, 242, 1993.
149. Wright, J. P., Exercise and the gastro-intestinal tract, *S. Afr. Med. J.*, 83, 50, 1993.
150. Soffer, E. E., Wilson, J., Duethman, G., Launspach, J., and Adrian, T. E., Effect of graded exercise on esophageal motility and gastroesophageal reflux in nontrained subjects, *Dig. Dis. Sci.*, 39, 193, 1994.
151. Gil, S. M., Yazaki, E., and Evans, D. F., Aetiology of running-related gastrointestinal dysfunction. How far is the finishing line?, *Sports Med.*, 26, 365, 1998.
152. Kaplan, J. P., Powell, K. E., Sikes, R. K., Shirley, R. W., and Campbell, C. C., Epidemiologic study of the benefits and risks of running, *J. Am. Med. Assoc.*, 248, 3118, 1982.
153. Hogan, D. B. and Cape, R. D., Marathoners over sixty years of age: results of a survey, *J. Am. Geriatr. Soc.*, 34, 121, 1984.
154. Kannus, P., Niittymaki, S., Jarvinen, M., and Lehto, M., Sports injuries in elderly athletes: a three-year prospective, controlled study, *Age Ageing*, 18, 263, 1989.
155. Kallinen, M. and Markku, A., Aging, physical activity and sports injuries. An overview of common sports injuries in the elderly, *Sports Med.*, 20, 41, 1995.
156. Rosenberg, I. H. and Miller, J. W., Nutritional factors in physical and cognitive functions of elderly people, *Am. J. Clin. Nutr.*, 55, 1237S, 1992.

157. Young, R. J., The effect of regular exercise on cognitive functioning and personality, *Br. J. Sports Med.*, 13, 110, 1979.
158. Molloy, D. W., Beerschoten, D. A., Borrie, M. J., Crilly, R. G., and Cape, R. D., Acute effects of exercise on neuropsychological function in elderly subjects, *J. Am. Geriatr. Soc.*, 36, 29, 1988.
159. Madden, D. J., Blumenthal, J. A., Allen, P. A., and Emery, C. F., Improving aerobic capacity in healthy older adults does not necessarily lead to improved cognitive performance, *Psychol. Aging*, 4, 307, 1989.
160. Rikli, R. E. and Edwards, D. J., Effects of a three-year exercise program on motor function and cognitive processing speed in older women, *Res. Q. Exerc. Sport*, 62, 61, 1991.
161. Hill, R. D., Storandt, M., and Malley, M., The impact of long-term exercise training on psychological function in older adults, *J. Gerontol.,* 48, P12, 1993.
162. Netz, Y. and Jacob, T., Exercise and the psychological state of institutionalized elderly: a review, *Percept. Mot. Skills*, 79, 1107, 1994.
163. Emery, C. F., Huppert, F. A., and Schein, R. L., Relationships among age, exercise, health, and cognitive function in a British sample, *Gerontologist*, 35, 378, 1995.
164. Okumiya, K., Matsubayashi, K., Wada, T., Kimura, S., Doi, Y., and Ozawa, T., Effects of exercise on neurobehavioral function in community-dwelling older people more than 75 years of age, *J. Am. Geriatr. Soc.*, 44, 569, 1996.
165. Blackwood, S. K., MacHale, S. M., Power, M. J., Goodwin, G. M., and Lawrie, S. M., Effects of exercise on cognitive and motor function in chronic fatigue syndrome and depression, *J. Neurol. Neurosurg. Psychiatry*, 65, 541, 1998.
166. Gomez-Pinilla, F., So, V., and Kesslak, J. P., Spatial learning and physical activity contribute to the induction of fibroblast growth factor: neural substrates for increased cognition associated with exercise, *Neuroscience*, 85, 53, 1998.
167. Ruuskanen, J. M. and Ruoppila, I., Physical activity and psychological well-being among people aged 65 to 84 years, *Age Aging*, 24, 292, 1995.
168. Berkman, L. F., Seeman, T. E., Albert, M., Blazer, D., Kahn, R., Mohs, R., Finch, C., Schneider, E., Cotman, C., McClearn, G., Nesselroade, J., Featherman, D., Garmezy, N., McKhann, G., Brim, G., Prager, D., and Rowe, J., High, usual and impaired functioning in community-dwelling older men and women: findings from the MacArthur Foundation Research Network on Successful Aging, *J. Clin. Epidemiol.*, 46, 1129, 1993.
169. Seeman, T. E., Berkman, L. F., Charpentier, P. A., Blazer, D. G., Albert, M. S., and Tinetti, M. E., Behavioral and psychosocial predictors of physical performance: MacArthur studies of successful aging, *J. Gerontol. A Biol. Sci. Med. Sci.,* 50, M177, 1995.
170. Kendrick, Z. V., Nelson-Steen, S., and Scafidi, K., Exercise, aging, and nutrition, *Southern Med. J.*, 87, S50, 1994.
171. Chernoff, R., Effects of age on nutrient requirements, *Clin. Geriatr. Med.*, 11, 641, 1995.
172. Russell, R. M., Rasmussen, H., and Lichtenstein, A. H., Modified food guide pyramid for people over seventy years of age, *J. Nutr.*, 129, 751, 1999.
173. Anderson, G. H., Regulation of food intake, in *Modern Nutrition in Health and Disease*, 8th ed., Shils, M. E., Olson, J. A., and Shike, M., Eds., Lea and Febiger, Philadelphia, 1994, pp. 524-536.
174. Groff, J. L., Gropper, S. S., and Hunt, S. M., Energy balance and weight control, in *Advanced Nutrition and Human Metabolism*, 2nd Ed., West Publishing, Minneapolis, 1995, pp. 466-487.
175. Coulston, A. M. and Rock, C. L., Popular diets and use of moderate calorie restriction for the treatment of obesity, in *Obesity: Pathophysiology, Psychology and Treatment*, Blackburn, G. L. and Kanders, B. S., Eds., Chapman and Hall, North Potomac, MD, 1994, 185.
176. Harris, J. and Benedict, F., A biometric study of basal metabolism in man, Publication #279, Carnegie Institution, Washington, D. C., 1919.
177. Campbell, W. M., Crim, M. C., Young, V. R., and Evans, W. J., Increased energy requirement and changes in body composition with resistance training in older adults, *Am. J. Clin. Nutr.*, 60, 167, 1994.
178. Roberts, S. B., Young, V. R., Fuss, P., Heyman, M. B., Fiatarone, M., Dallal, G. E., Cortiella, J., and Evans, W. J., What are the dietary energy needs of elderly adults?, *Int. J. Obesity*, 16, 969, 1992.
179. National Research Council, Energy, in *Recommended Dietary Allowances*, 10th ed., National Academy of Sciences, Washington, D. C., 1989, pp. 24-38.
180. Goran, M. I. and Poehlman, E. T., Endurance training does not enhance total energy expenditure in healthy elderly persons, *Am. J. Physiol.*, 263, E950, 1992.

181. Arciero, P. J., Goran, M. I., Gardner, A. M., Ades, P. A., Tyzbir, R. S., and Poehlman, E. T., A practical equation to predict resting metabolic rate in older females, *J. Am. Geriatr. Soc.*, 41, 389, 1993.
182. Arciero, P. J., Goran, M. I., Gardner, A. M., Ades, P. A., Tyzbir, R. S., and Poehlman, E. T., A practical equation to predict resting metabolic rate in older men, *Metabolism*, 42, 950, 1993.
183. Arciero, P. J., Goran, M. I., and Poehlman, E. T., Resting metabolic rate is lower in women than in men, *J. Appl. Physiol.*, 75, 2514, 1993.
184. Starling, R. D., Toth, M. J., Carpenter, W. H., Matthews, D. E., and Poehlman, E. T., Energy requirements and physical activity in free-living older women and men: a doubly labeled water study, *J. Appl. Physiol.,* 85, 1063, 1998.
185. U.S. Department of Agriculture and Department of Health and Human Services, *Dietary Guidelines for Americans*, 3rd ed., Home and Garden Bulletin No. 232, U.S. Government Printing Office, Washington, D. C., 2000.
186. Expert Panel on Detection, Evaluation, and Treatment of High Blood Cholesterol in Adults, *Second Report of the Expert Panel on Detection, Evaluation, and Treatment of High Blood Cholesterol in Adults*, NIH Publication No. 93-3095, National Institutes of Health, Bethesda, MD, 1993.
187. U.S. Department of Agriculture, Human Nutrition Information Service, *The Food Guide Pyramid*, Home and Garden Bulletin No. 252, U.S. Government Printing Office, Washington, D. C., 1996.
188. Horber, F. F., Gruber, B., Thomi, F., Jensen, E. X., and Jaeger, P., Effect of sex and age on bone mass, body composition and fuel metabolism in humans, *Nutrition*, 13, 524, 1997.
189. Linscheer, W. G. and Vergroesen, A. J., Lipids, in *Modern Nutrition in Health and Disease*, 8th ed., Shils, M. E., Olson, J. A., and Shike, M., Eds., Lea and Febiger, Philadelphia, 1994, pp. 47-88.
190. National Research Council, Protein and amino acids, in *Recommended Dietary Allowances*, 10th ed., National Academy of Sciences, Washington, D.C., 1989, pp. 52-77.
191. Campbell, W. W., Crim, M. C., Young, V. R., and Evans, W. J., Increased protein requirements in elderly people: new data and retrospective reassessments, *Am. J. Clin. Nutr.*, 60, 501, 1994.
192. Campbell, W. W., Crim, M. C., Young, V. R., Joseph, L. J., and Evans, W. J., Effects of resistance training and dietary protein intake on protein metabolism in older adults, *Am. J. Physiol.*, 268, E1143, 1995.
193. Campbell, W. W. and Evans, W. J., Protein requirements of elderly people, *Eur. J. Clin. Nutr.*, 50, S180, 1996.
194. Vellas, B. J., Hunt, W. C., Romero, L. J., Koehler, K. M., Baumgartner, R. N., and Garry, P. J., Changes in nutritional status and patterns of morbidity among free-living elderly persons: a 10-year longitudinal study, *Nutrition*, 13, 515, 1997.
195. Millward, D. J., Fereday, A., Gibson, N., and Pacy, P. J., Aging, protein requirements, and protein turnover, *Am. J. Clin. Nutr.*, 66, 774, 1997.
196. Russell, R. M. and Suter, P. M., Vitamin requirements of elderly people: an update, *Am. J. Clin. Nutr.*, 48, 4, 1993.
197. Russell, R. M., New views on the RDAs for older adults, *J. Am. Diet. Assoc.*, 97, 515, 1997.
198. Blumberg, J., Nutrient requirements of the healthy elderly—should there be specific RDAs?, *Nutr. Rev.*, 52, S15, 1994.
199. Fielding, R. A., Exercise, free radical generation, and aging, *Aging*, 9, 12, 1997.
200. Institute of Medicine, *Dietary Reference Intakes: Calcium, Phosphorus, Magnesium, Vitamin D, and Fluoride*, National Academy Press, Washington, D. C., 1997.
201. Ruud, J. S. and Grandjean, A. C., Nutritional concerns of female athletes, in *Nutrition in Exercise and Sport*, 3rd ed., Wolinsky, I., Ed., CRC Press, Boca Raton, FL, 1998, pp. 431-448.
202. MacLaughlin, J. and Holick, M. F., Aging decreases the capacity of human skin to produce vitamin D_3, *J. Clin. Invest.*, 76, 1536, 1985.
203. Institute of Medicine, Food and Nutrition Board, *Dietary Reference Intakes for Thiamin, Riboflavin, Niacin, Vitamin B-6, Folate, Vitamin B-12, Pantothenic Acid, Biotin, and Choline*, National Academy Press, Washington, D.C., 1998.
204. Yates, A. A., Schlicker, S. A., and Suitor, C. W., Dietary Reference Intakes: the new basis for recommendations for calcium and related nutrients, B vitamins, and choline, *J. Am. Diet. Assoc.*, 98, 699, 1998.
205. Ribaya-Mercado, J. D., Russell, R. M., Sahyoun, N., Morrow, F. D., and Gershoff, S. N., Vitamin B-6 requirements of elderly men and women, *Am. J. Clin. Nutr.*, 121, 1062, 1991.

206. Brants, H. A., Brussaard, J. H., Bouman, M., and Lowik, M. R., Dietary intake among adults with special reference to vitamin B-6, *Eur. J. Clin. Nutr.*, 51, S25, 1997.
207. Madigan, S. M., Tracey, F., McNulty, H., Eaton-Evans, J., Coulter, J., McCartney, H., and Strain, J.J., Riboflavin and vitamin B-6 intakes and status and biochemical response to riboflavin supplementation in free-living elderly people, *Am. J. Clin. Nutr.*, 68, 389, 1998.
208. Jacob, R. A., and Bowen, P. E., Biological characteristics of the antioxidant micronutrients, vitamin C, vitamin E, and the carotenoids: an update, *J. Am. Diet Assoc.*, 96, 693, 1996.
209. Heseker, H., Antioxidative Vitamine und Katarakte im Alter, *Z. Ernahrungswiss*, 34, 167, 1995.
210. Tessier, F., Moreaux, V., Birlouez-Aragon, I., Junes, P., and Mondon, H., Decrease in vitamin C concentration in human lenses during cataract progression, *Int. J. Vitam. Nutr. Res.*, 68, 309, 1998.
211. Lyle, B. J., Mares-Perlman, J. A., Klein, B. E., Klein, R., and Greger, J. L., Antioxidant intake and risk of incident age-related nuclear cataracts in the Beaver Dam Eye Study, *Am. J. Epidemiol.*, 149, 801, 1999.
212. Ames, B. N., Micronutrients prevent cancer and delay aging, *Toxicol. Lett.*, 102, 5, 1998.
213. Brown, L. M., Swanson, C. A., Gridley, G., Swanson, G. M., Silverman, D. T., Greenberg, R. S., Hayes, R. B., Schoenberg, J. B., Pottern, L. M., Schwartz, A. G., Liff, J. M., Hoover, R., and Fraumeni, J. F., Jr., Dietary factors and the risk of squamous cell esophageal cancer among black and white men in the United States, *Cancer Causes Control*, 9, 467, 1998.
214. Correa, P., Malcom, G., Schmidt, B., Fontham, E., Ruiz, B., Bravo, J. C., Bravo, L. E., Zarama, G., and Realpe, J. L., Review article: Antioxidant micronutrients and gastric cancer, *Aliment. Pharmacol. Ther.*, 12, 73, 1998.
215. Head, K. A., Ascorbic acid in the prevention and treatment of cancer, *Altern. Med. Rev.*, 3, 174, 1998.
216. Lee, I. M., Antioxidant vitamins in the prevention of cancer, *Proc. Assoc. Am. Physicians*, 111, 10, 1999.
217. Prasad, K. N., Kumar, A., Kochupillai, V., and Cole, W. C., High doses of multiple antioxidant vitamins: essential ingredients in improving the efficacy of standard cancer therapy, *J. Am. Coll. Nutr.*, 18, 13, 1999.
218. Schorah, C. J., Micronutrients, vitamins, and cancer risk, *Vitam. Horm.*, 57, 1, 1999.
219. Zhang, S., Hunter, D. J., Forman, M. R., Rosner, B. A., Speizer, F. E., Colditz, G. A., Manson, J. E., Hankinson, S. E., and Willett, W. C., Dietary carotenoids and vitamins A, C, and E and risk of breast cancer, *J. Natl. Cancer Inst.*, 91, 547, 1999.
220. Kanter, M., Free radicals, exercise and antioxidant supplementation, *Proc. Nutr. Soc.*, 57, 9, 1998.
221. Meydani, S. N., Meydani, M., Rall, L. C., Morrow, F., and Blumberg, J. B., Assessment of the high-dose, short-term supplementation with vitamin E in healthy older adults, *Am. J. Clin. Nutr.*, 60, 704, 1994.
222. Meydani, M., Evans, W. J., Handelman, G., Biddle, L., Fielding, R. A., Meydani, S. N., Burrill, J., Fiatarone, M. A., Blumberg, J. B., and Cannon, J. G., Protective effect of vitamin E on exercise-induced oxidative damage in young and older adults, *Am. J. Physiol.*, 264, R992, 1993.
223. Meydani, S. N., Meydani, M., Blumberg, J. B., Leka, L. S., Siber, G., Loszewski, R., Thompson, C., Pedrosa, M. C., Diamond, R. D., and Stollar, B. D., Vitamin E supplementation and *in vivo* immune response in healthy elderly subjects. A randomized controlled trial, *J. Am. Med. Assoc.*, 277, 1380, 1997.
224. National Research Council, Fat-soluble vitamins, in *Recommended Dietary Allowances*, 10th ed., National Academy of Sciences, Washington, D. C., 1989, pp. 78-114.
225. National Research Council, Water-soluble vitamins, in *Recommended Dietary Allowances*, 10th ed., National Academy of Sciences, Washington, D. C., 1989, pp. 115-173.
226. Carr, A. C. and Frei, B., Toward a new recommended dietary allowance for vitamin C based on antioxidant and health effects in humans, *Am. J. Clin. Nutr.*, 69, 1086, 1999.
227. Clarkson, P. M., Micronutrients and exercise: anti-oxidants and minerals, *J. Sports Sci.*, 13, S11, 1995.
228. Clarkson, P. M. and Haymes, E. M., Exercise and mineral status of athletes: calcium, magnesium, phosphorus, and iron, *Med. Sci. Sports Exerc.*, 27, 831, 1995.
229. Escanero, J. F., Villanueva, J., Rojo, A., Herrera, A., del Diego, C., and Guerra, M., Iron stores in professional athletes throughout the sports season, *Physiol. Behav.*, 62, 811, 1997.

230. Konig, D., Weinstock, C., Keul, J., Northoff, H., and Berg, A., Zinc, iron, and magnesium status in athletes—influence on the regulation of exercise-induced stress and immune function, *Exerc. Immunol. Rev.*, 4, 2, 1998.
231. Rosenzweig, P. H. and Volpe, S. L., Iron, thermoregulation, and metabolic rate, *Crit. Rev. Food Sci. Nutr.*, 39, 131, 1999.
232. O'Keefe, S. T., Gavin, K., and Lavan, J. N., Iron status and restless legs syndrome in the elderly, *Age Ageing*, 23, 200, 1994.
233. National Research Council, Trace elements, in *Recommended Dietary Allowances*, 10th ed., National Academy of Sciences, Washington, D. C., 1989, pp. 195-246.
234. Weaver, C. M. and Rajaram, S., Exercise and iron status, *J. Nutr.*, 122, 782, 1992.
235. Salonen, J. T., Nyyssonen, K., Korpela, H., Tuomilehto, J., Seppanen, R., and Salonen, R., High stored iron levels are associated with excess risk of myocardial infarction in eastern Finnish men, *Circulation*, 86, 803, 1992.
236. Meyers, D. G., Strickland. D., Maloley, P. A., Seburg, J. K., Wilson, J. E., and McManus, B. F., Possible association of a reduction in cardiovascular events with blood donation, *Heart*, 78, 188, 1997.
237. Underwood, B. A., Perspectives from micronutrient malnutrition elimination/eradication programmes, *Bull. World Health Organ.*, 76, 34, 1998.
238. Nielsen, P. and Nachtigall, D., Iron supplementation in athletes. Current recommendations, *Sports Med.*, 26, 207, 1998.
239. Tripp, F., The use of dietary supplements in the elderly: current issues and recommendations, *J. Am. Diet. Assoc.*, 97, S181, 1997.
240. Kleiner, S. M., Water: an essential but overlooked nutrient, *J. Am. Diet. Assoc.*, 99, 200, 1999.
241. Taylor, P. N., Wolinsky, I., and Klimis, D. J., Water in exercise and sport, in *Macroelements, Water, and Electrolytes in Sports Nutrition*, Driskell, J. A. and Wolinsky, I., Eds., CRC Press, Boca Raton, FL, 1999, pp. 93-108.
242. Rolls, B. J. and Phillips, P. A., Aging and disturbances of thirst and fluid balance, *Nutr. Rev.*, 48, 137, 1990.
243. Phillips, P. A., Bretherton, M., Johnston, C. I., and Gray, L., Reduced osmotic thirst in healthy elderly men, *Am. J. Physiol.*, 261, R166, 1991.
244. O'Neill, P. A. and McLean, K. A., Water homeostasis and aging, *Med. Lab. Sci.*, 49, 291, 1992.
245. Mack, G. W., Weseman, C. A., Langhans, G. W., and Scherzer, W., Body fluid balance in dehydrated healthy older men: Thirst and renal osmoregulation, *J. Appl. Physiol.*, 76, 1615, 1994.
246. Stout, N. R., Kenny, R. A., and Baylis, P. H., A review of water balance in aging in health and disease, *Gerontology*, 45, 61, 1999.
247. Hoffman, N. B., Dehydration in the elderly: insidious and manageable, *Geriatrics*, 46, 35, 1991.
248. Kenney, W. L., Control of heat-induced vasodilation in relation to age, *Eur. J. Appl. Physiol.*, 57, 120, 1988.
249. Meischer, E. and Forney, S. M., Responses to dehydration and rehydration during heat exposure in young and older men, *Am. J. Physiol.*, 257, R1050, 1989.
250. Chernoff, R., Thirst and fluid requirements, *Nutr. Rev.*, 52, S3, 1994.
251. Schaefer, D. C. and Cheskin, L. J., Constipation in the elderly, *Am. Fam. Physician*, 58, 907, 1998.
252. Slavin, J. L., Implementation of dietary modifications, *Am. J. Med.*, 106, 46S, 1999.
253. Kromhout, D., Bosschieter, E. N., and de Lezenne, C., Dietary fiber and 10-year mortality from coronary heart disease, cancer, and all causes: the Zutphen Study, *Lancet*, 2, 518, 1982.
254. Rimm, E. B., Ascherio, A., Givanucci, E., Spiegelman, D., Stampfer, M. J., and Willett, W. C., Vegetable, fruit and cereal fiber intake and risk of coronary heart disease among men, *J. Am. Med. Assoc.*, 275, 447, 1996.
255. Mensink, G. B., Relationships between nutrient intake, nutritional status and activity levels in an elderly and in a younger population: a comparison of physically more active and more inactive people, *Z. Gerontol.*, 22, 16, 1989.
256. Chatard, J. C., Boutet, C., Tourney, C., Garcia, S., Berthouze, S., and Guezennec, C. Y., Nutritional status and physical fitness of elderly sportsmen, *Eur. J. Appl. Physiol.*, 77, 157, 1998.
257. Allison, M. and Keller, C., Physical activity in the elderly: benefits and intervention strategies, *Nurse Pract.*, 22, 53, 1997.

258. National Research Council, Water and electrolytes, in *Recommended Dietary Allowances*, 10th ed., National Academy of Sciences, Washington, D. C., 1989, pp. 247-261.
259. Frye, S. L., Fluids, hydration, and performance concerns of all recreational athletes, in *Nutrition for the Recreational Athlete*, Jackson, C. G. R., Ed., CRC Press, Boca Raton, FL, 1995, pp. 137-152.
260. Convertino, V. A., Armstrong, L. E., Coyle, E. F., Mack, G. W., Sawka, M. N., Senay, L. C., Jr., and Sherman, W. M., American College of Sports Medicine. Position stand on exercise and fluid replacement, *Med. Sci. Sports Exerc.*, 28, I, 1996.
261. Hultman, E., Harris, R. C., and Spriet, L. L., Work and exercise, in *Modern Nutrition in Health and Disease*, Shils, M. E., Olson, J. A., and Shike, M., Eds., Lea and Febiger, Philadelphia, 1994, pp. 663-685.
262. Hu, F. B., Stampfer, M. J., Manson, J. E., Rimm, E. B., Colditz, G. A., Rosner, B. A., Speizer, F. E., Hennekens, C. H., and Willett, W. C., Frequent nut consumption and risk of coronary heart disease in women: prospective cohort study, *Br. Med. J.*, 317, 1341, 1998.
263. Lichtenstein, A. H., Trans fatty acids, plasma lipid levels, and the risk of developing cardiovascular disease. A statement for healthcare professionals from the American Heart Association, *Circulation*, 9, 2588, 1997.
264. Ascherio, A. and Willett, W. C., Health effects of trans fatty acids, *Am. J. Clin. Nutr.*, 66, 1006S, 1997.
265. Zock, P. L. and Katan, M. B., Trans fatty acids, lipoproteins, and coronary risk, *Can. J. Physiol. Pharmacol.*, 75, 211, 1997.
266. Nelson, G. J., Dietary fat, trans fatty acids, and risk of coronary heart disease, *Nutr. Rev.*, 56, 250, 1998.
267. Ascherio, A., Katan, M. B., Zock, P. L., Stampfer, M. J., and Willett, W. C., Trans fatty acids and coronary heart disease, *N. Engl. J. Med.*, 340, 1994, 1999.
268. American Society for Clinical Nutrition and American Institute of Nutrition, ASCN/AIN Task Force on Trans Fatty Acids, Position paper on trans fatty acids, *Am. J. Clin. Nutr.*, 63, 663, 1996.
269. Kritchevsky, D., Trans fatty acids and cardiovascular risk, *Prostaglandins Leukot. Essent. Fatty Acids*, 57, 399, 1997.
270. Shapiro, S., Do trans fatty acids increase the risk of coronary artery disease? A critique of the epidemiologic evidence, *Am. J. Clin. Nutr.*, 66, 1011S, 1997.
271. Meunier, P., Prevention of hip fractures by correcting calcium and vitamin D insufficiencies in elderly people, *Scand. J. Rheumatol. Suppl.*, 103, 75, 1996.
272. Feit, J. M., Calcium and vitamin D supplements for elderly patients, *J. Fam. Pract.*, 45, 471, 1997.
273. Swain, R., An update of vitamin B12 metabolism and deficiency states, *J. Fam. Pract.*, 41, 595, 1995.
274. Buchman, A. L., Vitamin supplementation in the elderly: a critical evaluation, *Gastroenterologist*, 4, 262, 1996.
275. Reid, I. R., The roles of calcium and vitamin D in the prevention of osteoporosis, *Endocrinol. Metab. Clin. North Am.*, 27, 389, 1998.
276. Vieth, R., Vitamin D supplementation, 25-hydroxyvitamin D concentrations, and safety, *Am. J. Clin. Nutr.*, 69, 842, 1999.
277. Monsen, E.T., Dietary reference intakes for the antioxidant nutrients vitamin C, vitamin E, selenium, and carotenoids, *J.Am. Diet. Assoc.*, 100, 637, 2000.

Part II

Nutritional Concerns of Athletes in Specific Groups

CHAPTER 6

Nutritional Concerns of Olympic and Elite Athletes

Ann C. Grandjean, Jaime S. Ruud, and Kristin J. Reimers

CONTENTS

I. INTRODUCTION

Dietary habits of Olympic athletes have always been of considerable interest. Throughout history, athletes have pursued optimal performance by eating specific foods and using substances thought to have ergogenic properties. Early writings on the training and dietary regimens of well-known ancient athletes are among the most fascinating texts to survive from antiquity.[1,2]

A significant body of research on nutrition and performance enhancement has accumulated during the second half of the 20th century. Based on that research, recommendations on amounts of nutrients to consume, foods to include or avoid, timing and types of meals and snacks, and types of supplements to use, abound. Some recommendations are based on research, others empirical wisdom, while still others appear to have limited bases.

Olympic athletes devote many years to intense training in hopes of one day being the best in the world. With a life-long dream at stake, Olympic hopefuls must be in top physical and mental condition. It is assumed, therefore, that Olympic athletes follow a diet that epitomizes people's

0-8493-8199-1/00/$0.00+$.50

perception of healthful. Research on Olympians and other elite athletes has revealed that their eating habits vary greatly. Some are extremely regimented with regard to their diet and follow a nutrition program to the letter. Others only worry about the basics — adequate energy, adequate protein, plenty of fluids. Some are very resistant to making changes in their diet, especially if they are convinced the nutrition program they are following will give them a competitive edge, while others will basically eat whatever is available with little concern of negative impact. All in all, Olympians reflect humankind. Some are obsessive about their diets, others very relaxed.

Upon learning that the diet of many accomplished athletes includes meat, milk, desserts, ice cream, chips, snack foods, and quick-service restaurant foods in addition to the assumed eaten poultry, fish, fruits, vegetables, rice, and pasta, many ask, "Well, if they don't eat a perfect diet how do they win gold medals and national titles and break world records?"

The truth is, the diets consumed by elite athletes are as varied as the athletes themselves. There is no such thing as a "perfect" diet. A variety of eating patterns can provide the energy and nutrients an athlete requires. In conversations with Olympic champions, there are several striking similarities. With few exceptions, the most common similarity, whether they medaled in 1939 or 1996, is that trial and error was the method by which they determined the nutrition program that worked best. This is not to say that they didn't receive guidance along the way, but the best nutrition program for any athlete is one that is tailored to meet individual needs and lifestyle. And trial and error is a necessary step to a tailor-made nutrition program.

II. ENERGY AND MACRONUTRIENT INTAKES AND RECOMMENDATIONS

A. Energy

Meeting energy needs is the foundational component of an athlete's diet, and a factor that impacts nutritional adequacy. Case in point, elite swimmers are known for their intense workouts. They spend anywhere from 2 to 5 hours a day (6 days a week) in the pool and then another hour in the weight room. To maintain energy levels, they must eat constantly, even when they are not hungry. It is not uncommon to see male swimmers eating as much as they can in an effort to maintain their weight. In contrast, female swimmers may have more weight-related issues and thus limit food intake.[3] Trappe et al.[4] measured the energy expenditure of elite female swimmers during high volume training using the doubly labeled water method. Energy intake averaged 3136 ±227 kcal/d and estimates of energy expenditure averaged 5593 ±495 kcal/d. The swimmers were able to maintain their body weight, despite the estimated difference between energy intake and energy expenditure. The researchers speculated that the negative energy balance was due to under reporting of food intake or under eating at the time of the study. While these are logical and obvious explanations, other potential explanations must be considered. One is that these athletes have become "energy efficient," expending less energy than estimated by indirect methods. Inexact standards and equations must also be considered for the discrepancies, or at least partial cause of error. Additionally, some female athletes have energy requirements that are truly lower than non-athletic peers, which must be considered when calculating energy requirements. These hypotheses are reviewed elsewhere.[5]

Training for cycling, particularly distance road events, requires a great deal of energy, and cyclists must balance energy intake and energy expenditure on a daily basis. Saris et al.[6] studied cyclists competing in the Tour de France, one of the most strenuous of all endurance competitions. The mean energy intake for the cyclists was 5903 kcal/d, very close to their estimated mean energy expenditure (6071 kcal/d).

Ten male cyclists volunteered for a study conducted by Garcia-Roves et al.[7] Energy intake of the 10 cyclists averaged 5617 kcal/d for the three 24-hour periods for which food and fluid intake was determined by weighing and measuring. These athletes were competing in the Tour of Spain, a three-week cycling event that covers approximately 3600 km without a rest day. The average distance covered for each stage is 170 km. Energy expenditure was not estimated.

A study by Frentsos and Baer[8] can help exemplify the potential impact of the training program. Six repeat competitors in the Hawaiian Ironman Triathlon reportedly trained close to 11 hours per week. Assuming 1 day of rest, this is less than 2 hours of training a day and the triathletes' average energy intake was 2318 kcal/d. On the other hand, a typical training week for triathletes studied by Burke et al.,[9] was 13 km swimming, 323 km cycling, and 75 km running. Their average daily energy intake was 4095 kcal/d, approximately 77% higher than the triathletes studied by Frentsos and Baer.[8] Factors other than training must be considered as potentially contributing to the difference. For example, subjects in the Burke et al.[9] study were all male and averaged 25 years of age, while four males and two females participated in the Frentsos and Baer[8] study and averaged 31 years of age. The athletes studied by Burke et al.[9] were reported to average 59 kcal/kg bw, indicative of an exceptional level of activity.[10] Energy expenditure was not reported on a per kg basis by Frentsos and Baer,[8] making true comparisons impossible.

As shown in Tables 6.1 and 6.2, the energy intake of elite athletes can be staggering or rather modest, depending on the type and intensity of the training program. Offshore sailing is an Olympic sport that can be physiologically and psychologically demanding based on the class of the boat, type of race, number of crew, and wind conditions.[11]

Bigard et al.[12] studied the nutrient intake of elite sailors during a solitary long-distance offshore race. Total daily energy intake averaged 4429 kcal/d ranging from 10.71 to 24.15 MJ/d. Despite high-energy intakes, body weight decreased significantly (1.31 ± 0.32 kg (range 3.5 to 0.1 kg)) during the race, which the authors attributed to disrupted fluid and/or energy balance.

On the other end of the spectrum are aesthetic (gymnastics, figure skating, surfing) and weight-class sports (lightweight rowing, wrestling, judo) where concerns about body weight and appearance are common. Many athletes strive to keep body weight low throughout the season by restricting energy intake. Body weight affects a ski jumper's distance. Of the studies shown in Table 6.1, the ski jumpers studied by Rankinen et al.[13] had the lowest energy intake reported. The ski jumpers averaged 1816 kcal/d. While their energy intake was low, the ski jumpers' diets were reported to have been nutrient dense. Nutrient dense, low-energy diets are not always the case with female athletes who must maintain a low body weight for their sport.

The lowest energy intake reported in Table 6.2 was the 1571 kcal/d consumed by artistic gymnasts studied by Jonnalagadda et al.[14] While the vitamin E intake of these artistic gymnasts was the lowest of all the nutrients analyzed, averaging less than 50% of the RDA,[10] intakes of calcium and zinc were also less than optimal. Less than optimal nutrient intake often accompanies low energy diets.

Felder et al.[15] reported marginal energy intakes in elite female surfers and zinc intakes below recommended levels. The mean energy intake of the surfers during competition was 2263 kcal/d, which was less than estimated energy requirements. Surfers, like many athletes who compete internationally, travel to competitions held all over the world. Felder et. al.[15] concluded that surfers' energy intakes were suboptimal because of obstacles the athletes faced while competing and traveling. Food choices were limited and thus, the athletes were unable to meet energy and nutrient needs. This topic will be covered in greater detail in the section on dietary concerns in this chapter.

Reports on dietary intakes of elite athletes reveal that energy intake reported as an absolute value varies not only between sport groups and between sub-populations of athletes from the same sport, but also for the same athlete at different times of training and competition. This must be remembered when considering group means or the diet of an individual athlete. Although mean energy intakes of male figure skaters studied by Grandjean[16] and Ziegler[17] were similar, 2533 kcal/d and 2325 kcal/d, respectively, a wider variance was reported for professional soccer players (2629 kcal/d) studied by Maughan[18] and Olympic soccer players (3952 kcal/d) studied by Rico-Sanz et al.[19] This may be due in part to differences in body size, playing position, and level of competition.

Table 6.1 Energy and Macronutrient Intake of Male Athletes

			Energy		Protein			CHO			Fat		
Sport	(Ref)*	Number Athletes	Kcal/d	Mj/d	g/d	g/kg	% en	g/d	g/kg	% en	g/d	g/kg	% en
Australian Football	(1)	40	3155[1a]	13.2	139	1.6	18	415	4.8	52	104	1.3	29
Australian Football	(2)	56	3395	14.2	126	1.5	15	373	—	44	141	—	38
Cycling	(3)	9	4269	17.9	160	2.2	15	471	6.5	43	196	2.7	41
Cycling	(4)	10	5617[4a]	23.5	202	3	15	841	13	60	159	2.4	26
Distance Running	(3)	11	3107	13.0	124	1.8	16	420	6.1	53	106	1.5	29
Figure Skating	(3)	7	2533	10.6	103	1.8	16	336	5.8	52	88	1.5	31
Figure Skating	(5)	12	2325	9.75[5a]	94	—	16	308	—	53	82	—	32
Gymnastics	(6)	4	3310	13.96[6a]	151	2.6	18	357	6.1	43	141	2.4	38
Hockey	(3)	8	3468	14.5	156	1.9	18	343	4.2	39	155	1.9	39
Judo	(3)	7	3159	13.2	114	1.5	14	358	4.9	45	127	1.7	36
Jumpers	(7)	4	2863	12.07[7a]	104	1.5	15	359	5.2	54	99	1.4	31
Long-distance running	(7)	8	3628	15.27[7a]	139	2.3	15	429	7.1	52	131	2.2	32
Marathon	(2)	19	3570	14.9	128	2.0	15	487	—	52	128	—	32
Middle-distance running	(7)	4	3437	14.47[7a]	131	2.1	15	382	6.2	49	139	2.2	36
Sailing	(8)	11	4429[8a]	18.5	—	—	15	—	7.3	51	—	—	35
Ski Jumping	(9)	18	1816[9a]	7.6	—	1.3	18	—	—	52	—	—	28
Soccer	(10)	8	3952	16.51[0a]	142	2.3	14	526	8.3	53	142	—	32
Soccer	(11)	26	2629[11a]	11.0	103	1.3	16	354	—	51	93	—	32
Sprinting	(7)	10	2653	11.17[7a]	102	1.5	15	340	5.1	54	90	1.4	30
Swimming	(6)	3	5938	24.96[6a]	320	4.3	22	484	6.5	33	315	4.3	48
Throwers	(7)	2	3591	15.07[7a]	134	1.3	15	429	4.1	55	119	1.1	30
Throwing	(6)	6	5353	22.46[6a]	265	2.4	20	450	4.1	34	277	2.5	47
Triathlon	(12)	4	2318	9.71[2a]	90	—	15	344	4	59	57	—	18
Triathlon	(2)	25	4095	17.2	134	2.0	13	627	—	60	127	—	27
Weightlifting	(3)	21	3758	15.7	178	1.9	19	372	4.2	39	165	1.8	38
Weightlifting	(2)	19	3640	15.2	156	1.9	18	399	—	43	155	—	39
Weightlifting	(6)	10	4597	19.26[6a]	257	3.2	22	431	5.4	38	205	2.6	40

[a] calculated value; 1 mJ = 239 kcal

*References

1. Schokman, C. P., H. E. Rutishauser, and R. J. Wallace, Pre- and post-game macronutrient intake of a group of elite Australian football players. *Int. J. Sport Nutr.* 9, 60, 1999.
2. Burke, L. M., Gollan, R. A., and Read, S. D., Dietary intakes and food use of groups of elite Australian male athletes. *Int. J. Sport Nutr.* 1:378, 1991.
3. Grandjean, A. C., Reimers, K. J., and Ruud, J. S., Dietary habits of Olympic athletes, in *Nutrition in Exercise and Sport,* Wolinsky, I., Ed., CRC Press, Boca Raton, FL, 421, 1998.
4. Garcia-Roves, P. M., Terrados, N., Fernandez, S. F., and Patterson, A. M., Macronutrient intake of top level cyclists during continuous competition—change in the feeding pattern. *Int. J. Sport Med.* 19:61, 1998.
5. Ziegler, P. J., Khoo, Chor San, Kris-Etherton, P. M., Jonnalagadda, S. S., Sherr, B., and Nelson, J. A., Nutritional status of nationally ranked junior US figure skaters. *J. Am. Diet. Assoc.* 98:809, 1998.
6. Chen, J. D., Wang, J. F., Li, K. J., Zhao, Y. W., Wang, S. W., Jioa, Y., and Hou, X. Y., Nutritional problems and measures in elite and amateur athletes. *Am. J. Clin. Nutr.* 49:1084, 1989.
7. Sugiura, K., Izumi, S., and Kobayashi, K., Nutritional intake of elite Japanese track-and-field athletes. *Intl. J. Sport Nutr.* 9:202, 1999.
8. Bigard, Andre-Xavier, Guillemot, Pierre-Yves, Chauve, Jean-Yves, Duforez, F., Portero, P., Guezennec, and Charles-Yannick, Nutrient intake of elite sailors during a solitary long-distance offshore race. *Int. J. Sport Nutr.* 8:864, 1998.
9. Rankinen, T., Lyytikainen, S., Vanninen, E., Penttila, I., Rauramaa, R., and Uusitupa, M., Nutritional status of the Finnish elite ski jumpers. *Med. Sci. Sports Exerc.* 30:1592, 1998.
10. Rico-Sanc, J., Frontera, W. R., Mole, P. A., Rivera, M. A., Rivera-Brown, A., and Meredith, C. N., Dietary and performance assessment of elite soccer players during a period of intense training. *Int. J. Sport Nutr.* 8:230, 1998.
11. Maughan, R., J., Energy and macronutrient intakes of professional football (soccer) players. *Br. J. Sport Med.* 31:45, 1997.
12. Frentsos, J. A. and Baer, J. T., Increased energy and nutrient intake during training and competition improves elite triathletes' endurance performance. *Int. J. Sport Nutr.* 7:61, 1997.

Table 6.2 Energy and Macronutrient Intake of Female Athletes

			Energy		Protein			CHO			Fat		
Sport	(Ref)*	Number Athletes	Kcal/d	Mj/d	g/d	g/kg	% en	g/d	g/kg	% en	g/d	g/kg	% en
Artistic Gymnasts	(1)	8	1571	—	68	—	17	276	—	70	25	—	15
Cycling	(2)	10	3009	12.6	100	1.7	13	409	7.1	53	111	1.9	31
Distance Running	(2)	9	2142	9.0	82	1.6	15	275	5.4	50	74	1.4	30
Figure Skating	(2)	8	1866	7.8	66	1.4	14	248	5.3	52	69	1.5	33
Figure Skating	(3)	16	1674	7.0[3a]	66	—	16	241	—	58	53	—	29
Gymnastics	(4)	5	2298	9.6[4a]	94	2.1	16	242	5.4	42	106	2.4	42
Judo	(2)	4	1966	8.2	62	1	12	264	4.4	53	77	1.2	34
Jumpers	(5)	4	1982	8.3[5a]	82	1.5	16	244	4.5	51	72	1.3	33
Long-distance running	(5)	7	2720	11.4[5a]	109	2.4	16	337	7.2	51	98	2.1	33
Middle-distance running	(5)	4	2764	11.6[5a]	111	2.3	16	335	7.1	50	106	2.2	34
Sprinters	(5)	11	2393	10.0[5a]	89	1.7	15	305	5.8	53	86	1.6	33
Surfing	(6)	10	2263	9.5	76	—	14	326	5.7	57	66	—	26
Swimming	(4)	3	4595	19.2[4a]	230	3.5	26	405	6.2	35	248	3.8	49
Swimming	(7)	6	2472	10.3[7a]	90	1.4	15	334	—	53	94	—	32
Tennis	(2)	9	2040	8.5	80	1.4	15	279	4.8	54	68	1.2	29
Throwers	(5)	8	2617	11.0[5a]	93	1.4	14	336	5.1	54	94	1.4	32
Throwing	(4)	6	4446	18.6[4a]	208	2.5	19	386	4.6	35	230	2.7	47

[a] Calculated value; 1 mJ = 239 kcal

*References

1. Jonnalagadda, S. S., Benardot, D., and Nelson, M., Energy and nutrient intakes of the United States National Women's Artistic Gymnastics team. *Int. J. Sport Nutr.* 8:331, 1998.
2. Grandjean, A. C., Reimers, K. J., and Ruud, J. S., Dietary habits of Olympic athletes, in *Nutrition in Exercise and Sport,* Wolinsky, I., Ed., CRC Press, Boca Raton, FL, 421, 1998.
3. Ziegler, P. J., Khoo, Chor San, Kris-Etherton, P. M., Jonnalagadda, S. S., Sherr, B., and Nelson, J. A., Nutritional status of nationally ranked junior U.S. figure skaters. *J. Am. Diet Assoc.* 98:809, 1998.
4. Chen, J. D., Wang, J. F., Li, K. J., Zhao, Y. W., Wang, S. W., Jioa, Y., and Hou, X. Y., Nutritional problems and measures in elite and amateur athletes. *Am. J. Clin. Nutr.* 49:1084, 1989.
5. Sugiura, K., Izumi, S., and Kobayashi, K., Nutritional intake of elite Japanese track-and-field athletes. *Intl. J. Sport Nutr.* 9:202, 1999.
6. Felder, J. M., Burke, L. M., Lowdon, B. J., Cameron-Smith, D., and Collier, G. R., Nutritional practices of elite female surfers during training and competition. *Int. J. Sport Nutr.* 8:36, 1998.
7. Vallieres, F., Tremblay, A., and St-Jean, L., Study of the energy balance and the nutritional status of highly trained female swimmers. *Nutr. Research.* 9:699, 1989.

The elite Puerto Rican Soccer players studied by Rico-Sanz et al.[19] were younger and smaller in stature than elite Scottish soccer players surveyed by Maughan.[18]

The studies reviewed in this section exemplify why reporting energy in absolute numbers is of limited value; the relationship of intake to body size, which is one of the major factors impacting energy requirements, cannot be made. Presenting data as energy per kg body weight allows for more-meaningful comparisons.

B. Carbohydrate

Numerous studies have examined the effects of the timing and amounts of carbohydrate on performance in subjects of varying training levels. These studies, reviewed elsewhere, help elucidate the carbohydrate requirements of athletes.[20–22] While athletes participating in prolonged (>60 minutes) intense exercise (65%–70% VO_{2max}) are advised to consume a diet containing approximately 8 to 10 g CHO/kg bw/d,[22] it has been shown that there are no deleterious effects on training capability or high-intensity performance on 5g CHO/kg bw/d.[23]

It is still commonly recommended, however, that athletes in non-endurance sports consume 55–65% of total energy as carbohydrate and endurance athletes, 65–70%. Interestingly, the vast majority of the group averages reported in Tables 6.1 and 6.2 are below those recommendations. Overall, mean intakes ranged from 33% to 60% for groups of elite male athletes with only four of the 27 groups averaging 55% or more of energy from carbohydrate. For the studies on elite female athletes, the mean intakes ranged from 35% to 70%, with three of the 17 groups studied averaging more than 55%. Considering carbohydrate intake as percent of energy is of limited value and, when working with elite athletes, inappropriate. Carbohydrate intake based on lean body mass would be ideal, but, short of that, calculating for body size (g/kg) is more meaningful than as percent of energy.

Few events are as physically demanding as a stage race. The carbohydrate intakes of the 10 male cyclists surveyed by Garcia-Roves[7] and colleagues during the Tour of Spain ranged from 684 to 1113 gm (3-day average) for a g/kg bw range of 10.4–14.1. The group means, shown in Table 6.1, reveal that overall carbohydrate supplied an average of 60% of energy. Triathletes studied by Frentsos and Baer[8] consumed an average of 59% of energy from carbohydrate. However, on a body weight basis, the average was only 4 g/kg, or approximately 30% of the average 13g/kg consumed by the cyclists in the Garcia-Roves[7] study. By contrast, Grandjean et al.[16] reported a mean carbohydrate intake of 43% of energy, with an average of 6.5 g/kg/d for nine nationally ranked male cyclists. It must be kept in mind that the cyclists studied by Grandjean[16] were in pre-season training, whereas data collected in the Garcia-Roves[7] study was during competition. Frentsos and Baer[8] reported only that all subjects were actively training and competing at the time of the study.

C. Protein

For many years, the consensus was that athletes require no more protein than nonathletes. More-sophisticated research indicates otherwise.[24,25] Research[24] not only suggests that athletes have increased protein requirements than the general population, it indicates that strength athletes need between 1.4 and 1.8 g/kg bw/d and endurance athletes between 1.2 and 1.4 g/kg bw/d. As with carbohydrate, using percent of energy as a guideline for protein requirements is flawed. At 1.5 g of protein/kg bw, an 80-kg athlete consuming 2800 kcals would need 17% of energy to be provided by protein, while an 80-kg athlete consuming 3200 kcals would need 15% of energy from protein. An 80-kg athlete participating in a high-energy sport, and thus consuming 5000 kcals, would need less than 10% of energy from protein. The athlete's weight is a more reliable reference point on which to base protein needs than is percent of energy intake.

It should be noted that the estimated protein requirements for athletes make two important assumptions: adequate calorie intake, and a diet providing both animal and plant proteins. Negative energy balance will increase protein requirements because of increased protein use as an energy substrate.

Biological value of the protein consumed also affects requirements. Recommendations for protein are based on studies in which the subject consumed approximately 65% of their protein as animal protein. The strict vegetarian will have a higher per kg bw requirement for protein than the athlete who eats meat, fish, eggs, or dairy products. This is due mainly to differences in the digestibility and amino acid composition of plant protein versus animal protein. Sugiura, et al.,[25] studying 62 nationally ranked Japanese track and field athletes concluded that, when consuming a diet high in plant protein, Japanese athletes may require more than 2.0/kg/d.

As can be seen in Tables 6.1 and 6.2, most authors reported the amount of protein consumed on the basis of body weight. The mean intake was 1.0 gram or greater for all of the athletic groups shown, with intakes of 1.5g or greater in 82% of the groups.

D. Fat

Mean fat intakes as percent of energy from studies shown in Tables 6.1 and 6.2 ranged from 18% to 48% for male athletes and 15% to 49% for female athletes. The Sub-Committee on Nutrition of the United Nations recommends 15% of energy as the lower limit of fat intake for most adults.[26,27]

The lower limit recommended for women of reproductive age is 20% of energy. The upper limit of fat intake recommended is 30% of energy for sedentary individuals, and, for active people, 35%.[26,27]

The Dietary Guidelines for Americans suggest that individuals consume no more than 30% of their energy from fat.[28] However, this recommendation targets the generally sedentary U.S. population and is meant to decrease risk of heart disease and some cancers. While most athletes do consider their future health, they are also interested in the role of dietary fat in performance. Among athletes with high energy needs, a fat intake greater than 30% is often necessary to meet energy requirements.

Fat phobia has been one of the less desirable results of the emphasis on decreasing fat. Some athletes strive to reduce both body fat and dietary fat to unrealistic and sometimes unhealthy levels. Severely restricting fat and/or energy intake can lead to a continuum of nutrition-related health problems including nutritional deficiencies, amenorrhea, and osteoporosis, not to mention decrements in performance. While fat phobia occurs in both male and female athletes, associated problems appear to occur more often in female athletes. Amenorrhea and osteoporosis are covered in greater detail elsewhere in this volume.

III. SUPPLEMENTS

It is not possible to estimate, with any degree of accuracy, the percentage of elite athletes who take dietary supplements. Surveys of athletes at varying levels of participation, as well as recreational exercise enthusiasts, report dietary supplement use to range from less than 20% up to 100%.[6,14-16,29-32]

Limited reports exist regarding the rationale for supplement use by elite athletes. However, athletes queried have reported they use supplements to compensate for poor nutrition and lifestyle, to compensate for tiredness and loss of appetite due to heavy training, and in response to respiratory infections and excess alcohol consumption.[9,33] Increasing strength, muscle mass, anaerobic energy, aerobic energy, mental arousal, general well-being, post-exercise recovery, and reducing body fat, pain, or inflammation are also among the reasons given for supplement use.[30]

IV. DIETARY CONCERNS

Factors that affect food intake of Olympians and Olympic hopefuls include food availability, food preferences, and economic factors; basically the same factors that affect the food intake of most humans. In addition, elite athletes must also ensure that their diet supports their training and enhances their performance where possible.

The many hours and stress of hard training can suppress appetite and make it difficult to follow a routine eating schedule. Training for several hours a day leaves little time for preparing and eating meals, a dilemma shared by professional and collegiate athletes as well. As a result, small meals and/or snacks often become an essential part of a nutrition program for the busy athlete.

A. Travel

In addition to long training hours, travel is another disruption for athletes who compete nationally and internationally.[15,34] Food intake often depends on local restaurant facilities and, thus, access to familiar foods may be limited. This can be a dilemma, especially for athletes who have trouble maintaining body weight. Eating atypical foods for long periods of time may have negative psychological and physical effects. Consuming foods and beverages not normally consumed can contribute to diarrhea, constipation, gas, or nausea. Food-borne illness is another chief concern. A review of traveler's diarrhea stated that up to 60% of athletes traveling abroad may be affected.[35]

Traveler's diarrhea can be caused by food or water that contains bacteria, viruses, or parasites. It is estimated that bacterial enteropathogens cause at least 80% of traveler's diarrhea with *Escherichia coli* and shigella being the two most common agents.[36] Clinical features of traveler's diarrhea include frequent loose stools and abdominal cramps, sometimes accompanied by nausea, vomiting, or the passage of bloody stools. Since contaminated food and water can cause traveler's diarrhea, athletes need to be cautious of what they eat and drink and to apply stringent food hygiene rules. Prevention of the problem involves selecting eating establishments that are well known or recommended by coaches or other individuals who have been to the area before and who are aware of food safety issues. Information on immunization requirements and recommended prophylactic precautions should also be established well in advance of travel. This advice is readily available from travel agents, airlines, and embassies.

Foods such as fruits that can be peeled and vegetables that have been thoroughly washed with boiling water, are usually safe food choices. As a general rule, athletes should drink only bottled water, juices, or soft drinks directly from sealed containers. Ice can be a source of pathogens.

Oral prophylactic drugs can be used to help prevent traveler's diarrhea. Depending on the duration of the trip, these drugs are generally taken on the first day of arrival and continued for 1 or 2 days after departure. However, when used for an extended period of time, the disadvantages of prophylaxes may outweigh the benefits. Certain probiotic organisms, such as lactobacillus, offer a non-drug approach. Lactobacillus GG has been shown to be effective in stimulating antibody production against rotavirus,[37,38] and to reduce the duration of diarrhea.[39]

In situations where pureness of the water is uncertain, care must be taken not to swallow water when taking a bath or shower or when brushing teeth. Using bottled water while brushing teeth decreases risk. Athletes participating in sports that are held in natural waters, such as canoeing, kayaking, or windsurfing, need to be cautious about swallowing water during training and events.

B. Overtraining

Gould et al.[40,41] surveyed 296 athletes and 46 coaches who participated in the 1996 Olympics Games held in Atlanta, Georgia. Overtraining was one of several factors athletes identified as having hurt their Olympic performance.

It's been reported that overtraining syndrome affects mainly endurance athletes.[42] It is unclear if this is due to a higher risk in endurance athletes or lack of studies in athletes participating in anaerobic sports. Individuals who do not adapt to the stress of training or do not allow for adequate rest and recovery are at greatest risk. However, an individual athlete will tolerate different levels of training, competition, and stress at different times, and overtraining for one athlete may be insufficient training for another. Athletes will often ignore fatigue, heavy muscles, and depression, all symptoms of overtraining, but will complain about under performance. Sleep disturbances, weight loss, and loss of appetite are also among the numerous symptoms of overtraining.

Rest, not to be confused with total inactivity, is the primary treatment modality for an athlete diagnosed with overtraining syndrome. Preventive strategies include close monitoring of training program, rest between training sessions, full hydration, and proper nutrition.[42,43]

V. CONCLUSION

It was once thought that the nutritional needs of athletes, with the exception of energy, varied little from those of nonathletes. Several decades of research has proven otherwise. While we know decidedly more about the impact of nutrition on performance, sports nutrition as a discipline is still in its infancy. To continue the evolution of sports nutrition, researchers must continue to be precise in their measures and exact in their reporting, allowing for more targeted recommendations. Nowhere in sport is this more necessary than at the elite level.

REFERENCES

1. Messinesi, X. L., *A Branch of Wild Olive. The Olympic Movement and the Ancient and Modern Olympic Games.* Exposition Press, New York, 1973.
2. Kieran, J., Daley, A., and Jordan, P. *The Story of the Olympic Games: 776 B.C. to 1976.* J.B. Lippincott, Philadelphia, 1977.
3. Applegate, E. A., Baumgartner, B., Clarkson, P. M., Grivetti, L. E., Haislett, N., McDonald, R. B., Mills, B., and Oerter, A., Gold medal roundtable: athlete presentations, audience questions, and summary statements. *J. Nutr.* 127,886S, 1997.
4. Trappe, T. A., Gastaldelli, A., Jozsi, A. C., Troup, J. P., and Wolfe, R. R., Energy expenditure of swimmers during high volume training. *Med. Sci. Sports Exerc.,* 29,950, 1997.
5. Grandjean, A.G., Ruud, J.S., and Reimers, K.R.., Nutrition and the female athlete, in *Encyclopedia of Sports Medicine: Women in Sport*, Drinkwater, B. Ed., Blackwell Science, Oxford, UK, 2000, 120-131.
6. Saris, W. H. M., van Erp-Baart, M. A., Brouns, F., Westerterp, K. R., and ten Hoor, F., Study on food intake and energy expenditure during extreme sustained exercise: The Tour de France. *Int. J. Sports Med.*, 10, S26, 1989.
7. Garcia-Roves, P. M., Terrados, N., Fernandez, S. F., and Patterson, A. M., Macronutrient intake of top level cyclists during continuous competition-change in the feeding pattern. *Int. J. Sports Med.* 19, 61, 1998.
8. Frentsos, J. A. and Baer, J. T. Increased energy and nutrient intake during training and competition improves elite triathletes' endurance performance. *Int. J. Sport Nutr.* 7, 61, 1997.
9. Burke, L. M., Gollan, R. A., and Read R. S. D., Dietary Intakes and Food Use of Groups of Elite Australian Male Athletes. *Intl. J. Sports Nutr.* 1, 378, 1991.
10. Food and Nutrition Board, National Research Council (1989) *Recommended Dietary Allowance*, 10th ed., National Academy Press, Washington D.C., 179.
11. Shepherd, R. J., The biology and medicine of sailing. *Sports Med.* 9, 86, 1990.
12. Bigard, Andre-Xavier, Guillemot, Pierre-Yves, Chauve, Jean-Yves, Duforez, F., Portero, P., Guezennec. C.-Y., Nutrient intake of elite sailors during a solitary long-distance offshore race. *Int. J. Sport Nutr.* 8, 364, 1998.
13. Rankinen, T., Lyytikainen, S., Vanninen, E., Penttila, I., Rauramaa, R., and Uusitupa, M., Nutritional status of Finnish elite ski jumpers. *Med. Sci. Sports Exerc.,* 30, 1592, 1998.
14. Jonnalagadda, S. S., Benardot, D., and Nelson, M., Energy and nutrient intakes of the United States National Women's Artistic Gymnastics team. *Int. J. Sport Nutr.* 8, 331, 1998.
15. Felder, J. M., Burke, L. M., Lowdon, B. J., Cameron-Smith, D., and Collier, G. R., Nutritional practices of elite female surfers during training and competition. *Int. J. Sport Nutr.* 8, 36, 1998.
16. Grandjean, A. C., Reimers, K. J., and Ruud, J. S., Dietary habits of Olympic athletes, in *Nutrition in Exercise and Sport*, 3rd ed., Wolinsky, I., Ed., CRC Press, Boca Raton, FL, 1998, 421-430.
17. Ziegler, P. J., Khoo, Chor San, Kris-Etherton, P. M., Jonnalagadda, S. S., Sherr, B., and Nelson, J. A., Nutritional status of nationally ranked junior U.S. figure skaters. *J. Am. Diet. Assoc.*, 98, 809, 1998.
18. Maughan, R. J., Energy and macronutrient intakes of professional football (soccer) players. *Br. J. Sports Med.* 31, 45, 1997.
19. Rico-Sanc, J., Frontera, W. R., Mole, P. A., Rivera, M. A., Rivera-Brown, A., and Meredith, C. N., Dietary and performance assessment of elite soccer players during a period of intense training. *Int. J. Sport Nutr.* 8, 230, 1998.
20. Sherman, W. M., Brodowicz, G., Wright, D. A., Allen, W. K., Simonsen, J., and Dernback, A., Effects of 4 h pre-exercise carbohydrate feedings on cycling performance. *Med. Sci. Sports Exerc.*, 21, 598, 1989.
21. Sherman, M. W., Carbohydrate feedings before and after exercise. in *Perspectives in Exercise Science and Sports Medicine*, Vol. 4: Ergogenics — Enhancement of Performance in Exercise and Sport. William C. Brown, Publ., Ann Arbor, MI, 1991.
22. Jacobs, K. A. and Sherman, W. M., The efficacy of carbohydrate supplementation and chronic high-carbohydrate diets for improving endurance performance. *Int. J. Sport Nutr.* 9, 92, 1999.
23. Sherman, W. M., Doyle, J. A., Lamb, D. R., and Strauss, R. H., Dietary carbohydrate, muscle glycogen, and exercise performance during 7 d of training, *Am. J. Clin. Nutr.* 57, 27, 1993.
24. Lemon, P.W.R., Effects of exercise on dietary protein requirements. *Int. J. Sports Nutr.* 8,426, 1998.

25. Sugiura, K., Izumi, S. and Kobayashi, K., Nutritional intake of elite Japanese track-and-field athletes. *Int. J. Sports Nutr.* 9, 202, 1999.
26. FAO Food and Nutrition Paper 57. Fats and oils in human nutrition. FAO, Rome, 1994.
27. Beaton, G., Prevention and the role of nutrition. *ACC/SCN News*, No. 14:14, 1997.
28. U.S. Department of Agriculture and U.S. Department of Health and Human Services, *Nutrition and Your Health: Dietary Guidelines for Americans*, 4th ed., Home and Garden Bulletin No. 232, 1995.
29. Sobal, J. and Marquart, L. F., Vitamin/mineral supplement use among athletes. A review of the literature. *Int. J. Sport Nutr.* 4, 320, 1994.
30. Armstrong, L. E. and Maresch, C. M., Vitamin and mineral supplements as nutritional aids to exercise performance and health. *Nutr Rev.* 54, S149, 1996.
31. van Earp-Baart, A. M. J., Saris, W. M. H., Binkhorst, R. A., Vos, J. A. and Elvers, J. W. H., Nationwide survey on nutritional habits in elite athletes, Part II. Mineral and vitamin intake. 10, S11, 1989.
32. Rosen, O., Sundgot-Borgen, J. and Maehlum, S., Supplement use and nutritional habits in Norwegian elite athletes. *Scand. J. Med. Sci. Sports.* 9, 28, 1999.
33. Burke, L. M. and Read, R. S. D., A study of dietary patterns of elite Australian football players. *Can. J. Spt. Sci.*13,15, 1988.
34. Grandjean, A. G. and Ruud, J. S., The traveling athlete, in *Encyclopedia of Sports Medicine: Nutrition in Sport*, Maughan, R.J., Ed., Blackwell Science, Oxford UK., 2000, 484–491.
35. Grantham, P., Traveler's diarrhea in athletes. *Phys. Sportsmed.* 11, 65, 1983.
36. DuPont, H. L. and Ericsson, C. D., Prevention and treatment of traveler's diarrhea. *N. Engl. J. Med.* 328, 1821, 1993.
37. Kaila M., Isolauri E., Soppi E., Virtanen E., Laine S. and Arvilommi H., Enhancement of the circulating antibody secreting cell response in human diarrhea by a human Lactobacillus strain. *Pediatr. Res.* 32:141, 1992.
38. Kaila M., Isolauri E., Saxelin M., Arvilommi H. and Vesikari T., Viable versus inactivated lactobacillus strain GG in acute rotavirus diarrhea. *Arch. Dis. Child.* 72:51, 1995.
39. Isolauri E., Juntunen M., Rautanen T., Sillanaukee P. and Koivula T., A human Lactobacillus strain (*Lactobacillus casei* sp strain GG) promotes recovery from acute diarrhea in children. *Pediatrics.* 88:90, 1991.
40. Gould, D., Greenleaf, C., Guinan, D., Medbery, R., Strickland, M., Lauer, L., Chung, Y. and Peterson, K., Factors influencing Atlanta Olympian performance. *Olympic Coach.* 8:9, 1998.
41. Gould, D., Greenleaf, C., Guinan, D., Medbery, R., Strickland, M., Lauer, L., Chung, Y. and Peterson, K., Effective and ineffective coaching lessons learned from Atlanta. *Olympic Coach.* 9:2 1999.
42. Budgett, R. Fatigue and under performance in athletes: the overtraining syndrome. *Br. J. Sports Med.* 32:107, 1998.
43. Panel Statement. Overtraining: the challenge of prevention. *Olympic Coach.* 8, 4, 1998.

CHAPTER 7

Nutritional Concerns of Vegetarian Athletes

Mauro DiPasquale

CONTENTS

I. INTRODUCTION

Vegetarian is derived from the Latin *vegetus*, meaning whole, sound, fresh, lively. The original definition of "vegetarian" was "with or without eggs or dairy products" and that definition is still used today by the Vegetarian Society. However, most vegetarians in India exclude eggs from their diet, as did those in classical Mediterranean lands.

More and more people are becoming vegetarians. For some, becoming a vegetarian is a statement to promote animal rights or to save the environment, while for others it's simply a choice they make for various other reasons including health and just fitting in with "alternative" lifestyles.

In general, people have distorted ideas on just what a vegetarian is. The word sometimes evokes visions of hippies with peace signs painted on various parts of their bodies carrying signs and demonstrating against the killing of animals. That caricature, like most, is untrue. Vegetarians are merely people in all walks of life who, for moral and other reasons, simply do not eat red meat or, to some extent or another, other animal foods.

0-8493-8199-1/00/$0.00+$.50

II. TYPES OF VEGETARIANS

Vegetarians generally abstain from eating red meat and usually forgo eating poultry, fish, and other seafood. Depending on the type of vegetarian, the forbidden foods may also include any food of animal origin. While there are many different kinds of vegetarians, the following two basic types are the most common.

1. Lacto-ovo vegetarian. The most common form of vegetarianism avoids consuming animal flesh but allows dairy products and eggs with a diet of vegetables, fruits, nuts, seeds, legumes, and grains. Vegetarians may also avoid milk products but consume eggs (lacto vegetarian) or vice versa (ovo vegetarian).
2. Vegan. This type of vegetarian excludes all animal products including diary, eggs, and even honey. Their diet is derived exclusively from plants and is based on grains, vegetables, legumes, fruits, seeds, and nuts. Their entire protein intake is in the form of plant protein. Some vegans also refuse to eat yeast products. As well, the strict vegan avoids any products derived from animals such as leather, wool, fur, down, silk, ivory, and pearl. Additionally, cosmetics and household items that contain animal ingredients or that are tested on animals are avoided.

Dietary vegans are people who follow a vegan diet, but do not necessarily exclude non-food uses of animals.

While these two types are the most common, there are many other types and classifications for vegetarian eating. For example, a fruitarian is even stricter and avoids any plant products except those parts of the plant that are cast off or dropped from the plant and that do not involve the destruction of the plant itself. For example, fruits can be picked without killing the plant while vegetables such as celery and carrots cannot.

As well, there are a number of confusing terms used for different kinds of vegetarians. Pescatarian is a vegetarian, usually lacto-ovo, who also eats fish. A semi-vegetarian eats less meat than the average person does. A pseudo-vegetarian claims to be a vegetarian, but isn't. For example, they may eat less meat than the average person or they may eat dairy foods, eggs, chicken, and fish but no other animal flesh. This term is often used by true vegetarians to describe semi-vegetarians and pescatarians.

In addition to these somewhat confusing terms, there are several others that are also in use that describe variable eating patterns. For example, a "vegetable consumer" means anyone who consumes vegetables, but may not necessarily be a vegetarian. An "herbivore" means eating grass and/or plants but again may not necessarily qualify as a vegetarian. A "plant-eater" mainly eats plants, but may not necessarily qualify as a vegetarian.

As the term implies, "non meat eater" does not eat meat. Most commonly used definitions do not consider fish, fowl, or seafood to be "meat." Animal fats and oils, bonemeal, and skin are not considered meat.

At present there are more vegetarians than ever because more and more people, including athletes, are experimenting with vegetarian diets.

There are several reasons that an individual may choose to become a vegetarian. Health benefits are one of the reasons. Those that turn to the vegetarian lifestyle for health reasons often perceive plant foods to be beneficial because they are high in dietary fiber and generally lower in saturated fat than animal foods. And they are correct.

Studies have shown that vegetarians are at less risk for high blood pressure, coronary heart disease, stroke, diabetes, obesity, constipation, lung cancer, gallstones, and alcoholism. Also, while the data is not as strong, it appears that vegetarians are at lower risk for breast cancer, diverticular disease of the colon, colonic cancer, calcium kidney stones, osteoporosis, dental erosion, and dental caries[1,2]

Vegetarian diets are frequently purported to reduce cancer risk. Diets rich in the carotenoids, including beta-carotene (the plant form of vitamin A) and vitamin C may reduce the risk of certain cancers.[3] Additionally, reducing fat in the diet may reduce cancer risk. Diets high in fiber-rich foods, especially vegetables from the cabbage family, may reduce the risk of cancers of the colon and rectum. The FDA, in fact, has authorized several health claims on food labels relating low-fat diets high in some plant-derived foods with a possible reduced risk of cancer.

While the FDA acknowledges that high intakes of fruits and vegetables rich in beta-carotene or vitamin C have been associated with reduced cancer risk, it believes the data are not sufficiently convincing that either nutrient by itself is responsible for the association. Nevertheless, since most fruits and vegetables are low-fat foods and may contain vitamin A (as beta-carotene) and vitamin C, the agency authorized a health claim relating diets low in fat and rich in these foods to a possibly reduced risk of some cancers.

Although cardiovascular disease and cancer are found less in the vegetarian population, the reduced incidence of disease cannot be attributed solely to dietary factors. Vegetarians as a group tend to be more conscious of overall good health practices, including regular exercise, abstinence from the use of tobacco products, and avoidance of excessive alcohol intake.

Nevertheless, health benefits are not the only reason vegetarian diets attract followers. Some give up meat because they feel it's unethical to eat mammals or, depending on the kind of vegetarian, any living animal or simply anything living, whether plant or animal.

Certain people, such as Seventh-day Adventists, choose a vegetarian diet because of religious beliefs. Some believe it's a better use of the earth's resources to eat low forms on the food chain; that is, to eat plant foods rather than the animals that eat plant foods. Additionally, some people eat plant foods simply because they are less expensive than animal foods.

Some individuals, such as teenagers, become vegetarian out of genuine concern for animal welfare or because they do not like the taste or texture of meat.

III. THE NUTRITIONAL QUALITY OF VEGETARIAN DIETS

While the nutritional quality of the foods eaten by lacto-ovo vegetarians is quite high and almost on par nutritionally with that eaten by those who eat red meat, the more restrictive the vegetarian diet, the more difficult it is to get the necessary nutrients. In cases of vegans, the diet must be very carefully planned so that athletes can get their full quota of high quality protein and other macro and micronutrients. As the diet becomes much more restrictive (in fruitarians, for example), it becomes impossible to meet the nutritional demands of high level athletic activity.

On the other hand, if appropriately planned, vegan diets, though restrictive, can provide adequate nutrition even for competitive athletes, including those in the power sports such as bodybuilding, powerlifting, and Olympic lifting.

One of the main concerns for vegetarian athletes is to obtain enough high quality protein in their diets to meet their increased protein needs. Protein deficiencies may be more of a problem with vegans than with lacto-ovo vegetarians who eat eggs, milk, yogurt, cheese, and other dairy foods, since these foods are excellent sources of high quality protein, but this can be accomplished if they choose wisely among the various plant proteins.

The key for strict vegetarians or vegans is to eat a variety of grains that have complementary amino acids. For example, beans and rice are an example of mixing legumes (peas and beans) and grains. Also, tofu is an excellent addition to a vegetarian diet. Tofu is a high-quality plant protein that contains all essential amino acids and offers the bonus of phytochemicals that protect against heart disease and cancer.

Vegetarian Food Guide — Four Basic Foods Groups

It's not difficult for most people to become vegetarians. Vegetarian foods make up much of the U.S. Department of Agriculture and Department of Health and Human Services' Food Guide

Pyramid, which recommends 6 to 11 daily servings of bread, cereal, rice, and pasta. Daily intakes advised for other foods are: 3 to 5 servings of vegetables; 2 to 4 servings of fruits; 2 to 3 servings of milk, yogurt, and cheese; and 2 to 3 servings of meat, poultry, fish, dried beans, eggs, and nuts. The guide advises using fats, oils, and sweets sparingly. Looking at the food pyramid, it's easy to see that an ovo-lacto vegetarian and even vegans (except for the dairy servings) can easily fulfill each category in the food pyramid.

For vegans, the four food groups of meat, dairy, grains, and fruits/vegetables are replaced by the four food groups of grains, legumes, vegetables, and fruits.

Let's examine these groups in more detail.

- **Whole grains**: This group includes bread, rice, pasta, hot or cold cereal, corn, millet, barley, bulgur, buckwheat groats, and tortillas. Build a meal based on a dish of whole grains as these foods are rich in fiber and other complex carbohydrates, as well as protein, B vitamins and zinc.
- **Vegetables**: Vegetables contain many nutrients such as vitamin C, beta-carotene, riboflavin and other vitamins, iron, calcium, and fiber. Dark green, leafy vegetables such as broccoli, collards, kale, mustard and turnip greens, chicory, or bok choy are especially good sources of these important nutrients. Dark yellow and orange vegetables such as carrots, winter squash, sweet potatoes, and pumpkin provide extra beta-carotene. Include generous portions of a variety of vegetables in the diet.
- **Legumes**: Beans, peas, and lentils are all good sources of fiber, protein, iron, calcium, zinc, and B vitamins. This group also includes chickpeas, beans, soymilk, tofu, tempeh, and textured vegetable protein.
- **Fruit**: Fruits are rich in fiber, vitamin C, and beta-carotene. Be sure to include at least one serving each of fruits that are high in vitamin C — citrus fruits, melons, and strawberries are all good choices. Choose whole fruit over juices, which don't contain as much healthy fiber. Juices may be preferable for those who need to take in a lot of calories but are getting enough fiber.

For lacto-ovo vegetarians, the incorporation of egg and/or milk products can make a world of difference as far as accessibility to first-quality protein and fewer problems with most micronutrient intakes.

Supplying Required Nutrients

Vegetarians who eat no meat, fish, poultry, or dairy foods face the greatest risk of nutritional deficiency. On the other hand, no matter which diet is chosen, it's important to plan that diet so that it not only matches vegetarian needs, but also provides the nutrients needed to remain healthy.

Nutrients most likely to be lacking and some non-animal sources of these nutrients are presented in Table 7.1.

Table 7.1 Possible Nutrient Deficiencies and Non-Animal-Based Food Sources

Nutrients	Food sources
Vitamin B12	Fortified soy milk and cereals
Vitamin D	Fortified margarine and sunshine
Calcium	Tofu, broccoli, seeds, nuts, kale, bok choy, legumes, greens, calcium-enriched grain products, and lime-processed tortillas
Iron	Legumes, tofu, green leafy vegetables, dried fruit, whole grains, and iron-fortified cereals and breads, especially whole wheat
Zinc	Whole grains, whole-wheat bread, legumes, nuts, and tofu

IV. NUTRITIONAL CONSIDERATIONS OF VEGETARIANS

While choosing to be a vegetarian is a personal decision, it's important to know that the vegetarian way of eating can cause some macronutrient and micronutrient deficiencies. Therefore, it is vital to realize that the decision to become a vegetarian is also accompanied by a need to learn how to eat the right foods to ensure getting a healthy share of all the necessary nutrients. It is important to know enough to create a diet with no deficiencies. The degree of care depends on the type of vegetarian diet adopted.

Being a vegetarian doesn't guarantee improved health. Depending on the type of vegetarian diet, one of the various protein supplements can be utilized and additional vitamins and minerals can be added. For instance, if dairy products are eliminated, it may be necessary to supplement the diet with calcium, magnesium, and vitamin D.

Several studies on both vegetarian men and women have shown that, compared with non-vegetarians, they ingested less calcium, iron, zinc, and vitamin B12.[4,5] Most subjects in these studies ate less than half the RDA for B12, a vitamin crucial for healthy red blood cells and nerve fibers. Since vitamin B12 is found only in animal products, such as red meat, fish, shellfish, eggs, and milk, strict vegetarians must increase their consumption of foods, such as soy milk, that are fortified with this vitamin.

French researchers caution that a strict vegan diet may lead to deficiency of important vitamins that are critical to eyesight. In a case report,[6] a French patient lost most of his eyesight resulting from following a strict vegan diet. The patient did not supplement with vitamins, leading to B12 deficiency. This vitamin is important in maintaining the health of nerves, including the optic nerve, which transmits signals from the eye to the brain. The researcher also found the patient had below normal levels of B1, B12, A, C, D, E, zinc, and selenium.

V. VEGETARIAN ATHLETES

Since vegetarian athletes need more of some of the critical nutrients, they must be especially careful that their diets fulfill these needs. Thus, as vegetarian styles of eating become more popular among athletes, the risk of poorly planned diets leading to nutrient insufficiencies and deficiencies increases. Inadequate dietary intakes of iron and zinc have been observed in athletes who have eliminated meat. Marginal iron or zinc status may adversely affect exercise performance, while frank iron or zinc deficiency definitely decreases exercise performance.

For athletes, while it is possible to obtain all essential nutrients by eating a completely plant-based diet, it requires critical planning and execution. Athletes must also learn that it's not enough to just cut meats out of the diet. These foods have many essential nutrients that are more difficult to get elsewhere. Realistically, however, it may be difficult for vegetarian athletes, especially vegans, to get the nutrients they need. Also, because vegan diets are typically high in fiber, it may be difficult to take in enough food to satisfy energy requirements.

Additionally, there are special considerations regarding age and gender of the vegetarian athlete. Amenorrhea may be more common among vegetarian than nonvegetarian female athletes.[7] Efforts to maintain normal menstrual cycles might include increasing energy and fat intake, reducing fiber, and reducing strenuous training. When vegetarian female athletes are properly nourished, especially with adequate calories, their menstrual cycle function should be comparable to that of matched non-vegetarian women.

Vegetarian diets have been shown to result in decreases in the levels of anabolic hormones even in lacto-ovo vegetarians.[8] Male endurance athletes on a lacto-ovo vegetarian diet exhibited lower total testosterone levels than those using a diet mixed with meat.[9] As well, another study showed that, in older men, the consumption of a meat-containing diet contributed to greater gains in fat-free mass and skeletal muscle mass with resistance training than did a lacto-ovo vegetarian diet.[10]

A plant-based diet facilitates high-carbohydrate intake, which can be essential to supporting prolonged exercise. A well-planned vegetarian diet can provide athletes with adequate amounts of all known nutrients, although the potential for sub-optimal iron, zinc, trace element, and protein intake exists if the diet is too restrictive.

This concern, however, exists for all athletes, vegetarian or non-vegetarian, who have poor dietary habits. Athletes who consume diets rich in fruit, vegetables, and whole grains receive high amounts of antioxidant nutrients that help reduce the oxidative stress associated with heavy exertion. Whereas athletes are most often concerned with performance, vegetarian diets also seem to provide long-term health benefits and a reduction in risk of chronic disease.

The bottom line is that, if the decision to become a vegetarian is not a choice made because of moral or ethical principles, it may be more realistic and productive for athletes to include some meat in their diet.

Common Vitamin and Mineral Deficiencies

It's important to remember that vegetarians have special nutritional needs and concerns. Thus, vegetarians must be careful to receive their daily quota of the macronutrients, essential fatty acids, and vitamins and minerals.

Because vegans don't eat dairy products or eggs, they are at higher risk for having deficiencies of calcium, vitamin B12, and vitamin D. These nutrients, while abundant in dairy products, are less available in plant sources. Calcium is found in fortified foods, green leafy vegetables, beans, and tofu products.

Vitamin D can be a problem for vegans with low sun exposure. However, exposure to the sun on limited parts of the body for 10 to 15 minutes a day is enough to supply the daily requirement of vitamin D.

Because vitamin B12 is found only in animal products, vegans must obtain it from fortified foods or from nutritional supplements. The American Dietetic Association strongly recommends supplement use to ensure the proper quantity of B12.

VI. SPECIFIC NUTRITIONAL NEEDS OF VEGETARIANS

Lack of calories is common with vegans because of the bulk of food that must be consumed, since plant foods are generally less dense calorically and a lot of fiber is consumed. Additionally, lacto-ovo vegetarians and vegans can face some nutrient deficiencies.

Getting enough dietary protein is generally not a problem with lacto-ovo vegetarians because both eggs and dairy products are nutritionally dense and contain first-quality protein. However, vegans, especially those who exercise vigorously or take part in sports, have to be extremely careful in planning their diets so as to supply enough energy, since plant foods tend to be nutritionally less dense. Also, vegans have to mix proteins so that an overall amino acid balance is achieved.

Considering the importance of dietary protein, especially for athletes, this topic deserves in-depth attention.

A. Protein

The quantity of protein in the diets of athletes, while important, is rarely a concern, regardless of whether they are meat eaters or non-meat eaters. Increased dietary intake can be accomplished easily by both choosing high protein foods or by supplementing with protein powders, Nevertheless, the quality of protein can pose a problem. Well-processed soybean protein is equal in quality to animal protein. However, other legumes do not contain a full complement of the essential amino acids required for the efficient manufacture of protein by the human body.

Previous vegetarian dietary guidelines recommended that a variety of plant protein sources (such as grains and beans) be combined simultaneously at one meal to complement each other and provide a complete protein source. Current research supports the notion that by eating a variety of legumes, as well as all other food groups throughout the day, one can obtain the full array of essential amino acids required for efficient protein metabolism.

Thus, by combining various plant proteins and making use of soybean protein, most vegetarians can easily get an adequate level of dietary protein. Vegetarian athletes, on the other hand, may find that combining complementary proteins at one meal may be beneficial.

Ensuring Adequate and High Quality Protein

The mixture of proteins from grains, legumes, seeds, nuts, and vegetables provides a complement of amino acids, enabling deficits in one food to be made up by another. At present, it is felt that, for most vegetarians, not all types of plant foods need to be eaten at the same meal, since the amino acids are combined in the body's protein pool.

In general, proteins of animal origin contain adequate amounts of the essential amino acids and hence, they are known as first-class proteins. On the other hand, many proteins of vegetable origin are relatively deficient in certain amino acids, notably lysine and the sulfur-containing amino acids. However, soy protein has been shown to be nutritionally equivalent in protein value to proteins of animal origin and, thus, can serve as the sole source of protein intake if desired.

The essential amino acid lysine is consistently at a much lower concentration in all major plant-food protein groups than in animal foods. Since lysine is the limiting amino acid, the addition of limited amounts of lysine to cereal diets improves their protein quality. Studies in Peru and Guatemala have demonstrated that growing children benefited by this addition.[11] In addition, the sulfur-containing amino acids are distinctly lower in legumes and fruits, and threonine is lower in cereals than in proteins of animal origin.

Complementary Proteins

There are important differences among and between food products of vegetable and animal origin, including the concentrations of proteins and indispensable amino acids they contain. The concentration and quality of the protein in some foods of vegetable origin may be too low to make them adequate as sole sources of proteins. In some of the poorer parts of the world, diets are based predominantly on a single plant (e.g. corn), and they frequently lead to malnutrition.

Foods of plant origin contain many amino acids, but single food items usually do not contain all the essential amino acids in adequate amounts to support good health. Vegetarian diets are planned so that the amino acid content is adequate to support good nutritional health. Amino acids are the building blocks of protein, the nutrient that is supplied in the greatest quantity by meat, fish, poultry, eggs, milk, and cheese. The mainstays of strict vegetarian diets, vegetables, whole grains, legumes, nuts, and seeds, which do not contain an optimal balance of essential amino acids when eaten separately. Therefore, the vegetarian must combine foods that complement each other, thus providing the body with the right amino acid mix. Mixtures of plant proteins can serve as a complete and well-balanced source of amino acids for meeting human physiological requirements.[12] However, combining the right foods is necessary to obtain the necessary levels of both the essential or indispensable and conditionally indispensable amino acids. The addition of eggs and/or dairy products with meals or snacks greatly improves the overall protein quality of the vegetarian diet.

Fortunately, the amino acid deficiencies in a protein can usually be improved by combining it with another so that the mixture of the two proteins will often have a higher food value than either one alone. For example, many cereals are low in lysine, but high in methionine and cysteine. On the other hand, soybeans, lima beans, and kidney beans are high in lysine but low in methionine and cysteine. When eaten together, these types of proteins give a more favorable amino acid profile.

Rice, the staple food for more than half of the world's population, is inadequate in its amino acid content when it is the sole protein source, but when combined with another type of plant protein such as legumes, a complete protein mixture is formed. A mixture of red beans or black-eyed peas and rice is an example of complementary protein foods, as is a peanut butter sandwich (peanuts are legumes while the wheat of the bread is a grain). Other examples are corn tortillas with refried beans, and tofu with fried rice.

Soybeans, which are low in sulfur-containing amino acids, can be combined with cottonseed, peanut and sesame flour, and cereal grains, which are deficient mainly in lysine. In general, oil-seed proteins, in particular, soy protein, can be used effectively in combination with most cereal grains to improve the overall quality of the total protein intake. A combination of soy protein, which is high in lysine, with a cereal that contains a relatively good concentration of sulfur-containing amino acids results in a nutritional complementation; the protein quality of the mixture is greater than that for either protein source alone.

Nutritional Responses to Combining Two Dietary Proteins

Various nutritional responses are observed when two dietary proteins are combined. These have been classified by Bressani et al.[13] into one of four types.

1. No protein complementary effect is achieved. For example, this occurs with combinations of peanuts and corn, where each of the protein sources has a common and quantitatively similar lysine deficiency and both are also deficient in other amino acids.
2. Combinations are made of two protein sources that have the same limited amino acid, but in quantitatively different amounts. Corn and cottonseed flour, for example, are both limited in lysine, but cottonseed is relatively less inadequate than is corn.
3. A true complementary combination, because there is a synergistic effect on the overall nutritive value of the protein mixture; the protein quality of the best mix exceeds that of each component alone. This type of response occurs when one of the protein sources has a considerably higher concentration of the most limiting amino acid in the other protein. An example of this response is observed when corn and soy flour are mixed so that 60% of the protein intake comes from corn and the remainder from soy protein.
4. Both protein sources have a common amino acid deficiency. The protein component giving the highest value is the one containing a higher concentration of the deficient amino acid. Combinations of some textured soy proteins and beef protein follow this type of response.

These nutritional relationships have been determined from rat bioassay studies. However, the more limited results available from human studies with soy and other legumes confirm the applicability of this general concept in human nutrition. This knowledge helps to understand and evaluate how nutritionally effective combinations of plant protein foods can be achieved.

Even when combinations of plant protein foods are used, there is still the concern of timing of ingestion of complementary proteins. Is there a need to ingest different plant proteins at the same time, or within the same meal, to achieve maximum benefit and nutritional value from proteins with different, but complementary, amino acid patterns? This concern may also extend to the need to ingest a significant amount of protein at each meal, or whether it is sufficient to consume protein in variable amounts at different meals and even different days, as long as the average daily intake meets or exceeds the recommended or safe protein intakes.

According to FAO/WHO/UNU,[14] estimates of protein requirements refer to metabolic needs that persist over moderate periods of time. However, the body does not store much protein outside of a scant free amino acid pool, and begins certain catabolic processes in the post-absorptive phase (after a meal) making the ingestion of regular amounts of protein critical for maximizing the anabolic effects of exercise.

There is a limited database that we can consult to make a definitive conclusion on the timing of consumption of complementary proteins or of specific amino acid supplements for proteins that are deficient in one or more amino acids. Earlier work in rapidly growing rats suggested that delaying the supplementation of a protein with its limiting amino acid reduces the value of the supplement.[15,16] Similarly, the frequency of feeding of diets supplemented with lysine in growing pigs affects the overall efficiency of utilization of dietary protein.[17] Studies in human adults showed that overall dietary protein utilization was similar whether the daily protein intake was distributed among two or three meals.[18,19]

In general, especially under conditions where intakes of total protein are high, it may not be necessary to consume complementary proteins at the same time. Separation of the proteins among meals over the course of a day would still permit the nutritional benefits of complementation.

However, in athletes trying to maximize protein synthesis and muscular hypertrophy, it is necessary to have a full complement of amino acids present for every meal to maximize the anabolic effects of exercise. With the presence of the full complement of amino acids, there is a meal-related decrease in proteolysis and increase in protein synthesis.[20]

The decrease in whole-body proteolysis is closely associated with the rise in plasma insulin concentrations following meal ingestion. This suggests that the transition from tissue catabolism to anabolism is the result, at least in part, of decreased whole-body proteolysis. This meal-related decrease in proteolysis is independent of the dietary amino acid composition or content. In contrast, the rate of protein synthesis was sustained only when the meal complete in all amino acids was provided, indicating a predominant control of protein synthesis by amino acid availability. Therefore, it appears important for athletes to consume meals that contain an optimal mixture of amino acids.

B. Fats

Lower levels of fats in most plant foods can result in impaired endurance performance. This takes in includes plant oils containing monosaturated fatty acids such as olive oil, and polysaturated fatty acids such as many of the seed oils.

Essential Fatty Acids

This is an essential fat in the diet. Omega-3 fats are associated with lower risks of heart disease due to their anti-blood-clotting effects. Omega-3 fatty acid deficiency is only a concern to vegetarians if foods such as tofu, nuts, and seeds are excluded from the diet.

Diets that do not include fish or eggs lack the long-chain n-3 fatty acid docosahexanoic acid (DHA). Lack of some of the essential fatty acids, especially DHA and EPA, can be made up in part by consuming more alpha-linolenic acid from vegetable oils, especially flax oil. On the other hand, because of limited formation of DHA and EPA from alpha-linolenic acid, the use of DHA and EPA supplements is a common practice among athletes.

C. Fiber

Vegetarian diets are generally high in both soluble and insoluble fiber. A small amount of soluble fiber before or during exercise may be beneficial by preventing rapid highs and lows in blood sugar. However, some athletes are sensitive to fiber before exercise, especially major competitions. If stomach or intestinal cramps, or diarrhea are experienced before exercise, limiting high fiber foods such as legumes, whole grain products, bran products, and dried fruit in the meal preceding exercise may eliminate this distress. Sensitive athletes may need to reduce their fiber intake 24 to 36 hours before competition. Regular meal times and bowel habits also prevent exercise-induced intestinal complications.

It is also important to consider that adequate fiber intake is easily met and often exceeded by vegetarian athletes who have high calorie intakes. Sometimes, trying to eat a high calorie diet containing excess fiber can cause discomfort. Cyclists, for example, participating in a simulated Tour de France had difficulty maintaining adequate energy intake of 8,000 to 10,000 calories when whole grains and high fiber food were selected.[21] Therefore, those athletes with high calorie intakes should not be overly concerned about fiber and should select a variety of high carbohydrate foods that are low in fiber (white bread, pasta, white rice, potatoes without skin, and fruit juice).

D. Minerals

While the macronutrients may not pose much of a problem for vegetarians, there can be problems with some of the micronutrients, especially certain vitamins and minerals. The "usual suspects" are iron and zinc for all vegetarians; calcium, vitamin B12, and vitamin D for vegans.

Micronutrients are important for building and repairing of body tissues, blood, energy production, healthy bones, and an adequate immune system. Prolonged restricted diets often bring about inadequate micronutrient intake and status. This can ultimately result in bone loss, anemia, impaired immune function, poor athletic performance, and reduced recovery from injuries.

Iron

Iron deficiency is likely the most common problem seen in vegetarians. Vegetarian diets reduce the availability of iron even if it is adequately supplied in the food. That's because non-meat sources of iron (nonheme iron) are not efficiently absorbed. Also, many vegetarians aren't meticulous about planning their meals.

The bottom line is that, although dietary intake of iron is typically above recommended amounts in vegetarians, serum ferritin concentrations and other iron-status indicators are often lower than those in nonvegetarians.[22]

Iron deficiency can lead to anemia and as such can seriously affect athletic performance. Women of childbearing age and teenagers have higher iron requirements and are particularly at risk. In addition, many women are continually on a weight reduction diet, which further compounds their deficiencies.

In addition to iron lost in sweat, women also lose iron through menstruation. Twenty to 30% of average American women may be deficient in iron stores in the body. Female athletes represent a higher number, up to 60%.

Even though many women may have adequate dietary iron intake, most of their iron comes from foods that contain a form of iron that has low availability in the body. These foods may be breakfast cereals and bars, fat-free and low-fat snacks, or other foods that contain high fiber. Some foods, such as legumes, contain compounds (phytates) that bind iron in the gut and prevent it from being absorbed. Fruits enhance the absorption and availability of iron. For vegetarians, it's best to take some fruit or supplemental vitamin C with the recommended daily iron supplement.

Zinc

Zinc is another mineral that can be in short supply for vegetarians. As with iron, zinc is not as readily available from plant-based foods as from meats. Zinc bioavailability from some plant sources is limited by their contents of fiber and/or phytates. Although fractional absorption of zinc from plant-based diets can be similar to that from animal sources, the low zinc content of plant foods tends to result in a low net absorption and, as such, low total intake.

Zinc is an essential trace mineral that is important for insulin and enzyme formation and function, immune system function, and in protein synthesis and carbohydrate metabolism. Deficiencies are common due to zinc-depleted soils and food processing. In athletes, zinc is lost during sweating and in the urine.

Zinc, which is needed for a strong immune system, is found almost exclusively in meat, although oysters are an especially rich source. An exception is whole grains; however, once they are refined they lose their zinc content. Wheat germ is one of the best zinc sources; and adding a tablespoon or two to hot cereals, casseroles, soups, or blender drinks can increase zinc intake.

Calcium

Adequate dietary calcium is a prerequisite for maximizing peak bone mass during the first three decades of life and for minimizing subsequent bone loss. Although many nutrients are important to bone health, calcium requires the most attention because it is the nutrient most likely to be deficient.

Taking in adequate amounts of dietary calcium can be a problem for everyone, but more so for those vegetarians who don't consume dairy products. For most of us, the liberal consumption of dairy products in the diet does the job.

Some plants provide absorbable calcium, but the quantity of vegetables required to reach sufficient calcium intake make an exclusively plant-based diet impractical for most individuals unless fortified foods or supplements are included.

The low calcium content of common plant sources, including most vegetables, fruit, and cereal grains, makes it difficult for most Americans to meet their requirements exclusively from these foods, even when the bioavailability of calcium from these sources is high and the larger serving sizes consumed by many vegetarians are taken into account. Therefore, it is prudent for individuals who choose not to eat dairy products to include calcium-fortified foods or supplements in their diet, with the possible exception of those rare individuals who carefully plan their diet around plant foods.

If calcium supplements are substituted for dairy products to meet calcium needs, attention to other nutrients may be needed because low calcium intakes have been associated with low intakes of magnesium and several vitamins, including riboflavin, B-6, B-12, and thiamin.

Calcium bioavailability from plant foods can be affected by their contents of oxalate and phytate, which are inhibitors of calcium absorption content. In general, calcium absorption is inversely proportional to the oxalic acid content of the food. Thus, calcium bioavailability is low from both American and Chinese varieties of spinach and rhubarb, intermediate from sweet potatoes, and high from low-oxalate vegetables such as kale, broccoli, and bok choy. A notable exception to this generalization is soybeans. Soybeans are rich in both oxalate and phytate, yet soy products have relatively high calcium bioavailability. In contrast, common dried beans, which are also rich in phytate, have substantially lower calcium bioavailability. Chinese vegetables (except for Chinese spinach) and calcium-set tofu are unusually rich sources of bioavailable calcium.

Calcium can be obtained from foods that are naturally rich in calcium, from fortified foods and beverages, from supplements, or from a combination of these sources. Calcium sources should be evaluated on the basis of both content and bioavailability of calcium.

Consumption of adequate dietary calcium can be accomplished within a variety of tastes and lifestyle choices. For most individuals in a western culture, liberal consumption of dairy products is the easiest approach and is the least restrictive with regard to consumption of protein, salt, or caffeine. On the other hand, those who choose to meet their calcium needs completely from plant sources need to be aware of not only the calcium content of plants but also the bioavailability of the calcium because other plant constituents can impede calcium absorption.

Also, depending on the protein and sodium content of the vegetarian diet, the calciuretic effect of a plant-based diet may not differ significantly from that of an omnivorous diet. It is important for those consuming diets free of animal products and others who avoid dairy products to adjust the protein and sodium content of their diets to maximize bone mass, or to use calcium-fortified foods or supplements.

E. Vitamins

Vegans risk vitamin B12 deficiency, which can result in irreversible nerve deterioration. The need for vitamin B12 increases during pregnancy, breast-feeding, and periods of growth. As well, elderly people should be especially cautious about adopting vegetarian diets because their bodies may absorb vitamin B12 poorly. Ovo-vegetarians and vegans may also have inadequate amounts of vitamin D.

Studies show that those using a vegetarian diet maintain higher antioxidant vitamin status (vitamin C, vitamin E, beta-carotene) than those using a predominantly meat-based diet.[23] These vitamins are derived from consumption of many carbohydrate-rich plant foods such as fruits and vegetables, cereals, legumes, and nuts.

VII. NUTRITIONAL SUPPLEMENTS AND THE VEGETARIAN ATHLETE

The most useful nutritional supplements for vegetarians are those in which they may be marginally deficient. Also, like most athletes, they would benefit by increasing dietary protein with the use of high quality soy protein for vegans and with one or more of whey, casein, egg, and soy protein in ovo-lacto vegetarians. There are also other nutritional supplements, such as creatine and some of the amino acids, which may be useful for enhancing performance.

There is one caveat to using nutritional supplements. Vegetarians need to carefully examine the ingredients of the various nutritional supplements to make sure they don't contain any of the ingredients that are not on their food list. For example, many meal replacement powders use a combination of soy and milk proteins. Also, there are many vitamin supplements that do not contain animal products.

Considering that many vegetarian diets exclude dairy foods, it is important to ensure adequate intake of calcium, as well as iron, riboflavin, and vitamin D. To make up for possible calcium deficiencies in these diets, calcium supplements should be used by all vegan athletes, especially women and children. Extra calcium should also be taken by vegan women during pregnancy and when breast-feeding.

A high quality vitamin supplement should be included in a vegetarian diet. This would include vitamin D, which may be needed if sunlight exposure is limited, since sunlight activates a substance in the skin and converts it into vitamin D. Vegan diets should include a reliable source of vitamin B_{12} because this nutrient occurs only in animal foods. Vitamin B12 deficiency can result in irreversible nerve deterioration.

If a diet is low in essential fatty acids, 1 tsp of flax seed oil or 2 Tbsp canola/soybean oil may be added to the diet.

Some supplements normally found in abundance in red meat may be OK for vegetarians to use since these supplements are synthesized and so contain no animal products. An example of this would be creatine monohydrate, although it is necessary to ascertain that the creatine mixes contain no added nutrients that may be of animal origin.

Creatine

The estimated daily need for creatine in humans is about 2 g, whereas the daily intake from meat and/or fish is about 1 g in the average American diet. The body makes up the deficit by producing creatine in the liver, kidney, and pancreas, using glycine and arginine as precursors. When dietary supply is low, the body steps up its production of creatine, but may not completely compensate, especially among vegetarians, who have a reduced body creatine pool.

Creatine stores vary greatly among individuals, and, apart from diet, the reasons are unclear. Athletes with low stores might be most apt to benefit from supplementation. Creatine supplementation of 20 g per day for at least 3 days has resulted in significant increases in total Cr for some individuals but not others, suggesting that there are "responders" and "nonresponders." These increases in total concentration among responders is greatest in individuals who have the lowest initial total Cr, such as vegetarians.[24]

On average, muscle creatine levels increase an average of 20% after 6 days of supplementing at 20 g/day ("rapid creatine loading"). These higher levels can be maintained by ingesting as low as 2 g/day thereafter. A similar, but slower, 20% rise in muscle creatine levels occurs by ingesting 3 g/day for 1 month, the "no-load" method.

The use of nutritional supplements and certain foods in and around training can maximize the anabolic effects of exercise and make a significant difference in an athlete's degree of lean body mass and strength. These supplements include:

- The amino acids, including the branched-chain amino acids, glutamine, and arginine, used both before and during training
- The ephedra, caffeine, aspirin stack prior to training
- Post-exercise meal replacement supplement used within an hour of training

VIII. CONCLUSIONS AND RECOMMENDATIONS

While the nutritional quality of the foods eaten by lacto-ovo vegetarians is quite high and almost on par with that eaten by the rest of society, the more restrictive the vegetarian diet, the more difficult it is to get the nutrients needed. In cases of vegans, the diet must be very carefully planned so that athletes can get their full quota of high quality protein and other macro and micronutrients. As the diet becomes much more restrictive (in fruitarians for example), it becomes impossible to meet the nutritional demands of high level athletic activity.

Vegetarian athletes, by carefully planning their diets, can meet their nutritional needs, although the vegetarian diet may not be the best diet for these athletes. The areas of concern, covered in this chapter, are protein and fat intake as far as the macronutrients, micronutrients, or iron and zinc, and, for those who are vegans, calcium, vitamin B12, and vitamin D.

However, the key to any healthful diet — vegetarian or non-vegetarian — is adherence to sound nutrition principles. It's important for the vegetarian diet to include many different foods, since no one food contains all the nutrients required for good health. The wider the variety, the greater the chance of getting the nutrients needed. With a plant-based daily diet, eating a variety of foods and sufficient calories for energy needs will help ensure adequate intakes of necessary macro- and micronutrients.

With the array of fruits, vegetables, grains, and spices available in U.S. grocery stores and the availability of vegetarian cookbooks, it's easy to devise tasty vegetarian dishes utilizing a variety of foods including whole grains, vegetables, fruits, legumes, nuts, seeds and, if allowed, dairy products and eggs.

There's much to learn about vegetarians and the vegetarian way of life. The more you know the better prepared you will be in handling your special needs, especially if exercise and sports are part of your way of life. Although, for most vegetarians, the basic fundamentals of proper nutrition can easily be mastered, there is still the basic concern that a vegetarian diet, especially a strict vegan one, is not the best diet for most competitive athletes.

While a well-crafted vegan diet may supply all the vitamins, minerals, carbohydrates, protein, and fluids normally required, it may not be the optimal diet for a high level athlete. Therefore, unless there are moral or religious reasons to contend with, athletes, specifically power athletes, should include egg and milk products in their diets, and, if possible, red meat.

REFERENCES

1. Gillman, M.W., Cupples, L.A., and Gagnon, D., et al. Protective effects of fruits and vegetables on development of stroke in men. *JAMA* 1995; 273(14): 1113-1117.
2. Manson, J.E., Willett, W.C., and Stampfer, M.J., et al.: Vegetable and fruit consumption and incidence of stroke in women, abstract. *Circulation* 1994; 89(2):932.
3. Slattery, M.L., Benson, J., Curtin, K., Ma, K.N, Schaeffer D, and Potter, J.D. Carotenoids and colon cancer. *Am J Clin Nutr* 2000; 71(2):575-82.
4. Alexander, D., Ball, M.J., and Mann, J., Nutrient intake and haematological status of vegetarians and age-sex matched omnivores, *Eur. J. Clin, Nutr.*, 1994, 48(8): 538-46.
5. Helman, A.D. and Darnton-Hill, I. Vitamin and iron status in new vegetarians. *Am J Clin Nutr* 1987; 45(4):785-9
6. Milea, D., Cassoux, N., and LeHoang, P. Blindness in a strict vegan. *N Engl J Med* 2000; 23;342(12):897-8
7. Barnard, N.D., Scialli, A.R., Hurlock, D., Bertron, P. Diet and sex-hormone binding globulin, dysmenorrhea, and premenstrual symptoms. *Obstet Gynecol* 2000; 95(2):245-50.
8. Dupont, A, Prevost, J; Caron, S; and Sevigny, J. Influence of diet on plasma steroids and sex hormone-binding globulin levels in adult men. Belanger, A., Locong, A., Noel, C. and Cusan, L.; *J Steroid Biochem* 1989, 32 (6) 829-33.
9. Raben, A., Kiens, B., and Richter, E.A, et al. Serum sex hormones and endurance performance after a lacto-ovo vegetarian and a mixed diet. *Med Sci Sports Exerc* 1992;24(11):1290-97.
10. Campbell, W.W., Barton, M.L., Jr, Cyr-Campbell, D., Davey, S.L., Beard, J.L., Parise, G., and Evans, W.J. Effects of an omnivorous diet compared with a lacto-ovo vegetarian diet on resistance-training-induced changes in body composition and skeletal muscle in older men. *Am J Clin Nutr* 1999;70(6):1032-9.
11. Graham, G.G., Lembcke, J., Lancho, E., and Morales, E. Quality protein maize: digestibility and utilization by recovering malnourished infants. *Pediatrics* 1989; 83(3);416-21.
12. Young, V.R. and Pellett, P.L. Plant proteins in relation to human protein and amino acid nutrition. *Am. J. Clinic. Nutr. 1994* 59(5 Suppl):1203S-1212S.
13. Bressani, R, Elias L.G., and Gomez Brenes, R.A.. Improvement of protein quality by amino acid and protein supplementation. In: Bigwood, E.J., Ed. *Protein and Amino Acid Functions*. Vol. 11. Oxford, UK: Pergamon Press, 1972; 475-540.
14. Food and Agriculture Organization/World Health Organization/United Nations University. Energy and protein requirements. Report of joint FAO/WHO/UNU expert consultation. Geneva: World Health Organization. 1985. (WHO Tech rep ser no. 724)
15. Geiger, E. The role of the time factor in feeding supplementary proteins. *J. Nutr.* 1948; 36:813-9.
16. Geiger, E. Experiments with delayed supplementation of incomplete amino acid mixtures. *J. Nutr.* 1947; 34:97-111.
17. Batterham, E.S., O'Neill, G.H. The effect of frequency of feeding on the response by growing pigs to supplements of free lysine. *Br. J. Nutr.* 1978;39:265-70.
18. Taylor, Y.S.M., Young, V.R., Murray, E., Pencharz, P.B., and Scrimshaw, N.S. Daily protein and meal patterns affecting young men fed adequate and restricted energy intakes. *Am J Clin Nutr* 1973; 26:1216-22.

19. Scrimshaw, N.S., Behar, M., Wilson, D., Viteri, F., Arroyave, G., and Bressani, R. *American Journal of Clinical Nutrition*, Volume 9, 1961: All-vegetable protein mixtures for human feeding. *Nutrition Reviews* 1989; 47(11):346-9.
20. Nissen, S. and Haymond, M.W. Changes in leucine kinetics during meal absorption: effects of dietary leucine availability. *Am. J. Physiol.* 1986; 250(6 Pt 1):E695-701.
21. Brouns, F., Saris, W.H., Stroecken, J., Beckers, E., Thijssen, R., Rehrer, N.J., and ten Hoor, F. Eating, drinking, and cycling. A controlled Tour de France simulation study, Parts I and II. *Int J Sports Med* 1989;10 Suppl 1:S32-48
22. Haddad, E.H., Berk, L.S., Kettering, J.D., Hubbard, R.W., and Peters, W.R. Dietary intake and biochemical, hematologic, and immune status of vegans compared with nonvegetarians.*Am. J. Clin. Nutr.* 1999; 70(3 Suppl):586S-593S.
23. Rauma, A.L., and Mykkanen, H. Antioxidant status in vegetarians versus omnivores. *Nutrition* 2000 Feb;16(2):111-9.
24. Demant, T.W. and Rhodes, E.C. Effects of creatine supplementation on exercise performance. *Sports Med.* 1999; 28(1):4960.

CHAPTER 8

Nutritional Concerns of Physically Disabled Athletes

Jayanthi Kandiah

CONTENTS

I. INTRODUCTION

In the U.S. alone, as many as 2–3 million athletes with disabilities compete annually in recreational and organized sports.[1-3] The range of activities for these athletes includes badminton, athletics, archery, basketball, bocce, cycling, fencing, swimming, kayaking, lawn bowling, shooting, table tennis, tennis, volleyball, water polo, weight lifting, and skiing.[4] Athletes who train regularly and compete for 1 or more hours per day have nutritional needs that go beyond those of a nonathlete. An athlete's ability to perform is dictated not only by the type of sport, duration of the activity, and type of muscles utilized, but also by the diet.

Although the Special Olympics and Paralympic Games have been actively involved in encouraging and hosting international competitions for developmentally disabled athletes, there is still insufficient nutrition research available on developmentally disabled athletes.[5-8] The present review will discuss health and nutritional concerns of two groups of physically disabled athletes, namely, competitive athletes with cerebral palsy and spinal cord injury.

0-8493-8199-?/00/$0.00+$.50

II. GENERAL HEALTH CONSIDERATIONS FOR THE DISABLED

The limited mobility brought about by either functional (neuromuscular dysfunction, poor body- or motor control) or environmental situations, oftentimes places athletes with cerebral palsy (CP), vision impairment, spinal cord injury (SI), and amputations at a higher risk for cardiovascular disease,[9-12] obesity,[13] osteoporosis,[14,15] and malnutrition.[16] Nutrient deficiencies and mortality are further aggravated in this population when disabled athletes have complexity in feeding, communication, metabolic disorders, altered growth patterns, or drug-nutrient interactions and inappropriate care.

III. NUTRITIONAL CONCERNS OF ATHLETES WITH CEREBRAL PALSY

Two major medical classifications of CP observed among individuals are spastic and athetoid CP. The majority (70%) have a tendency to have spastic CP, where the muscles are taut, causing limited activity. Twenty to 30% have athetoid CP, where the muscles are in constant motion and muscle movements increases under stressful and emotional situations.[17] Based on the differences in medical classifications and level of physical activity, energy needs vary between spastic and athetoid CP. Obesity is often an issue with nonambulatory spastic individuals, while an increase in energy requirement is observed in athetoid CP.[18] If CP individuals are on drug therapy that causes lethargy and lesser motor activity, caloric needs are further altered. Since physical growth varies from one type of CP to another, energy recommendations are based on kcal/cm height.[17] Continuous involuntary movement in athetosis has been shown to increase resting metabolic rate by approximately 500 kcal/d (2100 kJ).[18]

Due to the unavailability of reference standards for the assessment of anthropometrics in CP athletes, a combination of measurements are in use and comparisons are made with norms developed for healthy individuals.[18-20] Because of a multitude of factors, CP athletes are more susceptible to major metabolic bone diseases such as osteopenia and fractures. Kandiah[5] found that, from a pool of 19 Paralympic CP athletes, 63% consumed an average of less than 800 mg calcium/day. Mean daily intake of calcium in female CP athletes ranged from 446–638 mg/day.[5] In a more recent study by Kandiah,[8] female CP athletes had not only low dietary intake of calcium, but also of zinc, folate, and iron. Decreased consumption of milk, abstinence from animal foods, which provide heme-iron, and limited intake of dark green leafy vegetables were the prime contributors of nutrient deficiencies. Additionally, elite Paralympic CP swimmers and track and field athletes had greater than 30% of their total calories from fat, with saturated fat contributing 14% and 12% in diets of males and females, respectively.[8]

IV. NUTRITIONAL CONCERNS OF ATHLETES WITH SPINAL CORD INJURY (WHEEL CHAIR ATHLETES)

Spinal cord injury (SCI) is categorized by level of the injury to the spinal cord nerve roots, which may necessitate wheel chair confinement. Although reference standards for the assessment of anthropometrics in SCP are nonexistent, knee height measurements are frequently used to estimate body height, and sling chair or wheelchairs (weight of equipment subtracted) to estimate weight.

Because of decreased activity and the risk of cardiovascular diseases in newly diagnosed SCI athletes, researchers suggest initial reduction of dietary fat to less than 20% of total calories.[4,21] With regular endurance activity and an increase in high-density lipoprotein levels, composition of the diet should be 20% fat, 68% carbohydrate, and 12% protein. Of the 20% of caloric intake consumed as fat, 15% should be from mono- and polyunsaturated fats, with only 5% from saturated fat.[21]

Besides cardiovascular disease, SCI athletes commonly experience osteoporosis that may stem from high dietary intake of fat, increased excretion of urinary calcium associated with decreased activity, and long-term immobilization of the lower extremities.[19] Because poor mobility of the lower extremities makes the athlete vulnerable to fractures from minor trauma or muscle spasms, adequate dietary calcium intake should be recommended and wheelchairs should be well padded. Since SCI athletes retain increased concentrations of calcium in their kidneys and bladder that can result in renal stones, selection of a calcium supplement is of utmost importance. Rice et al.,[14] showed calcium citrate malate to be a more bioavailable calcium source than any other calcium supplement.[14] Other nutrient deficiencies observed among the SCI population are iron, vitamin C, beta carotene, thiamin, copper, and folate.[23]

V. SPECIAL MEDICAL CONDITIONS

Athletes with physical disabilities experience similar types of injuries as able-bodied athletes. Common injuries include muscle strains, lacerations, elbow tendinitis, upper respiratory tract infections, and blisters.[1,24-27] Burnham[25] reported that 23% of all wheelchair athletes are prone to shoulder injuries and carpel tunnel syndrome.[25] Most of the above mentioned injuries can be prevented with proper training techniques; efficient biomechanics; the use of appropriate protective clothing, padding, and equipment; proper acclimatization strategies; good nutrition, and adequate hydration.[28]

Besides injuries, special medical conditions (e.g., cardiac concerns, hypo- and hyperthermia, and drug–nutrient interactions) pose the most risk for athletes with disabilities. Compared with other athletes, those with SCI have higher heart rates and lower blood pressure.[29] According to investigators[27, 30] athletes can improve their blood pressure and race time through a process referred to as autonomic dysreflexia (AD).[27,30] AD is extremely dangerous, as it is usually caused by a distended bladder, an infection, or an obstructed colon. When stressors like dehydration, fatigue, anxiety, or illness are coupled with AD, the situation frequently results in the death of the athlete.

Unlike CP athletes, SCI individuals with spinal lesions above the sixth thoracic level (T6) are more sensitive to temperature regulation disorders, dehydration, severe osteoroposis, and development of pressure sores.[31] Depending on the intensity and duration of the activity, thermoregulatory dysfunction caused by hypo- or hyperthermia, dehydration, gastrointestinal disorders, and bladder infections in SCI and CP athletes could be overcome by proper use of attire, replacement of fluids, nutrients, and electrolytes.[32,33]

Use of prescription drugs is a common occurrence in CP and SCI athletes. Many of the medications have mild to severe side effects that can either interfere with proper nutrition or complicate and exacerbate existing conditions.[3] For example, long-term usage of anticonvulsant drugs for the treatment of seizures in CP athletes causes constipation; osteomalacia, megaloblastic anemia, and hypertrophy of the gums. In SCI athletes, prescribed skeletal muscle relaxants or use of over-the-counter anti-inflammatory medications such as ibuprofen and aspirin may lead to renal damage and intestinal distress. Other medications (e.g., antibiotics) may cause less severe side effects such as nausea, vomiting, anorexia, and dry mouth in both CP and SCI athletes.

VI. CONCLUSIONS

In spite of the many functional and environmental limitations, physically disabled athletes are a very dedicated group of individuals whose eating habits are not unique. Unfortunately, at the present time, there are no reference standards for the assessment of anthropometrics, hardly any research on the relationship between nutrition and performance, and only some research on quality strength and conditioning. Although there is limited research on drug nutrient interactions, extensive research in all areas is warranted so that specific recommendations can be made to enhance athletic performance in this population.

REFERENCES

1. Ferrara, M.S., Buckley, W.E., McCann, B.C., Limbird, T.J., Powell, J.W., and Robol, R., The injury experience of the competitive athlete with disability: Prevention implications, *Med. Sci. Sports Exerc.*, 24, 184, 1992.
2. Laskowski, E.R., Strength training in the physically challenged population, *Strength Cond.*, 16, 66, 1994.
3. Stopka, C.B., An overview of common injuries to individuals with disabilities, *Palaestra*, 12, 44, 1996.
4. DePauw, K.P., and Gavron, S.J., Sport opportunities for athletes with disabilities, *Disability and Sport*, Human Kinetics, Champaign, IL, 1995.
5. Kandiah, J., Calcium and iron intakes of disabled elite athletes, in *Sports Nutrition—Minerals and Electrolytes*, Kies, C. and Driskell, J.A., Eds., CRC Press, Boca Raton, FL, 1995, chap.9.
6. Kandiah, J., Nutritional assessment of paralympic athletes with cerebral palsy, *FASEB J.*, A489, 1996.
7. Kandiah, J., Dietary intake and nutrition knowledge of elite disabled athletes, *INFORM-AOCS*, #94, Denver, CO, 1993.
8. Kandiah, J., Nutritional assessment of US paralympic athletes with cerebral palsy. *Int. J. Biosocial Med. Res.*, 95, 145, 1996.
9. Gisler, W.O., Jousse, A.T., Wynne-Jones, M., and Breithaupt, D., Survival in traumatic spinal cord injury, *Paraplegia*, 21, 364, 1983.
10. LaPorte, R.E., Brenes, G., and Dearwater, S., HDL cholesterol across a spectrum of physical activity from quadriplegia to marathon running, *Lancet*, 1, 1212, 1983.
11. Lee, C.T., and Price, M., Survival from spinal cord injury, *J. Chronic. Dis.*, 35, 487, 1982.
12. United States Committee on Veterans Administration Affairs, Relationship between the amputation of an extremity and the subsequent development of cardiovascular disorders, U.S. Government Printing Office, Washington, D.C., 1979.
13. Taylor, S.B., and Shelton, J.E., Caloric requirements of a spastic immobile cerebral palsy patient: a case report, *Arch. Phys. Med. Rehabil.*, 76, 281, 1995.
14. Rice, H.B., Ponichetera-Mulcare, J.A., and Glaser, R.M., Nutrition and the spinal cord-injured individual, *Clin. Kinesiol.*, 54, 21, 1995.
15. Shepard, R.J. Benefits of sports and physical activity for the disabled: implications for the individual and for society, *Scand. J. Rehab. Med.*, 23, 51, 1991.
16. Lee, B.Y., Agrawal, N., Corcoran, A., Thoden, W.R., and Guercio, A.D., Assessment of nutritional and metabolic status of paraplegics, *J. Rehabil. Res. Dev.*, 22, 11, 1985.
17. Sherill, C., Mushett, C., and Jones, J.A., Cerebral palsy and the CP athlete in *Training Guide to Cerebral Palsy Sports*, Jones, J.A., Ed., Human Kinetics, Champaign, IL, 1988,9.
18. Johnson, R.K., Goran, M.I., Ferrara, M.S., and Poehlman, E.T., Athetosis increasing resting metabolic rate in adults with cerebral palsy, *J. Am. Diet. Assoc.*, 1995, 95, 145.
19. Chumiea, W.C, and Roche, A.F. Nutritional anthropometric assessments of non-ambulatory persons using recumbent techniques, *Am. J. Phys. Anthrop.*, 1984, 63, 146.
20. Brotherhood, J.R., Nutrition and sports performance, *Sports Med.*, 1984, 1, 350.
21. Peck, D.M., and McKeag, D.B., Athletes with disabilities: removing medical barriers, *Phys. Sports Med.*, 1994, 22, 59.
22. Daniel, M., and Gorman, D., Nutritional considerations for the wheelchair athlete, *Sport N Spokes*, 1983, 9, 8.
23. Kofsky, P.R., Shepard, R.J., Davis, G.M., and Jackson, R.W., Fitness classification tablesfor lower limb disabled individuals in *Sports and the Disabled Athlete*, Sherill, C., Ed. Human Kinetics, Champaign, IL, 1986, 147.
24. Burnham, R.S., Shoulder pain in wheelchair athletes, *Am. J. Sports Med.*, 1993, 1, 238.
25. Burnham, R.S., and Steadward, R., D., Nerve entrapments in wheelchair athletes, *Arch. Phys. Med. Rehab.*, 1994, 75, 519.

26. Curtis, K.A., Prevention and treatment of wheelchair athletic injuries, *Athl. Ther. Today*, 1997, 2, 19.
27. Peck, D.M., and McKeag, D.B., Athletes with disabilities: removing barriers, *Phys. Sports Med.*, 1994, 2, 59.
28. Stopka, C.B., Management of common injuries in individuals with disabilities: evaluation, treatment and rehabilitation, *Palaestra*, 1996, 12, 32.
29. Stopka, C., Sports medical concerns for conditioning athletes with disabilities, *Strength Cond.*, 1998, 2, 1998.
30. Sherill, C., *Adapted Physical Activity, Recreation and Sport*, 5th ed., WCB/McGraw-Hill, Boston, MA, 1998.
31. Shepard, R.J., Sports medicine and the wheelchair athlete, *Sports Med.*, 1988, 4, 226.
32. Gisolfi, C.V., and Duchman, S.M., Guidelines for the optimal replacement beverages for different athletic events, *Med. Sci. Sports Exerc.*, 1992, 24, 672.
33. Fike, S., Kanter, M., and Markely, E., Fluid and electrolyte requirements of exercise, in *Sports Nutrition*, 2nd ed., Bernardot, D., Ed., American Dietetic Association, Chicago, Il, 1992, p 38.

CHAPTER 9

Nutritional Concerns of Athletes with Chronic Medical Conditions

Brent J. Shriver and L. Mallory Boylan

CONTENTS

0-8493-8199-?/00/$0.00+$.50

I. INTRODUCTION

An exercise program's impact on the health of many individuals with chronic disease or conditions is often a positive one. However, exercise has the potential in some cases to worsen a condition or be very detrimental to health. Individuals should consult their physicians before embarking on any type of exercise program or undertaking any strenuous activity. Professional guidance regarding duration, intensity, type of activity, and appropriate precautions for the chosen activity should be sought by anyone planning to exercise. While this chapter provides some information on such topics as risks, benefits, precautions, and guidelines relating to exercising in individuals with selected chronic medical conditions, professional advice should be considered vital for each person as to their specific exercise program.

II. INFORMATION ON EXERCISE FOR PERSONS WITH TYPE I OR INSULIN DEPENDENT DIABETES MELLITUS (DM)

A. Benefits

For the majority of people with type I diabetes, the impact of an appropriate exercise program on health should be a positive one. Benefits may include the following:[1-4]

- Improved cardiovascular fitness and a decrease in risk factors such as hypertension, hyperlipidemia, and obesity (increase in lean body mass and decrease in percent body fat).
- Increased insulin sensitivity and efficiency of glucose uptake by cells are noted, but this does not directly translate into improvement in long term blood glucose control.
- Increased strength and flexibility.
- Improved psychosocial well-being and sense of self esteem.

B. Risks

Detrimental effects of some activities are possible in individuals with diabetes, so each person should seek professional advice regarding precautions to take for each specific activity. In some cases, some activities would not be recommended, but most people with type I diabetes can safely participate in the sport activity of their choice.

Problems that may occur or be exacerbated by activity may include the following:[1-4]

- Hypoglycemia and possible increased risk of injury or death in some activities if hypoglycemia impairs judgment or state of consciousness.
- Hyperglycemia after strenuous exercise may occur in people who are underinsulinized.
- Hyperglycemia and worsening of ketosis may occur in those with poor glycemic control or insufficient insulin.
- In those with proliferative retinopathy, exercise may induce retinal or vascular hemorrhage. Heavy lifting should be avoided.
- Those with peripheral neuropathy or vascular disease are at increased risk for soft-tissue or joint damage in the feet and legs, especially during jogging, running, prolonged walking, or step exercises, or any activity stressing the legs and feet.

- Individuals with autonomic neuropathy have a decreased capacity for high-intensity exercise as the condition causes a decrease in maximum heart rate and aerobic capacity. This condition may also make it more difficult for the person to be aware of symptoms of dehydration and hypoglycemia. Postural hypotension post exercise may also develop in those with autonomic neuropathy. Type, intensity, and duration of exercise must be carefully controlled if these problems are to be avoided, but most activity is not contraindicated.
- Exercise may cause proteinuria in some people with diabetes.
- Individuals with diabetes may have a greater rise in blood pressure during exercise than that which occurs in those without diabetes.
- In people who have developed cardiovascular disease, exercise may exacerbate cardiovascular ischemia and arrhythmias.

C. Metabolic Effects of Exercise in Those With Type I DM

Insulin has a key role in regulating metabolic homeostasis during exercise.[5] Ideally, the individual with diabetes should have a low but adequate plasma insulin level and would be able to maintain normoglycemia during and after the event. This goal may be challenging to reach and is influenced by many variables.

One variable that influences the effect of exercise on blood glucose (BG) is the person's state of diabetes control at the time of the event. When insulin levels are inadequate, and self monitoring of blood glucose (SMBG) prior to the event reveals BG values of 250 to 300 mg/dL or greater, exercise can result in further elevation of BG and accelerated ketone body production. The elevation of BG under these conditions may be due to factors such as decreased exercise-induced muscle glucose uptake, as this process is insulin dependent. Also, high levels of counter-regulatory hormones may promote gluconeogenesis, and BG may rise due to this hepatic glucose production and release.

When people with poor diabetes control exercise, they also increase free fatty acid (FFA) mobilization, as the insulin they lack dampens this effect.[1,6,7] The high plasma FFA levels result in additional use of FFA by the muscle. A sevenfold rise in FFA uptake by leg muscle in diabetics in poor control as compared to three- to fourfold increased uptake by leg muscle in subjects without diabetes has been noted. In a ketotic state, exercise promotes greater conversion of FFA to ketone bodies.[1] Due to this exercise induced rise in BG and ketones, individuals whose diabetes is in poor control should avoid exercise until adequate BG management has been attained. As resynthesis of glycogen in muscle after exercise is insulin dependent, people who are under insulinized will also be able to only minimally replace their glycogen stores in the post-event period.

A more common scenario found in those whose diabetes is well controlled or who have only mild to moderate hyperglycemia is a decrease in BG during exercise.[1,5] In contrast to persons without diabetes, whose insulin levels decrease during exercise, those taking subcutaneous insulin may experience no decline or even an elevation of insulin levels, leading to a decrease in BG and, in some cases, a hypoglycemic reaction. Insulin inhibits hepatic glucose output during exercise, and, as muscle glucose uptake increases, there is the possibility of hypoglycemia as BG is removed from circulation.

Following exercise that is prolonged or strenuous where glycogen stores have been depleted, there is an increased risk of hypoglycemia during the next 24 to 48 hours. This is due to a prolonged increase in glucose uptake to replenish glycogen stores in liver and muscle. Glucose tolerance is improved and insulin requirements are diminished, so adjustment in insulin dosage and food intake and SMGB are needed.

D. Factors that Influence Fuel Use During Exercise

Metabolism of fuels and their regulation during exercise necessitate a complicated endocrine response and are influenced by many factors.[2,8] Very intensive short-term anaerobic-type exercise such as sprinting will use mainly carbohydrate for fuel via glycolysis. The carbohydrate utilized is generally from blood and muscle stores.

For longer-duration events such as distance running, cross country skiing, and cycling, both carbohydrates and fats are important sources of energy, but the mix of fuel used varies with intensity and duration of activity.[8] In a continuous moderate exercise scenario, the energy for the muscular work is provided mainly from endogenous lipid and carbohydrate stores. As activity continues and muscle and liver glycogen stores decline, the percent of energy for exercise from lipid increases. If exercise continues to the point where glycogen in specific muscles is severely depleted, then fatigue sets in.

Metabolic control of diabetes does appear to influence fuel release and usage during exercise.[2] In a situation where too little insulin has been given, glucagon response is higher than normal, promoting an above-normal hepatic glucose output and ketogenesis. Catacholamine release is also exaggerated, leading to increased lipolysis, elevation of free fatty acids and ketones, increased glucose production, and decreased glucose utilization. Due to these abnormalities in energy nutrient metabolism, exercise is not recommended when diabetes is out of control.

E. Carbohydrates During Intense Training and Endurance Events

Carbohydrate is a critical fuel during exercise and an intense exercise bout can deplete most of the body's glycogen stores in the liver and exercised muscles. This leads to fatigue and decreased performance. Strenuous endurance training over repeated days can lead to depletion of glycogen stores. At least 48 hours are required to replete muscles' glycogen stores depleted by exercise, and a high dietary intake of carbohydrate is needed during this time period to replenish glycogen stores. Insulin is needed for glycogen to be synthesized from carbohydrate and carbohydrate intake needs to remain higher than usual in the post-exercise period. Frequent SMBG, carbohydrate counting, and insulin adjustment will be necessary to permit optimal glycogen resynthesis and maintenance of normoglycemia after an athletic event.[1]

It is well established that carbohydrate-containing beverages can enhance performance in athletics participating in high-intensity aerobic exercise. These carbohydrates can keep spare glycogen and decrease the risk of hypoglycemia. Benefit for those participating in exercise that is not intense is negligible. Adequate fluid intake is critical for the well being and performance of any athlete. For nondiabetic athletes, Katch and McArdle[8] suggest that, for prolonged high intensity aerobic exercise, a 50% sugar solution be ingested 20 to 30 minutes after the start of the exercise, followed by 8 oz. (235 ml) of a 5% solution every 15 minutes during the event. Sport drinks containing glucose polymers may be useful, as glucose polymers do not have as negative an effect on water uptake as do simple sugars. The athlete with diabetes also needs fluids and carbohydrate during exercise, but must consider many additional factors in trying to find a regime to enhance performance. Some trials and evaluations of factors which effect performance will be critical.

F. Precautions and Guidelines for Exercise

Some factors to consider are:

- *Blood glucose prior to the event.* Exercise should be avoided if BG is greater than 250 to 350 mg/dL or if ketones are present in the urine.[1,2] Ingest carbohydrates prior to exercise if BG is less than 100 mg/dL.[2] Amount and type of carbohydrate to ingest will need to be individualized through trial and evaluation of effects on BG and performance.
- *Insulin injection.* Exercise can increase mobilization of insulin from an injection site. Generally, if exercise is at least 40 minutes after injection of regular insulin, the insulin absorption is not affected, as more than half the insulin has already been mobilized.[9] After a subcutaneous injection of intermediate-acting insulin, no increase in major mobilization will occur 2.5 hours post injection.

Exercise where insulin has been injected into a site used in the physical activity in the periods described above can increase risk of hypoglycemia during the event. A non-exercising area such as the abdomen would be advisable in some events such as running or biking. In some types of events, alterations in dosage or type of insulin may be needed. Athletes will have to monitor BG before, during, and after the practice or event to determine, for example, if their usual insulin dosage needs to be decreased. Morning or afternoon activity may necessitate reducing, by 10% of the total insulin dose, insulins that peak at the time of the exercise. A 20% reduction in dosage may be needed for all-day activities. Each person will need to find the appropriate dosage reduction, which may vary with level of activity, duration of exercise, state of physical condition, diabetes control, and other individual factor BG during the event. Exercise increases the risk of hypoglycemia, which is detrimental to performance and, in certain circumstances, could lead to major injury or even death.

- *Blood glucose during the event.* Franz recommends a 15g increase in carbohydrate for 1 hour of moderate exercise if pre-event BG is 100 to 180 mg/dL.[1] For strenuous activity of 1 to 2 hours, an additional 25 to 50g of carbohydrate is recommended if BG is 100 to 180mg/dL, with 15g being recommended for those whose BG is over 180 mg/dL. Again, fluids are needed to prevent dehydration, so, in many cases, a carbohydrate-containing beverage is a good choice. SMBG, record keeping, and adjustments will be necessary to determine what works best for any individual in regard to alteration of insulin and carbohydrate.
  - A source of quick-acting carbohydrate should always be attainable for treatment of hypoglycemia if it does occur during the event.[1] In those with neuropathy or lack of ability to perceive symptoms of hypoglycemia, SMBG during practice will be critical to find a regime that minimizes the chance of hypoglycemia during an athletic event. Individuals taking alcohol, aspirin, or betablockers may be at increased risk of hypoglycemic episodes during exercise.
  - In people with type I DM who exercise regularly, Bell et al[10] evaluated the effect of a food bar containing carbohydrates with three different glycemic index values, one of which was uncooked corn starch, on blood glucose values during and after 30 to 60 minutes of exercise. The food bar, containing 104 kcal, or a snack of four peanut butter crackers containing 142 kcal, were consumed prior to exercise on 2 days each and BG was measured prior to, every 30 minutes during, and 2 hours post exercise. The BG values for the two treatments were not significantly different and the incidence of hypoglycemic episodes was similar. Hyperglycemia was more prevalent in the usual snack group. It must be noted that exercise intensity and duration were not controlled closely, but duration was generally fairly short term. The snacks were not isocaloric and grams of carbohydrate per snack were not reported in the study. The possibility that snack bars containing uncooked corn starch could be useful in some types and durations of exercise is yet to be evaluated. The uncooked cornstarch should provide a source for blood glucose lasting 6 hours or more. Again, this study did not evaluate the use of this bar in an endurance event, so its usefulness in many circumstances is not known.
- *Post-Event Blood Glucose.* As blood glucose levels may continue to decline after exercise, blood glucose should be monitored every 1 to 2 hours after the event. Adequate carbohydrate and insulin are needed for glycogen repletion, which may take up to 48 hours. Carbohydrate gram counting and BG records will need to be kept to determine carbohydrate needs and appropriate insulin carbohydrate ratio during the post event period. Total energy intake must be adjusted by type and duration of exercise to promote weight maintenance.
- Other
  - Carry proper identification regarding diabetes and any medications used.
  - Always obtain your physician's approval regarding appropriate intensity and duration of exercise.
  - Follow guidelines regarding fluid and electrolyte replacement for the specific sport in which you participate.
  - Make needed adjustment for factors such as heat or medications such as diuretics that could predispose one to dehydration and depletion of electrolytes.
  - Follow all rules of safety for any sport and use proper equipment.
  - Seek advice from your health care professionals regarding all aspects of participation in athletic events including risks such as those identified earlier in this chapter.
  - Seek a mentor who has diabetes and is an athlete in the sport of your choice, as he or she may have valuable insight to facilitate diabetes control and athletic performance.

III. INFORMATION ON EXERCISE FOR PERSONS WITH TYPE II DM

A. Benefit

Exercise is generally a helpful treatment modality for type II DM and the following benefits have been noted.[1,3,4]

- Cardiovascular conditioning and lowering of blood pressure with improvement in lipid profile such as increased HDL, and decreased LDL and triglycerides may occur.
- Weight loss may be induced in those who are obese, with an increase in muscle mass and a decrease in body fat. Subsequently, exercise may help promote maintenance of a desirable body weight. As obesity is associated with insulin resistance, weight loss may promote better glucose tolerance.
- Enhanced insulin sensitivity induced by exercise may improve glucose control and need for, or dosage of, medications may be reduced.
- Strength and flexibility are increased.
- Self esteem may be improved and psychosocial well-being may be enhanced.

B. Risks

- Hypoglycemia may occur during or post exercise in individuals controlling their DM with insulin or sulfonylurea compounds. Extreme caution is needed when participating in activities where hypoglycemia may impair judgment or state of consciousness that could result in possible serious injury or even death.
- The last six risks under type I DM would also apply to individuals with type II DM.

C. Metabolic Effects of Exercise on Those with Type II DM

As exercise increases insulin sensitivity and the rate of glucose metabolism, BG has been found to decrease by about 30 to 40 mg/dL during 45 minutes of moderate exercise in those with type II DM.[11] In obese subjects with type II DM, exercise that is intense and of sufficient duration to result in depletion of glycogen stores will result in increased glucose clearing for about 12 to 14 or more hours after the event.[12] In general, training promotes improved glucose tolerance in those with type II DM, and, while BG declines during exercise, the risk of hypoglycemia is similar for both a nondiabetic and a person with type II DM who is being treated only with diet.[1] The individual being treated with sulfonylureas or insulin may be at increased risk for hypoglycemia during exercise. Theoretically, medications that slow carbohydrate absorption could also increase risk of hypoglycemia. Medications that work as oral hypoglycemic agents by enhancing insulin sensitivity should not promote hypoglycemia.

D. Precautions and Guidelines for Exercise

Some factors to consider are:

- *Insulin usage.* Those with type II DM who take insulin should review the precautions and guidelines for type I diabetes. No guidelines appear to be available for the degree of hyperglycemia at which exercise should be avoided in type II DM, but exercise probably should be avoided if BG exceeds 300 mg/dL. While those with type II diabetes are not prone to diabetic ketoacidosis, nonketotic, hyperosmotic, hyperglycemic coma is possible and exercise under these circumstances would be unadvisable.
  - In an obese individual for whom one goal of exercise is weight reduction, care must be taken to balance carbohydrates needed for adequate performance and hypoglycemia prevention, with

avoidance of excessive consumption, which would deter weight loss. Thus, decreasing insulin should be considered along with increased carbohydrate with adjustments made based on SMBG.

- *Other oral hypoglycemic usage.* Because insulin may inhibit hepatic glucose production during exercise, those with higher than normal insulin levels during exercise due to sulfonyluria usage are at risk for hypoglycemia. Medication dosage reduction or increased carbohydrate intake may be needed to prevent exercise induced hypoglycemia.
  - Individuals taking medications that slow glucose absorption may also benefit from reducing their medication dosage for long-term high-intensity exercise events. While studies about this topic were not found in the literature, a substance that slows carbohydrate absorption would seem to have the possibility of having a negative impact on athletic performance.
  - Medications for type II DM that enhance insulin sensitivity should not cause any major increase in risk of hypoglycemia during exercise. Effects on performance have not been reported.
  - As most people with type II DM are adults, many of whom must take multiple medications, they should consult their health care provider regarding the potential of medications to increase hypoglycemia risk. Alcohol, high doses of salicytates, beta adrenergic blocking agents, and maybe some other medications increase risk of hypoglycemia during exercise.
- *Blood glucose, performance, and weight control.* Review the recommendations for those with type I DM as many aspects are pertinent to those with type II DM. An individualized program based on records of food intake, medications, and exercise intensity and duration, along with SMGB are critical to finding the proper balance of factors that will promote adequate DM control, good athletic performance, and promotion of health. Most people will need to do some trial-and-error experimenting to come up with the optimal program.
  - For most people with type II DM who are not taking DM medications, no additional carbohydrate is needed for mild, short-duration exercise.[1] For any athlete, long-term high-intensity events may require supplemental carbohydrate, fluid, and, in some cases, electrolytes, for optimal performance. People with DM should always monitor their BG and adjust carbohydrate intake if needed. Replacement of kilocalories burned during activity would be important to prevent weight loss in those at an acceptable body weight. Adequate carbohydrate will also be needed to restore glycogen in liver and exercised muscle following strenuous exercise. Medication adjustments may also be needed and SMBG is critical for up to 48 hours after an event.
- *Other.* Items listed under "other" for those with type I DM also pertain to those with type II DM.

IV. INFORMATION ON EXERCISE FOR PERSONS WITH HYPERTENSION

A. Benefits

The general benefits of exercise for people with essential hypertension are basically the same as those described earlier for individuals with type II diabetes mellitus. The reader is referred to this section for a complete listing of these benefits. This section of the chapter attempts to provide a more detailed examination of the relationship between exercise and blood pressure.

B. Risks

Risks associated with exercise for individuals with hypertension include the potential to suffer a heart attack or stroke during the exercise event.[13] Hypertension is often accompanied by comorbidities such as obesity, dyslipidemias, and coronary artery disease.[14] The potential risk must be evaluated in light of the individual's overall health status. A consultation with a physician is warranted for all non-exercisers before they embark on a physical fitness program.[15] This is especially true for individuals with hypertension, particularly when comorbidities are present. With the help of the physician, the hypertensive individual should be able to design a program of physical activity that reduces the potential risks and maximizes the health benefits.

C. Type of Physical Activity

Aerobic activity, also referred to as endurance training (ET), appears to have the greatest positive impact on blood pressure (BP).[16] Although strength training (ST) confers many health benefits, such as increasing the percentage of lean body tissue and improving strength and flexibility, it appears to do little to lower blood pressure.[17] Exercising BP can rise dramatically during ST, increasing the risk for heart attack or stroke. For this reason, it has been suggested that individuals with moderate to severe hypertension should avoid ST until the hypertension is reduced in severity through the use of pharmacological agents.[18] ST appears to be safe for individuals with mild to moderate hypertension and can be incorporated into a comprehensive physical fitness program.

D. Effects of Endurance Training on Blood Pressure

It has been estimated that approximately 15 to 30% of the adult population in the Western industrialized countries are afflicted with essential hypertension. This form of cardiovascular disease is a major contributor to both morbidity and mortality in these countries. Within the hypertensive segment of the population, those individuals with mild to moderate hypertension (diastolic BP between 90 and 104mm Hg and/or systolic BP between 140 and 159mm Hg) account for the vast majority of cases.[16] The available experimental data strongly suggest that regular participation in ET can improve BP in these individuals. On average, researchers report a reduction in diastolic or systolic BP of approximately 10mm Hg in response to ET.[19] These findings have led numerous researchers to suggest that ET should be the treatment of first choice for individuals with mild to moderate hypertension who are able to engage in physical activity. ET should only be added to the treatment regime of those individuals with severe hypertension after BP is brought under some degree of control with pharmacological agents.[20]

E. Intensity, Frequency, and Duration of Endurance Training

In individuals with mild to moderate hypertension it appears that low- to moderate-intensity physical (40–70% of VO_{2max}) is as effective as more-intense physical activity in reducing BP.[19] In addition, low to moderate physical activity markedly reduces the risk of exercise-related complications. Walking, jogging, swimming, cycling, and circuit training are examples of low- to moderate-intensity physical activities that have been shown to reduce BP in these individuals.[21–24] It has been suggested that two to three sessions of 1 hour in duration per week are optimal for achieving the reduction in BP.[22,24] Increasing the duration to more than 1 hour or the frequency to more than three times per week appears to confer little or no added benefit.[22] Hypertensive individuals should consult their physician before beginning any exercise program.

F. Interaction of Antihypertensive Pharmacological Therapy and Exercise

It seems obvious and logical that certain antihypertensive agents may influence the ability of individuals to perform physical activity, as well as having an effect on the physiological response to exercise. However, the scientific literature is almost completely devoid of such information.[22] It is essential that individuals receiving pharmacological therapy discuss this topic with their physician.

G. Nutrition and Exercise in Individuals with Hypertension

There is little evidence to suggest that the general dietary and nutritional recommendations for individuals with hypertension are any different from those for normotensive individuals engaged in the same types of physical activities. Consumption of a high-carbohydrate diet on a routine basis appears to be highly effective at promoting the replacement of glycogen reserves depleted by ET.

Therefore, individuals who engage in regular ET are urged to consume at least 50% of their caloric intake in the form of complex carbohydrates. Diets that are very high in carbohydrate content (>70% energy intake) have the potential to markedly increase postprandial blood triglyceride levels.[25] Therefore, hypertensive individuals with comorbidities such as dyslipidemias or coronary artery disease might be wise to avoid very-high-carbohydrate diets. Hypertensive individuals who are following a sodium-restricted diet can meet these goals for carbohydrate intake within the guidelines of the sodium-restricted diet by selecting unprocessed or minimally processed carbohydrate-rich foods that are naturally low in sodium.

Exercise markedly increases the rate of fluid loss from the body, both through the skin as sweat and as water vapor exhaled from the lungs. During exercise, the thirst response is usually preceded by some degree of fluid depletion. As a result, all individuals who exercise, particularly in hot or dry climates, are encouraged to consume fluids routinely during the exercise event rather than waiting for thirst to set in.[26] Because the thirst response becomes delayed as a consequence of the aging process, this may be particularly important for exercisers who are middle-aged or older.[27] In addition to water, a significant amount of electrolytes can be lost in sweat during prolonged ET. For this reason, use of sports drinks containing electrolytes has become quite common for athletes who regularly engage in ET that exceeds 1 hour in duration. There is little information concerning the suitability of these products for use by hypertensive individuals. Individuals who are receiving pharmacological therapy to control blood pressure should discuss potential influences of these drugs on fluid and electrolyte balance with their physician.

V. INFORMATION ON EXERCISE FOR INDIVIDUALS WITH CORONARY ARTERY DISEASE

A. Benefits

The general benefits of exercise for people with coronary artery disease are essentially the same as those described earlier for individuals with type II diabetes mellitus. The reader is referred to this section for a complete listing of these benefits. This section of the chapter attempts to provide a more detailed examination of the influence of exercise on this chronic medical condition.

B. Risks

Coronary artery disease (CAD), often referred to as atherosclerosis, is characterized by partial restriction of blood flow to the coronary arteries. This disease can vary widely in its severity and is often be accompanied by one or more comorbid conditions such as obesity, dyslipidemias, type II diabetes mellitus, and hypertension. The risk associated with exercise in individuals with CAD will be influenced by the severity of the disease and the number and extent of any comorbid conditions. Individuals with known CAD should not begin an exercise program without the advice of a physician who is familiar with their patient's overall physical health. As was the case with hypertension, the major risk is the chance of suffering an ischemic episode (heart attack or stroke) during the exercise event, especially in individuals with uncontrolled comorbid conditions such as hypertension.[13]

C. Type of Physical Activity

As it is for hypertension, ET appears to be the most beneficial form of physical activity for individuals with CAD.[28] However, the increase in lean muscle mass and other physiological changes produced by ST can assist individuals with CAD in controlling their weight.[17] Therefore, ST can be a valuable component of a comprehensive physical fitness program in these individuals.

Individuals with CAD who are also suffering from hypertension should follow the guidelines on strength training discussed in the earlier section on hypertension.

D. SPECIFIC BENEFITS OF ENDURANCE TRAINING IN INDIVIDUALS WITH CORONARY ARTERY DISEASE

Endurance training can have a number of positive effects that reduce the morbidity and mortality in individuals with CAD. Among these are decreases in systolic or diastolic blood pressure (see the previous section), a decrease in LDL cholesterol, an increase in HDL cholesterol, a decreased susceptibility of LDL to oxidation, and improvements in cardiopulmonary function.[29–31]

High circulating levels of LDL cholesterol (LDL-C) are a known risk factor for the development of CAD. A regular program of ET alone has been shown to lower LDL-C levels in previously sedentary individuals by as much as 11%.[32] In addition to the level of LDL-C in the blood, the concentration of oxidized LDL may also be an important risk factor in the development of CAD. Numerous studies have reported a reduction in the potential of LDL for oxidation, or the actual concentration of oxidized LDL in individuals participating in ET.[30, 32] The concentration of HDL cholesterol (HDL-C) in the blood appears to be inversely related to the risk of developing CAD. ET appears to be a highly effective mechanism for raising HDL-C levels.[29,32]

Regular ET has also been shown to improve a number of measures of cardiopulmonary function in individuals with CAD such as anaerobic threshold, peak aerobic capacity, and work efficiency.[31] ET has also produced similar improvements in cardiopulmonary function in individuals with CAD who are recovering from coronary artery bypass surgery.[33]

E. Intensity, Duration, and Frequency of the Physical Activity

Individuals with CAD should consult their physicians before beginning an exercise program. The physician can assist their patients in designing an appropriate exercise program that is based on the severity of their CAD and overall physical health. Most exercise programs for individuals with CAD or who are recovering from coronary artery bypass surgery restrict the intensity of the physical activity to less than 75% of initial maximal oxygen intake.

F. Nutrition and Exercise in Individuals with CAD

There is an almost-complete absence of any information in the literature regarding specific nutritional guidelines for individuals with CAD who engage in a program of regular physical activity or participate in athletic events. Diet modification is usually an important component in the integrated management of CAD. The physician, along with other members of the individual's health care team such as a registered dietitian or nurse practitioner, can assist the individual in developing a treatment plan that will meet his or her needs. Recommendations concerning exercise, diet, medication, and other aspects of the treatment plan should be based on the individual's overall health and the specific goals of the plan.

VI. SUMMARY

Physical activity offers many health benefits to individuals afflicted with chronic diseases such as diabetes mellitus, hypertension, and coronary artery disease. Regular aerobic activity can usually slow the progression of these diseases and even partially reverse it in many cases. In addition, physically fit individuals usually respond better to pharmacological intervention and recover faster after surgery. The presence of one of these chronic medical conditions and their associated diseases should not prevent an individual from engaging in some type of physical activity. The type of exercise program that is appropriate for any given individuals will be governed by their overall physical health. Therefore, anyone suffering from one or more of these chronic medical conditions should have a complete medical check-up before beginning any exercise program. Based on the results, the physician will be able to offer guidance on a suitable exercise program. As overall health improves, more-vigorous physical activity can often be incorporated into the exercise plan.

REFERENCES

1. Franz, M. Exercise and Diabetes Mellitus, in *Handbook of Diabetes Nutritional Management*, Powers, M.A., Ed., Aspen Publications, Rockville, MD, 1987.
2. Wasserman, D.H. and Zinman, B., Exercise in individuals with IDDM, *Diabetes Care*, 17, 924, 1994.
3. Berkowitz, K.J., The challenge of exercise: practical advice for implementation into clinical practice, *Nurse Prac. Forum*, 9, 53, 1998.
4. American Diabetes Association. Diabetes mellitus and exercise, *Diabetes Care*, 18, 28, 1995.
5. Wallberg-Henriksson, H. and Wahren, J., Effects of nutrition and diabetes mellitus on the regulation of metabolic fuels during exercise, *Am. J. Clin. Nutr.*, 49, 938, 1989.
6. Hagenfeld, L. and Wahren, J., Turnover of free fatty acids during recovery from exercise, *J. App. Physiol.*, 39, 247, 1975.
7. Wahren, J., Hagenfeldt, L., and Felig, P., Splanchnic and leg exchange of glucose, amino acids, and free fatty acids during exercise in diabetes mellitus, *J. Clin. Invest.*, 55, 1303, 1975.
8. Katch, F.I. and McArdle, W.D., in *Introduction to Nutrition Exercise, and Health, 4th edition*, Lea & Febiger, Philadelphia, PA, 1993.
9. Berger, M., Cuppers, H.J., Hegner, H., and Berchtold, P. Absorption kinetics and biologic effects of subcutaneously injected insulin preparation, *Diabetes Care*, 5, 79, 1982.
10. Bell, S.J., Kistler, J., Mullooly, C.A., Ovalle, K.B., Zilvitis, B., and Forse, R.A., Glycemic control during exercise in type I diabetes: comparison of a new medical food bar with usual care, *Diabetes Care*, 21, 1775, 1998.
11. Zinman, B. and Vranic, M., Diabetes and exercise, *Med. Clin. North. Am.*, 69, 145, 1985.
12. Devlin, J.T. and Horton, E.S., Effects of prior high-intensity exercise on glucose metabolism in normal and insulin resistant men, *Diabetes*, 34, 973, 1985.
13. Warner, J. G., Jr., Metzger, D. C., Kitzman, D. W., Wesley, D. J. and Little, W. C., Losartan improves exercise tolerance in patients with diastolic dysfunction and hypertensive response to exercise, *J. Am.. Coll. Cardiol.*, 33, 1567, 1999.
14. Dengel, D. R., Hagberg, J. M., Pratley, R. E., Rogus, E. M., and Goldberg, A. P., Improvements in blood pressure, glucose metabolism, and lipoprotein lipids after aerobic exercise plus weight loss in obese, hypertensive middle-aged men, *Metabolism*, 47, 1075, 1998.
15. Ketelhut, R. G., Endurance training in hypertension is effective. Which form of sports, frequency, and intensity of training? Should adjuvant chemotherapy be considered? *Fortschr. Med.*, 116, 26, 1998.
16. Gordon, N. F., Scott, C. B., Wilkinson, W. J., Duncan, J. J., and Blair, S. N., Exercise and mild essential hypertension. Recommendations for adults, *Sports Med.*, 10, 390, 1990.
17. Stone, M. H., Fleck, S. J., Triplett, N. T., and Kraemer, W. J., Health and performance-related potential of resistance training, *Sports Med.*, 11, 210, 1991.
18. Franz, I. W., Blood pressure response to exercise in normotensives and hypertensive, *Can. J. Sport Sci.*, 16, 296, 1991.
19. Hagberg, J. M. and Brown, M. D., Does exercise training play a role in the treatment of essential hypertension?, *J. Cardiovasc. Risk,* 2, 296, 1995.
20. Keul, J., Lehmann, M., and Dickhuth, H. H., Hypertension, the heart, and physical activity, *Z. Cardiol.*, 78 (Suppl. 7), 199, 1989.
21. Tanaka, H., Bassett, D. R., Jr., Howley, E. T., Thompson, D. L., Ashraf, M., and Rawson, F. L., Swimming training lowers the resting blood pressure in individuals with hypertension, *J. Hypertens.*, 15, 651, 1997.

22. Petrella, R. J. How effective is exercise training for the treatment of hypertension?, *Clin. J. Sport Med.*, 8, 224, 1998.
23. Harris, K. A. and Holly, R. G. Physiological response to circuit training in borderline hypertensive subjects, *Med Sci. Sports Exerc.*, 19, 246, 1987.
24. Meridith, I. T., Jennings, G. L., Esler, M. D., Dewar, E. M., Bruce, A. M., Fazio, V. A., and Korner, P. I., Time-course of the antihypertensive and autonomic effects of regular endurance exercise in human subjects, *J. Hypertens.*, 8, 859, 1990.
25. MacDonald, I. A., Carbohydrate as a nutrient in adults: ranges of acceptable intakes, *Eur. J. Clin. Nutr.,* 53 (Suppl. 1), S101, 1999.
26. Greenleaf, J. E., Problems: thirst, drinking behavior, and involuntary dehydration, *Med. Sci. Sports and Exerc.,* 24, 671, 1992.
27. Rolls, B. J. and Phillips, P. A., Aging and disturbances of thirst and fluid balance, *Nutr. Rev.*, 48, 137, 1990.
28. Moore, R. L. Cellular adaptations of the heart muscle to exercise training, *Ann. Med.*, 30 (Suppl. 1), 46, 1998.
29. Borodina, L. M., Kazemov, V. V., Kozlov, A. A., Saufiullina, Z. M., and Shalaev, S. V. The efficacy of physical exercises in correcting the lipid metabolic disorders in patients who have had a myocardial infarct, *Vopr. Kurortol. Fizioter. Lech. Fiz. Kult.*, 5, 9, 1998.
30. Sanchez-Quesada, J. L., Ortega, H., Payes-Romero, A., Serrat-Serrat, J., Gonzalez-Sastre, F., Lasuncion, M. A., and Ordonez-Llanos, J., LDL from aerobically-trained subjects shows higher resistance to oxidative modification than LDL from sedentary subjects, *Atherosclerosis*, 132, 207, 1997.
31. Lavie, C. J. and Miliani, R. V. Effects of cardiac rehabilitation and exercise training on peak aerobic capacity and work efficiency in obese patients with coronary artery disease, *Am. J. Cardiol.*, 83, 1477, 1999.
32. Vasankari, T. J., Kujala, U. M., Vasankari, T. M., and Ahotupa, M., Reduced oxidized LDL levels after a 10-month exercise program, *Med. Sci. Sports Exerc.*, 30, 1496, 1998.
33. Goodman, J. M., Pallandi, D. V., Reading, J. R., Plyley, M. J., Liu, P. P., and Kavanagh, T., Central and peripheral adaptations after 12 weeks of exercise training in coronary artery bypass surgery patients., *J. Cardiopulm. Rehabil.*, 19, 144, 1999.

Part III

The Sport

CHAPTER 10

The Training Table

Jacqueline R. Berning

CONTENTS

Human performance involves a number of factors including training, motivation, athletic ability, and diet. In addition, jet lag, unfamiliar playing fields, and changes in sleep habits and patterns are a few factors that hinder athletes who travel. No matter where athletes compete, it is important that they choose the proper fuel for optimal performance. Too often, athletes skip meals, eat insufficient amounts of carbohydrates, and compete in a state of dehydration. Training tables, both at home and on the road, need to supply not only the fuels needed by the exercise bout but also the nutrients required by the body for health. Athletes who consume, both at home and on the road, diets that are chronically repetitive and deficient in carbohydrates and fluid can experience a progressive depletion of glycogen stores and reduced nutritional status that may cause a drop in endurance, precision, speed, and health.

I. ATHLETES' NUTRITION KNOWLEDGE

Surveys of athletes reveal that, like their sedentary counterparts, they consume more fat than carbohydrates in their diet.[3,13] Furthermore, when given a nutrition-knowledge test, they scored well on the basic nutrition information, but did poorly when it came to choosing foods that were high in a specific amount. For example, when asked to name a nutritious carbohydrate, 63% of

0-8493-8199-1/00/$0.00+$.50

adolescent and college swimmers attending an Olympic training camp correctly named apple, while 38% chose French fries. When asked which food provides a good source of protein, 63% correctly chose chicken, but 37% chose oatmeal. Overall 62% of the swimmers in this study picked correct answers, while 38% were unable to select the proper balance of foods necessary for the energy demands of their sport. If athletes cannot make proper food choices, they cannot be expected to select a proper diet that is required for peak performance.

In other surveys of athletes between the ages of 13–20, several misconceptions were reported.[4] For example, over half of them believed that everyone should take a vitamin and mineral supplement, that vitamin E improves performance, that supplementing with the B vitamins gives a boost in energy, and that milk consumption the day of the competition impairs performance. A study of male track athletes, baseball, and football teams, found that only 28% could define glycogen loading. Sixty-nine percent did not know which foods were a good source of carbohydrates and 54% did not know the major vitamins.[10] A nutrition-knowledge questionnaire completed by adolescent gymnasts showed that over 50% of the girls could not define a complex carbohydrate and did not know that carbohydrates were an important source of energy for exercise. Instead, 75% of the girls erroneously believed that protein was the best source of energy for the exercising muscle. Volleyball players had difficulty with questions on food sources of quality protein, vitamin C, good sources of energy, carbohydrate loading, and caloric requirement for training. However, they were knowledgeable about the importance of eating a variety of foods, vitamin supplementation, and the differences between plant and animal fat.

It is not only this lack of nutrition information that may lead to an improper diet but the athletes also tend to have poor eating habits. It has been reported that 29% of 18–22-year-olds skip breakfast, with that number approaching 50% for the college and high school age group. Nearly a quarter regularly miss lunch and 86% of these individuals who do eat some food at noon choose a fast food restaurant. Add in the fact that an average family of four eats together fewer than five times per week and its easy to see why athletes make improper food choices.

II. THE OPTIMAL TRAINING TABLE

A suggested distribution of calories for most competitive athletes is 10–15% protein, 25–30% fat and 50–60% carbohydrate.[1] Endurance athletes, (triathletes, century bicyclists, marathoners and ultramarathoners) however, should be consuming 60–70% of their total calories in the form of carbohydrates because one of the limiting factors in prolonged human performance is glycogen depletion. Athletes who consume diets chronically deficient in carbohydrate can experience a progressive depletion of glycogen stores. This may cause a decrement in endurance, precision, and speed.

Recently, several diet plans based on lowering carbohydrate consumption and increasing protein intake have been promoted to athletes. The promoters of these diets have aligned themselves with well-known athletes or teams as endorsements. The scientific basis for a low-carbohydrate, high-protein diet is not supported by peer-reviewed research. As a matter of fact, consuming more protein at the expense of carbohydrate has been associated with the development of cardiovascular disease, dehydration, calcium loss, and renal dysfunction[14] and may decrease the ability of athletes to perform aerobic endurance exercise as well as anaerobic workouts. In a couple of studies performed by Sherman et al.[11,12] it was found that consuming carbohydrates 3 to 4 hours before exercise, as well as the hour before exercise, can enhance performance by filling muscle and liver glycogen stores. In addition, other researchers have found that feeding carbohydrates to athletes during exercise lasting an hour or longer aided their performance by providing glucose for the exercising muscles to use when they are running low on glycogen.[6,7] Recently J. Mark Davis and colleagues from South Carolina.[8)] found that, when they supplemented carbohydrates in a high-intensity exercise that lasted under 30 minutes, performance was enhanced as measured by sprint time and number of sprints performed. Another concern for athletes who follow a high-protein, low-carbohydrate diet is the inability to resynthesize muscle glycogen. Athletes who consume diets chronically deficient in carbohydrates can experience a progressive depletion of glycogen stores. Ivy et al.[9] found that, when athletes consumed about 100 grams of carbohydrates immediately post exercise, their ability to resynthesize glycogen was at a higher rate, allowing them to maximize glycogen stores in about 16 hours instead of 24 hours. Zawadski and colleagues.[15] found that if athletes consumed 100 grams of carbohydrates plus 25 grams of protein, muscle glycogen stores were resynthesized in about 12 hours, thus allowing athletes who have to give back-to-back performances the energy to meet the demands of the sport.

Another issue for athletes is the timing of the meals. Many athletes have to eat when food is available or when they are not training. Sometimes this can lead to skipped meals or long periods without eating. Common sense dictates that when athletes go for a long time without food, it will be hard to compete, let alone train. Athletes in heavy training or having multiple workouts should be eating about every 3 hours to maintain blood glucose levels and spare muscle glycogen.[2]

Since carbohydrates are the primary fuel for the exercising muscle, athletes or individuals who exercise daily and eat less carbohydrate may not have the energy to maintain a regular exercise routine or compete at the level expected. The recommended mix of energy for athletes is 12–15% of the total calories from protein, 20–25% from fat and 60% from carbohydrate. For all but the extreme cases, protein consumption at 15% of total energy is sufficient for athletes.[5] Often, protein is calculated based on body weight. Table 10.1 can be used to figure an athlete's specific protein requirement.

Table 10.1 Protein Requirements for All Levels of Athletes

Protein for sedentary adult—0.36 g of protein per pound of weight
Adult recreational exerciser—0.5–0.75 g of protein per pound of weight
Adult competitive athlete—0.6–0.8 g of protein per pound of weight
Adult building muscle mass—0.7–0.8 g of protein per pound of weight
Dieting athlete—0.7–1.0 g of protein per pound of weight
Growing teenage athlet—0.7–0.8 g of protein per pound of weight

Examples:

160-pound sedentary adult 160 × 0.36 = 58 g of protein per day
170-pound recreational exerciser 170 × 0.5 = 85 g of protein per day
150-pound growing teenager 150 × 0.7 = 105 g of protein per day

A. Practical Applications

The food guide pyramid for athletes, Figure10.1, not only offers an easy strategy for an individual to select a nutritionally balanced diet, but also provides a guide in planning training tables for teams who eat together on a regular basis. Foods are classified according to their nutrient content. By eating a variety of foods from each group every day, the athlete will obtain the needed nutrients for a nutritionally sound diet. During periods of heavy training, athletes should increase their consumption from the Grain, Fruit, and Vegetable Group. This will increase their carbohydrate intake and help minimize the gradual decline of muscle glycogen and the feeling of fatigue that occurs with heavy training.

Athletes who travel need to make sure that they make wise food choices on the road either by providing them with a nutritionally balanced meal or educating them on how to choose a balanced meal on the road. For example, at a suitable restaurant, the athletes should ask for a pasta meal within their budget. Usually, the manager or chef can accommodate them, especially if this request is made on a regular basis when the group is in town. Pasta meals, burritos with beans and rice, cold cereal with lowfat milk, baked potatoes, fruits, and vegetables can usually be found in restaurants and provide the easiest and cheapest source of carbohydrates.

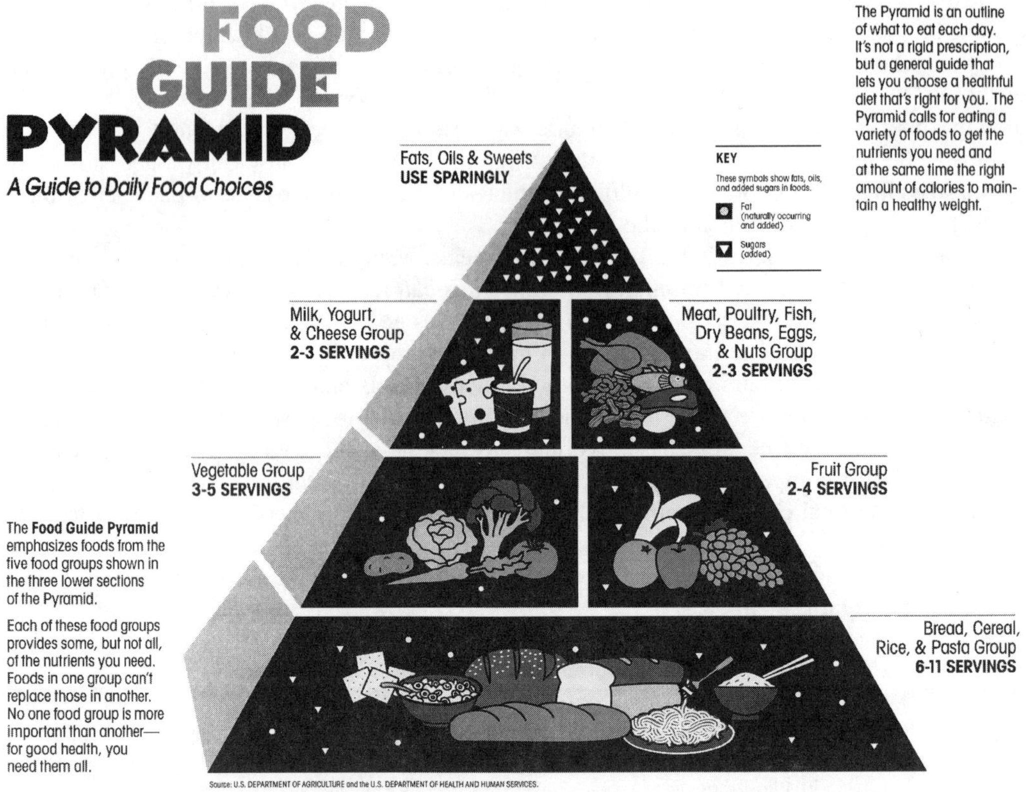
FOOD GUIDE PYRAMID
A Guide to Daily Food Choices
The Pyramid is an outline of what to eat each day. It's not a rigid prescription, but a general guide that lets you choose a healthful diet that's right for you. The Pyramid calls for eating a variety of foods to get the nutrients you need and at the same time the right amount of calories to maintain a healthy weight.
KEY
These symbols show fats, oils, and added sugars in foods.
Fat (naturally occurring and added)
Sugars (added)
Fats, Oils & Sweets
USE SPARINGLY
Milk, Yogurt, & Cheese Group
2-3 SERVINGS
Meat, Poultry, Fish, Dry Beans, Eggs, & Nuts Group
2-3 SERVINGS
Vegetable Group
3-5 SERVINGS
Fruit Group
2-4 SERVINGS
Bread, Cereal, Rice, & Pasta Group
6-11 SERVINGS
The Food Guide Pyramid emphasizes foods from the five food groups shown in the three lower sections of the Pyramid.
Each of these food groups provides some, but not all, of the nutrients you need. Foods in one group can't replace those in another. No one food group is more important than another—for good health, you need them all.
Source: U.S. DEPARTMENT OF AGRICULTURE and the U.S. DEPARTMENT OF HEALTH AND HUMAN SERVICES.

Figure 10.1 The Food Guide Pyramid offers a guide to a nutritionally balanced diet for both individuals and teams who eat together on a regular basis.

If the team or individual athletes stay in a hotel that offers food service, the coach or trainer should contact the catering manager and request high-carbohydrate meals within their budget. Table 10.2 gives guidelines for choosing meals while traveling. As long as the team or school is paying for the meals, they can demand the type and quality of food desired. They should be able to ask for special foods and get a reasonable price. The hotel or restaurant wants their business, but the team manager or representative must be able to tell the hotel or restaurant what they want for their meals. Athletes can also be taught how to order from the menu for better nutrition. For example, ordering à la carte might be more expensive, but it has the advantages of offering greater variety and possibly increasing the carbohydrate content of a meal by requesting substitutions, such as a baked potato instead of french fries, whole wheat bread for white bread, jelly instead of fat-laden pats of butter, and skim milk or fruit juice instead of calorie-dense soda pop. They can also ask for their salad dressing on the side to help control the amount of fat in the diet. These are ways in which athletes can make small changes when eating out that will make a significant difference in their nutritional status. All-you-can-eat buffets should be approached with caution. Some athletes regard buffet dining as a personal challenge, with the goal to get more than their money's worth by filling up their plates to overflowing. Athletes should be taught to survey the entire buffet line and then decide what foods are high in carbohydrate and low in fat and stick to those foods. If athletes fill up on nutritious foods first, they will get all the fuel and nutrients they need to compete and stay healthy. Table 10.3 lists key words to look for when reading a menu.

Table 10.2 Guidelines For Choosing Meals While Traveling

Breakfast

- Pancakes, waffles, french toast, bagels, muffins, cereal, fruit or juices for a high-carbohydrate breakfast
- Juice, dried fruit, fresh fruit, pretzels, and bagels are good snacks to pack when away from home
- Breakfast is the easiest meal at which to consume carbohydrate-rich foods
- Avoid high-fat choices such as bacon or sausage

Suggested Breakfast Menus	Total
Orange juice (1 cup) pancakes with syrup (3) banana sliced on pancakes (1)	547 calories, 90% carbohydrate
Apple Juice (6 ounces) Raisin Bran (1 large bowl) Low-fat milk (1 cup) Banana (1)	498 calories, 95% carbohydrate
Bran Muffin (1 large) Hot Cocoa (1 cup) Raisins or fresh fruit	310 calories, 69% carbohydrate
Plain English muffin (1) Strawberry jam (2 tablespoons) Egg (1 scrambled) Orange juice (1 cup) Low-fat yogurt (1 cup)	

Lunch

- Emphasize the bread in sandwiches rather than fillings
- Avoid hámburgers, fried fish, fried chicken, and french fries at fast-food restaurants
- Try baked potatoes, salads with fat-free dressing, plain hamburgers, chili, or plain burritos and tacos at fast-food restaurants as they have less fat
- Choose fruit juices or lowfat milk rather than soft drinks

Suggested Lunch Menus	Total
Large turkey sandwich on two slices of bread Low-fat fruited yogurt (1 cup) Orange Juice (1 cup)	1017 calories, 60% carbohydrate
Plain baked potato Chili (1 cup) Chocolate milkshake	916 calories, 62% carbohydrate
Vegetable soup (1 cup) Baked chicken (1 breast) Bread (1 slice) Applesauce (1 cup) Low-fat fruited yogurt (1 cup)	737 calories, 71% carbohydrate

Table 10.2 Guidelines For Choosing Meals While Traveling (Continued)

Dinner

- When on the road find a restaurant that offers pasta, baked potatoes, rice, breads, vegetables, and salads
- Order thick-crust pizza and double the amount of vegetable toppings like green peppers, mushrooms, onions, tomatoes, instead of pepperoni and sausage
- Try restaurants that offer Italian foods such as spaghetti, lasagna, breads, and salads
- Vegetable soups accompanied by crackers, bread, and muffins can add to a low-fat, carbohydrate-rich meal

Suggested Dinner Menus	Total
Minestrone soup (1 cup) Spaghetti (2 cups) Marinara sauce (2/3 cup) Parmesan cheese (1 tablespoon) Bread Sticks (2) Low-fat milk (1 cup)	977 calories, 68% carbohydrates
Turkey (4 ounces) Stuffing (1/2 cup) Mashed potatoes (1 cup) Peas (1 cup) Roll (1) Low-fat milk (1 cup)	960 calories, 55% carbohydrate
Lean Roast beef (3 ounces) Rice (1-1/2 cup) Corn (1 cup) Rolls (2) Low-fat milk (1-1/2 cup)	1320 calories, 60% carbohydrate

If athletes or athletic departments cannot afford all three meals at a hotel or restaurant, then they should choose breakfast for a team meal. With selections like cereal, both hot and cold; bagels; English muffins; pancakes; waffles; toast; fruit and fruit juices; as well as yogurt, breakfast can be an easy, inexpensive way to get carbohydrate-rich foods. If the budget does not allow restaurant meals or if the athletes are only on a day trip, any nearby grocery store will offer a great variety of foods that are cheaper and faster than eating in restaurants. Many grocery stores have a delicatessen or a soup and salad bar, and athletes can always pick up fresh fruits, vegetables, fruit juice, and low-fat dairy products as well as hot rotisserie chicken for an easy and nutritious meal on the road. In just about every grocery store, athletes can choose foods from all five food groups and come away with nutritious food choices that can enhance their performance.

Another way to urge athletes to make better food choices is to bring or pack a cooler with nutritious snacks for the road trip. Too often, when there is a long road trip where athletes travel by van or bus, they tend to consume candy, soda pop, chips, and fast foods. These types of foods can lead to increased fat content of the diet, which does not enhance athletic performance. To cut down on these types of foods, pack a cooler with high-carbohydrate foods. Table 10.4 lists examples of nutritious, high-carbohydrate snacks for athletes who travel.

B. Smart Food Choices at Fast-Food Restaurants

It's 7:00 p.m. and the team has just finished competing. They shower, dress, and pile into the team bus or vans. It's now 8:15 p.m. They are hungry, on a limited budget, and have a 2-hour drive home. Where can they stop to eat? Like many traveling teams and athletes, they stop at a fast-food

Table 10.3 Key Words to Look for When Selecting Nutritious Foods in Restaurants

Look Out For	Choose Instead
Fried, crispy, breaded, scampi style, creamed, buttery, au gratin, gravy	Marinara, steamed, boiled, broiled, tomato sauce, in its own juice, poached, charbroiled
Mexican	
Refried beans, chicken or bean burritos, tostados	Pot beans
Deep-fat-fried shells, flour tortillas	Baked or soft corn tortillas
Sour cream and guacamole	Salsa
Lots of chips	A few chips
Italian	
Pasta with cream sauces such as Alfredo	Pasta with marinara sauce
Pizza with extra cheese, pepperoni, or salami	Pizza with extra vegetables
Salads loaded with creamy dressing	Salads with dressing on the side
Buttery garlic toast	Bread with butter on the side
The dessert cart	Low-fat Italian ices and low-fat frozen yogurt
Chinese	
Deep-fried items such as egg rolls, wontons, and sweet and sour pork	Stir fry and steamed dishes, such as chicken and vegetables with rice
Burger Places	
Creamy salad dressings, high-fat extras such as potato salad	Salad bar using a low-fat or nonfat dressing
Fried burgers with extra cheese, mayonnaise, special sauce	Grilled burgers, no mayonnaise and go light on the cheese
French fries	Baked potato with toppings on the side
Milkshake	Juice or low-fat milk
Breakfast Cafes	
Large scoops of butter or margarine melting on pancakes, waffles, toast, English muffins, bagels	Butter or margarine on the side
Traditional breakfast fare such as eggs, bacon, ham and coffee	Fruit, fruit juices, and whole grain cereals, breads and muffins

restaurant. Although fast foods can be high in fat, low in carbohydrates, low in calcium, and low in vitamins C and A, athletes can make wise food selections by using Table 10.5. By making a few changes in their selection of foods at a fast-food restaurant, they can change a calorie-dense meal into a nutrient-dense meal. Try teaching these tips to athletes next time they step up to the counter at their favorite fast-food chain.

- Have athletes think about what they have already eaten and what they will eat later in the day. For example, if they have already had the deluxe meal combo, they might want to cut back and have a lighter meal for dinner.
- Make sure they include low-fat dairy products such as skim milk instead of soda pop and have them include at least two vegetables or fruits with each meal.
- Try limiting the amount of salad dressing or mayonnaise, or have them use fat-free choices when adding them to a salad or baked potato.
- Most fast-food chains offer lower-fat sandwiches such as grilled chicken. Even the plain hamburger or cheeseburger has less fat than the bigger burger smothered in cheese or sauce. Athletes could order two plainer items and get less fat than one regular burger.

Table 10.4 Packing the Cooler with Nutritious Foods

Water
Sports drinks
Fruit juices
Turkey sandwiches
Peanut butter sandwiches
Tuna sandwiches made with nonfat mayonnaise
Fresh fruit such as melons, apples, bananas, peaches, pears
Dried fruit such as raisins, apricots, and banana chips
Low-fat or nonfat yogurt
Vegetables such as carrots, celery, green peppers
String cheese
Energy bars
Cereal bars
Bagels, breads, rolls
Rice cakes
Bread sticks
Pretzels
Graham crackers
Animal crackers
Fig bars
Ginger snaps and vanilla wafers

- Try sharing an order of fries, a large sandwich, a baked potato, or an ice cream sundae with another teammate.
- Order the regular-size meal instead of supersizing it.

C. International Travel

While making wise food choices on the road is no easy task, trying to find familiar and nutritious food during international travel and competition is extremely difficult. Most athletes who travel internationally have problems finding enough food, let alone finding foods that are familiar and have been prepared in a way that doesn't present any potential food safety hazard.

Athletes who travel to other countries have a 50–50 chance of contracting traveler's diarrhea, a sometimes serious, always annoying, bacterial infection of the digestive tract. The risk is high because other countries' cleanliness standards for food and water are often lower than those of the United States and Canada. Another reason for the high incidence is that every region's microbes are different, and while individuals are immune to those in their own neighborhoods, traveling athletes have not had the chance to develop immunity to the pathogens in the places in which they are competing.

To protect the body against disease-causing organisms not found at home, the traveling athlete should drink only bottled water, even if just brushing their teeth. Many athletes make the mistake of using ice in their beverages when traveling abroad. They should drink only boiled, bottled, canned, or carbonated drinks without ice cubes. Most of the ice cubes made in foreign countries are made from local tap water and therefore may contain the microbes that could cause traveler's diarrhea. In addition to avoiding ice, athletes need to be careful not to swallow any water if they are swimming or showering, although swimming pools may be well chlorinated and are probably safe.

A meal at a fast-food restaurant doesn't need to be a dietary disaster. A typical fast-food meal is high in fat and low in carbohydrates, calcium, vitamin A, and vitamin C. It is difficult to choose a high-carbohydrate meal at a fast-food restaurant, but by making the food choices below, the carbohydrate content of the meal goes up as well as the nutrient density.

Table 10.5 Fast Food Choices

Breakfast	Lunch and Dinner
	McDonald's
Cheerios, Wheaties, hot cakes (no sausage), English muffin, apple, orange, or grapefruit juice, yogurt parfait	Grilled chicken sandwich, plain hamburger or cheeseburger, side salad with lite vinaigrette or reduced french dressing. Juice, milk, vanilla, chocolate or strawberry milkshake, or low-fat frozen yogurt cone
	Subway
	Turkey-breast or roast beef sub on whole wheat bread, watch the mayonnaise, side salad with low-calorie dressing or half the amount of regular dressing
	Hardees
Pancakes, no sausage or bacon, easy on the butter and syrup; oat bran muffin with orange juice	Regular cheeseburger or hamburgers; roast beef sandwich; hot ham and cheese sandwich; turkey club; grilled chicken breast sandwich; garden salad with low-calorie dressing, mashed potatoes with gravy (it's fat free); twist ice cream cone
	Taco Bell
	Bean burrito; regular or soft taco; chicken fajita; pinto beans and cheese; rice side order; lowfat milk; avoid extra cheese, added sour cream, guacamole
	Arby's
Blueberry muffin with orange juice; plain biscuit; cinnamon nut danish	Regular roast beef sandwich; grilled chicken deluxe; grilled chicken barbecue; turkey sub; anything from the light menu: roast turkey deluxe; roast chicken deluxe; roast beef deluxe sandwiches; baked potato instead of fries, easy on the toppings; garden salad; vegetable soup or chicken noodle soup.
	Wendy's
	Single hamburger; grilled chicken sandwich; jr. bacon cheeseburger; salads or baked potatoes, easy on the toppings and dressings Wendy's offers low-fat dressings or use half the amount of regular; a small Frosty has 2 grams fat.
	Pizza Hut
	Thicker crust pizza such as hand-tossed or pan pizza, ask for more vegetables on the pizza like green peppers and onions, avoid extra cheese, pepperoni and sausage; Best bets: veggie lover's pizza, supreme or super supreme, or pepperoni pizza; add a salad with low-fat dressing or use half the amount of regular; bread sticks are low in fat; hot ham and cheese sandwich; spaghetti

Table 10.5 Fast Food Choices (Continued)

Breakfast	Lunch and Dinner
	Burger King
Blueberry muffins and orange juice	Cheeseburger; hamburger; Whopper Jr; BK Broiler Chicken Sandwich; garden salad with low-calorie dressing or half the amount of regular dressing; worst choices: Double Whopper with cheese, Bacon Double Cheeseburger, fried chicken sandwich; french fries
	KFC
	Fried chicken with skin and fried coating removed; Chicken Little Sandwich; mashed potatoes with gravy (it's fat free); corn-on-the cob; garden salad with low-calorie dressing or half the amount of regular dressing; KFC Rotisserie chicken. Avoid fries, coleslaw and potato salad, which have at least 10 grams of fat for one serving.

D. Avoiding Traveler's Diarrhea

Since contaminated food and water can cause traveler's diarrhea, athletes need to be very careful of what they eat or drink. They should choose only restaurants that are well known or recommended by reliable people such as hotel managers, coaches, and athletes who have traveled in the area before. The U.S. Embassy is also a reliable place to get information about restaurants and water conditions. Also, whenever possible, athletes should avoid food sold on the street corners or in open-air markets. Caution should be taken at buffets, especially outdoors, and it should be certain that foods intended to be hot are served hot and that cold foods are kept refrigerated or on ice, and served cold.

Athletes also need to be careful about the amount and type of food eaten while traveling. Athletes should try to keep their eating habits close to normal if at all possible. If they are not usually big fruit eaters, they should not consume too much fruit while traveling. Eating too much of any food, even it is a food that they eat all the time, increases their risk of getting diarrhea. Also, many countries have their last meal of the day late in the evening. Having athletes wait to eat until late after competition may be devastating to the next day's performance. Try to stick to the same time of eating as when training at home.

Cooked foods are the best choice to avoid traveler's diarrhea. The cooking process kills most of the organisms that can cause diarrhea. Well-cooked vegetables and meats are good choices. Milk and milk products are a little bit more risky, because they require pasteurization and complete refrigeration. Milk products may be safe at first-class hotels, but if they have not been properly refrigerated or have been sitting on a buffet line without ice for over an hour, it is best to pass them by. Also, fruits that have to peeled in order to eat are good recommendations — oranges, grapefruit, and bananas are safe because the part consumed has been naturally protected by the skin. Athletes may want to pack some non-perishable foods from home to help on those days where they might suspect that food safety techniques have not been implemented.

E. Suggestions for Athletes with Traveler's Diarrhea

If athletes develop diarrhea, they should stop eating solid foods until the gas, cramps, and stomach pains go away. If available, drink large amounts of a sport drink or fluid-replacement drink or bottled water. Otherwise, try the BRAT diet. B is for bananas; R is for rice; A is for applesauce, and T is for toast. These types of foods are usually available in any country and they help in restoring muscle and liver glycogen that might have been depleted during the diarrhea. Carbonated beverages should be kept to a minimum. It is best not to take medication that might stop the diarrhea. The episodic bouts of diarrhea are the body's way of trying to get rid of the microbe that is causing the inflammation of the gastrointestinal tract. Taking medication may prevent the body from getting rid of the bacteria. If diarrhea persists for more than 48 hours, see a doctor.

F. Eating at all Day Events

Some athletic events such as swim or track meets, wrestling tournaments, volleyball and basketball tournaments, or double headers in baseball can last all day and competition may continue for several days. When athletes participate in a sport that lasts all day, they need to replenish carbohydrate stores and make sure they are well hydrated for peak performance. It is also important that athletes eat after competition to make sure they will have enough energy in their muscles for the next day's competition.

The same training-table principles used to plan the meals for the season can also apply to foods eaten at all-day competitions. If swimmers race at 10 a.m. and again in 2 hours, foods that are high in protein and fat will more than likely be in the swimmers' stomachs, causing some type of gastrointestinal distress as they get ready to race. The following guidelines have been recommended to help athletes make wise food choices at athletic events that last all day.

- If athletes have an hour or less between events or heats, they should stick with carbohydrate foods that are in liquid form, such as sports drinks. If they want something solid to eat they can try fruits like oranges, peaches, pears, and bananas. The more food they consume, the longer it will take to digest. The more athletes eat, even if it is carbohydrates and liquid, the longer it will take to digest, especially if they are nervous.
- If athletes have 2 to 3 hours between events or heats, they should add more-solid carbohydrates like bagels, hot or cold cereal with low-fat milk, or English muffins along with some type of fruit like apples, oranges, bananas, and peaches. They also need to make sure they are still drinking fluids, such as a sport drink, for rehydration and restoration of muscle glycogen.
- If athletes have 4 hours or more between events or heats, they can have a full meal, but it should be composed primarily of carbohydrates. For example, a turkey sandwich on two slices of whole grain bread, low-fat yogurt with fruit, and a sports drink, or they might try spaghetti with meat sauce, bread, a tossed salad with low-fat dressing and a sports drink as appropriate meal choices for this amount of time between events.

If athletes have a certain pre-game meal pattern that works, they should try to stick to it. Don't try new combinations of foods or different foods during the most important competition of their lives. Instead, try new foods and food combinations during training or a scrimmage to see if they are agreeable. Athletes who obtain food from concession stands need to be taught how to make the best food choices. Most concession stands are filled with high-fat, high-calorie foods that are not designed to maximize an athlete's performance. It is always wiser for athletes to pack a cooler from home with winning combinations than to rely on a concession stand.

III. SUMMARY

Because athletes have a high requirement for carbohydrates and have a difficult time making wise food choices, they need to learn wise strategies on how to eat better while traveling to and from competitions. First, it is important to learn that the food guide pyramid can be used as a guide in making food decisions as well as a menu guide for the training table. Second, if athletes can identify where they are going to eat or have a nutritious training table ready for them during the season and while traveling, it will help eliminate the nutrition pitfalls that athletes fall into during their careers. Last but not least, parents, coaches, trainers, and strength coaches, as well as athletes, must be good nutrition role models. It does no good to talk about the importance of good nutrition on athletic performance or to serve a well-balanced meal on a training table when a coach or trainer is on the sideline or pool deck drinking too much coffee or eating doughnuts. Athletes look up to coaches, trainers, strength coaches, and other athletes. To change athletes' eating habits, they must be educated so they have the knowledge to make wise food choices, opportunities to practice making good food choices at well-planned and -balanced training tables must be provided, and, most importantly, they must be given a good example to follow.

REFERENCES

1. American Dietetic Association, 1987, Nutrition for physical fitness and athletic performance for adults. *J. Am Diet Assoc.* 87; 933-939.
2. Bernadot, D. and Thompson, W.R., 1999, Energy from food for physical activity. Enough and on time. *ACSM's Health and Fitness Journal.*3.4):14-18.
3. Berning, J.R., Troup, J.P., VanHandel, P.J., Daniels, N., and Daniels, J.,1991, The nutritional habits of young adolescent swimmers. *Int. J. Sport Nutr.* 1;240-248.
4. Campbell, M.L. and McFadyen, K.L., 1984, Nutrition knowledge, beliefs, and dietary practices of competitive swimmers. *Can. Home. Econom. J.* 34;47.
5. Committee on Diet and Health. *Diet and Health: Implications for Reducing Chronic Disease Risk.* Washington, D.C.: National Academy Press, 1989.
6. Coyle, E.F., Coggan, A.R., Hemmert, M.K., Ivy, J.L., 1986, Muscle glycogen utilization during prolonged strenuous exercise when fed carbohydrate. *J. Am. Physio.* 61:165-172.
7. Coyle, E.F., Hagber, J.M., Hurley, B.F., Martin, W.H., Ehsani, A.A., and Holloszy, J.O., 1983, Carbohydrate feeding during prolonged strenuous exercise can delay fatigue. *J. Am. Physio.* 55; 230-235.
8. Davis, J.M., Jackson, D.A., Broadwell, M.S., Query, J.L., and Lambert, C.L., 1997, Carbohydrate drinks delay fatigue during intermittent, high-intensity cycling in active men and women. *Int. J. Sport Nutr.* 7:261-273.
9. Ivy, J.L., Lee, M.C., Brozinick, J.T., and Reed, M.J., 1988, Muscle glycogen storage after different amounts of carbohydrate ingestion. *J. Appl. Physiol.* 65.5):2018-2023
10. Shoaf, L.R., McClellan, P.D., and Birskovich, K,A., Nutrition knowledge, interests, and information sources of male athletes. *J. Nutr. Educ.*
11. Sherman, W.M., Peden, M.C., and Wright, D.A., 1991, Carbohydrate feedings 1 hour before exercise improves cycling performance. *Am. J. Clin. Nutr.* 54:866-870
12. Sherman, W.M., Brodowicz, G., Wright, D.A., Allen, W.K., Simonsen, J., Dernbach, A., 1989 Effects of 4-hour pre-exercise carbohydrate feedings on cycling performance. *Med. Sci. Sport Exerc.* 21; 598-604.
13. VanHandel, P.J., Cells, K.A., Bradley, P.W., and Troup, J.P., 1984 Nutritional status of elite swimmers, *J. Swim. Res.* 1;27-31.
14. Yuen, D.E. and Draaper, H.H., 1984, Effects of dietary protein on calcium metabolism in man. *Nutr. Abstr. Rev.* 54:447-49.
15. Zwadski, K.M., Yasppelkis, B.B., and Ivy, J.L., 1992, Carbohydrate protein complex increases the rate of muscle glycogen storage after exercise. *J. Appl. Physiol.* 72:1854-1859.

CHAPTER 11

Eating on the Road

David R. Ellis

CONTENTS

Evidence exists that the needs of athletes for some of the nutrients are different from individuals who are sedentary or moderately active.[1,2] Inadequate consumption of water, energy, complex carbohydrates, proteins, minerals (especially electrolytes), and vitamins can hinder athletic performance.[1-3] Other chapters in this book discuss the nutrient needs of athletes throughout their life cycle. This chapter addresses the practical issues of athletes eating while on the road, and the design and implementation of programs for feeding these athletes in travel situations.

I. THE SPORTS COMMUNITY AND TRAVEL

Applied sports nutrition works with a population group that has some unique needs, especially when traveling to compete. Like any enthusiastic community nutritionist, applied sports nutritionists learn the most about their clients once they gain their trust and become comfortable among them at home and on the road. On the road, applied sports nutritionists learn how overrated travel is and how unpredictable the best travel plans can become. The stress placed on the entire travel party can be enormous, especially for the student athlete. Applied sports nutritionists have an "eye" for looking at a travel itinerary and knowing how to anticipate and plan for the unpredictable.

0-8493-8199-1/00/$0.00+$.50

Something as simple as a snack planned at the airport prior to departure can become a significant advantage for one team over another. Planes frequently are delayed. On one occasion, the University of Wisconsin football team was flying to Tokyo to play in the Coca Cola Bowl. Both teams (Wisconsin and Michigan State) had to fly to Tokyo on the same plane. Both teams waited in an airport for a plane for 2 hours. One team purchased food at vending machines, while the other team, who had an experienced sports nutritionist along, had travel snacks and bottled water from their travel bags. These travel snacks were high in complex carbohydrates and nutrient-dense, and the foods from the vending machines likely were not. Likewise, a fast-food restaurant generally is not an appropriate place for athletes to eat when traveling to a competition.

There is no doubt that an athlete who has better energy levels and faster recovery, and who experiences less incapacitation due to illness or injury, has the ability to perform better physically than the competition. At home or on the road, an athlete who is conscious of the subtle, but very powerful, cumulative benefits of food is a good client for the applied sports nutritionist. A variety of travel circumstances involving athletes will be discussed in this chapter.

II. APPLIED "FUELING TACTICS"

Nutrition strategies for athletes are frequently referred to as "fueling tactics" because, at times, the strategies take on almost battle-like planning when working with a coaching staff to build a superior nutrition plan. Over the years, athletes, coaches, and trainers have become, in some cases, superstitious about "fueling" for competition. Anyone who works with fueling athletes for competition and travel quickly learns that success or failure during competition can immediately be attributed to the food and beverage consumed by the athletes. Radio or television broadcasters often remark "I wonder what they fed them today?" in a positive or negative light depending upon the performance of the team.

Coaches also like to evaluate performance against gross changes in body composition. They frequently talk about an athlete as being "too heavy" or "too light" to do the job. Applied sports nutritionists perform various anthropometric measurements (Figure 11.1) in evaluating body composition. Once an applied sports nutritionist begins to build a nutrition support service for a team, the magnitude of these issues as seen through the eyes of the athletes and coaches becomes immediately obvious. At this time, "fueling tactics" will take on greater meaning. The vast majority of what is known about travel nutrition has not been published and is frequently guarded as "trade secrets" passed along over the years.

A combination of time-tested experiences and research will ultimately yield sport-specific fueling tactics for travel that take into account the unique circumstances for team members in each sport. One set of rules will not work in all circumstances. It is best to have an experienced applied sports nutritionist travel with a team so that appropriate fueling tactics can be innovated and applied. Many teams do the same thing, year after year, out of habit, frequently simply leaving travel nutrition up to the athletes to fund. Ann Grandjean, of the International Center for Sports Nutrition, says it best: "Sometimes when I am out consulting with various professional teams, it is like walking back in time 10–15 years. Very little progress has been made with team nutrition services, most typically due to management not allocating any money for the services."[4] My own experiences consulting outside of college athletes have shown similar results. Even at elite levels of competition, it is not uncommon to find little or no nutrition support services beyond some free supplements provided by a corporate sponsor. Instead, the athletic trainer or strength coach is saddled with the extra responsibility. Sometimes these responsibilities fall on the shoulders of an administrative operations employee, or even the equipment manager.

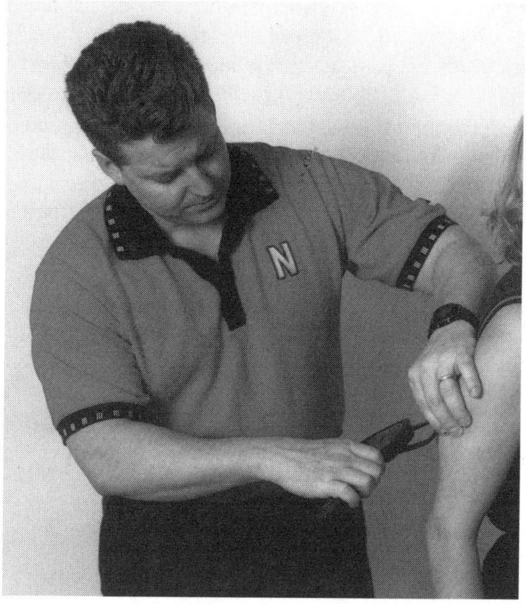

Figure 11.1 Various measurements are performed in evaluating body composition.

III. A TRUE COMMITMENT TO FUELING

Having a qualified professional on staff — and, hopefully, on the road — who is focused on coordinating the most appropriate fueling tactics is fast becoming a competitive advantage that will open doors for full-time applied sports nutritionists in the future. Below is an excerpt from the Knoxville, Tennessee, newspaper of July 10, 1998 titled "Vols Catch up with Huskers" written by John Adams, Sports Editor.[5]

> If you believe that the Tennessee Vols are only a few good meals from a national championship in football, then you should know about their new applied sports nutritionist.
>
> The applied sports nutritionist is Coach Carbohydrates. His arrival is encouraging to anyone with deep convictions about the correlation between winning and eating. "I fell into the right place at the right time" he says.
>
> He can thank Nebraska for that. As a few of you might remember, the Vols were a late-night snack for Nebraska in the Orange Bowl. In the subsequent post-game analysis (six months and counting), the 42–17 defeat has been attributed to coaching, blocking, tackling, running, catching, passing, conditioning, and eating.
>
> "It (nutrition) wasn't the reason we got beat like we did," (the University of Tennessee) strength and conditioning coach said, "but it was a contributing factor." And regrettably, it was totally ignored in this column. I assumed (the coach at Nebraska) might give the Cornhuskers a slight edge and I practically defied Nebraska's offensive line. But not in a single piece of pre-game correspondence did I alert the folks back home to the obvious nutritional advantage.
>
> Full-Time Nutritionist: Nebraska 1, Tennessee 0.

> Feel free to snicker. But after watching Nebraska win three of the last four National Championships (almost four out of five), I have devised a simple method for evaluating what's good and bad in college football. If Nebraska does it, it's good. If Nebraska doesn't do it, it's bad.
>
> Thanks to (the new applied sports nutritionist at Tennessee) it's not as bad as it used to be. He has a bachelor's degree in dietetics from (a Midwestern university), where he was an undersized defensive lineman, encouraged by his coaches to follow a high-fat, fast-gain diet. He has ignored their culinary advice this summer, during which he has become an integral part of (the University of Tennessee's) strength and conditioning program.
>
> (The coach) is committed to the quest. All freshman student-athletes will be steered toward a nutrition class this fall, and upperclassmen will be encouraged to do so as well. However, (the coach) realizes barbells are an easier sell than dinner bells.
>
> (The applied sports nutritionist) has provided one-on-one food counseling in 15-minute weekly meetings with each player. The early results are mixed. If not for the Orange Bowl, there might have been more teeth to pull. As any self-respecting nutritionist would tell you, that was a textbook mismatch in reserve carbohydrates.
>
> The Vols got tired so fast, even the least introspective among them must have wondered: "Was it something I ate?"

One year after Nebraska beat Tennessee in the Orange Bowl for the National Championship, Tennessee won the National Championship. One of the biggest changes Tennessee made was structuring the meals for the athletes, as opposed to just giving them the money to buy food while at the bowl game.

Athletes value a staff member whose job it is to look out for their nutritional well being. It is not uncommon for athletes to compare notes with their opponents on how things were handled leading up to a competition. Unfortunately, according to many coaches and athletes, there is a lack of commitment to feeding athletes due to "cost containment" measures mandated internally (administration) and externally (sports conference rules, etc.). Today, more than ever, it is easier to leave feeding up to the individual athlete than to use financial resources to have an experienced applied sports nutritionist plan the fueling tactics for the athletes.

Unfortunately, because many teams have given up on organizing feeding due to cost containment, athletes sometimes mix up their pre-game meals in a food blender in their hotel rooms. Cost containment has done more to elevate the utility of dietary supplements for athletes than any advertising campaign in any magazine. Nutritionists and others can preach "food first," but if costs dictate the extent of support services available to athletes, this trend will continue. If given the choice to eat food, take a pill, or mix up a power shake, the athlete would choose to eat.

> *If we want to disempower supplements in the eyes of athletes, we need to re-impower food by making a true commitment to feeding athletes.*

Unfortunately, this is more easily said than done. Even for teams that make the commitment to feed their athletes, the profit margins on which some hotels normally operate (especially in large markets) can challenge the common sense of even the staunchest applied sports nutritionist. If the team stays in an inexpensive hotel, meal arrangements, other than for the token continental breakfast, may not be possible at all. The training table on the road today competes with vending machines, fast foods, and dietary supplements. When traveling overseas, a fast-food chain can be a welcome sight for an athlete who cannot decipher the menu. Even when traveling in the U.S., when there is no plan or guidance, even the best-educated athletes will get their meals from the most convenient and inexpensive food supply available. Without guidance, athletes on the road will eat at any place within walking distance of the hotel.

IV. TIMING FOR CHANGE IS EVERYTHING

Athletic teams need to have someone facilitating a convenient way for players to eat appropriate meals, and sometimes this means bringing the meal to the site where the athletes are practicing. This approach saves the team the time required to go out to eat or pay "banquet" prices at the hotel. Frequently, coaches and athletes alike view travel as an opportunity to give the athletes money for food; athletes usually spend the money so sparingly that they have some left when they return home. It is not uncommon to see a softball or baseball team eating hot dogs at the concession stand, perhaps to save money for some important personal necessity. Sometimes the coaching staff facilitates this, because the idea of sacrificing some travel money for food is not popular with many team members who commonly express these feelings at team meetings. It takes strong commitment for the coaching staff to overcome this attitude, and not do what the athletes say they want, especially when the team has been successful doing the same thing year after year.

Timing is everything when initiating changes with a team. A great time to introduce something that might be perceived as a sacrifice or break from tradition is when a team is struggling and is looking to improve. When a team is on the brink of championship performance, but cannot quite win "the big one," is another time that change can be embraced with minimal resistance. However, coaches or administrators may perceive that any increases in the cost of doing business could be a risk for their dismissal. Applied sports nutritionists should not be surprised if they encounter this in athletic departments that are operating on limited funds. The potential for a love–hate relationship between the coach and the administrator is present, and often this pits what is best for the well being and performance of the athletes against cost containment. The applied sports nutritionist must pay attention to this struggle while designing the nutrition support service. If the applied sports nutritionist can cite examples where the nutrition commitment has been made in a successful and money-producing athletic program, this might help convince the coach and administrator to make a nutrition commitment to the athletes by putting a qualified professional in charge of the athletic nutrition support service.

An experienced, full-time, applied sports nutritionist will look over the travel itinerary and rationalize when, where, and what fueling tactics need to be implemented for an athlete or the team. In addition, the applied sports nutritionist can write menus for appropriate fueling tactics and communicate with qualified vendors about fulfilling the service of feeding the team appropriately before the team travels. It is not uncommon to find teams eating in planes, trains, and buses to stay on schedule and save money. Resourcefulness and being able to "think on your feet" are prerequisites to being able to help traveling athletes get appropriate meals. Otherwise, the overbooked travel staff encourages the team to eat fast food or airline food. Proper fueling tactics take planning and commitment.

V. RATIONALIZING WHEN AND WHERE TO FUEL

Experience helps one rationalize when and where to feed traveling athletes. It is not enough to just hope that suitable food and beverage will be available at or adjacent to your hotel, practice, or competition venue. An applied sports nutritionist must be able to get the team's travel itinerary soon enough to design a plan and put it into action.

To rationalize when to apply circumstantially correct fueling tactics, the applied sports nutritionist must be able to visualize the team traveling, while taking into account what the environmental and competitive duty cycle of work will be.

For example, applied sports nutritionists often joke that they feed every 4 hours when the athletes are awake. Based on our experience, that really is often the case. Athletes seem to feel and perform better when fed smaller, more frequent meals and snacks. This has been shown to be true in laboratory rats having a fixed daily protein intake.[6] The athletes learn that stuffing themselves is not necessary, as another meal or snack will be forthcoming. Starving athletes in anticipation of a big ceremonial pre-grame meal is an obsolete practice. Having a "sit-down" eating situation is not always possible or cost effective when feeding smaller meals and snacks frequently. Smaller, more frequent meals offer anxiety-prone athletes the opportunity to consume enough calories even though their appetites are diminished due to the ensuing competition.

Today's applied sports nutritionist must be knowledgeable, not only about when and how to initiate change, but to keep pace with the ever-changing rules that govern the benefits that athletes can receive from organizations like the National Collegiate Athletic Association (NCAA), Olympic federations, or high school athletic associations. The NCAA Division I Manual has about 10 pieces of legislation that impact feeding athletes at home or on the road. It is likely all these rules were voted on and approved by administrators who think of nutrition as three traditional meals per day for the athlete. That means they only allow money for three meals daily, which forces whoever is in charge to ultimately conform to that concept.

16.8.1.2.3 Meal-Allowance Limitation reads as follows:

> "All student-athletes on the same team must receive identical meal allowances on intercollegiate trips and during vacation periods when student-athletes are required to remain on the institution's campus for organized practice sessions or competition. Such allowances may not exceed the amount provided by the institution to institutional staff members on the away-from-campus trips and may not be provided for a particular meal if the student-athlete receives that meal (or its equivalent) from another source."[7]

Another cost containment-driven proposal about to be proposed for the NCAA Manual reads, "To permit an institution, at its discretion, to provide cash allowance (not to exceed U.S. $6) to student-athletes following home and away-from-home contests in lieu of a post-game meal or snack.[8]

Obviously, doing what is potentially best for the nutritional well being of the athletes has many obstacles to be navigated — conceptually and economically. The sooner the administrators who predominate in these rule-making committees, such as those of the NCAA, realize the effect these regulations have on their member institutions, the better for the student-athlete.

Wherever applied sports nutritionists feed the athletes, "hands on" management is required to accomplish the task, monitor the success of the effort, and plan for future innovation. This on-line quality management is often neglected when people who already have full-time jobs in the athletic department get nutrition responsibilities in addition to their other responsibilities. Often, these overextended staff members cannot supervise or attend the meal they have arranged for their athletes. This could result in pizza and chicken wings being delivered to a hotel room for a basketball team because the operations administrator wanted to make the athletes happy while he or she went out to dinner with the coaching staff. Too often, this type of convenient solution is utilized rather than having a qualified professional supervise the eating activities of the team.

VI. DETERMINING HOW MUCH STRUCTURE

Every sport has its own culture that evolves from year to year. As a group, athletes tend to conform to team leaders and the coach. An applied sports nutritionist needs to understand the cultural dynamics of the team and its leaders and then make some decisions as to how much structure should be tolerated when feeding the athletes at home or on the road. The size of the team seems to influence the threshold or structure that some teams can tolerate. Athletic teams that have a small to medium number of athletes, such as soccer and volleyball, may want to eat in the community in which they are playing. Some teams with a small number of athletes, like golf, may just leave the decisions up to the resourcefulness of their athletes while traveling. Sports that compete frequently, like the Major League Baseball, National Basketball Association, and National Hockey League, also tend to leave feeding up to the athletes. Some athletes in the professional ranks even travel with family members and may stay at hotels separate from the team. An applied sports nutritionist has to be flexible and stay focused when designing fueling tactics for these types of athletes.

When helping a team show up for a competition well-fueled, rested, and, hopefully, relaxed, don't expect complete success. Someone will always believe that food at the fast-food restaurant has more nutritional value than the team meal. The applied sports nutritionist should not overreact to these individuals. The majority of athletes appreciate structure when it comes to eating on the road as opposed to their having to figure out when and what to eat. Even the athletes who want to have meal money to spend as they desire get tired of ordering room service, fighting crowds at local restaurants, or getting food from fast-food establishments, concession stands, vending machines, and supplements. Coaches tend to support structured meals if:

- The meal plans are organized and ready when the team arrives (early or late).
- The meals offer variety and the best quality possible from the vendor.
- The majority of the athletes are happy.

Coaches know that when the food is good, the entire attitude of the team seems to be uplifted. A room full of happy athletes dining is not a quiet room. The athletes are relaxed and laughing. Conversations lighten up for a short time from the tension of the ensuing competition. Coaches realize that every minute that athletes are kept on schedule and relaxed helps them be well rested and probably better able to listen to and retain the last-minute details of the strategy for the game. When athletes have trouble getting food or do not like the food, they will complain. Whether the team wins or loses, one of the happiest persons on the trip home from the competition is the applied sports nutritionist who has completed working through days and weeks of consecutive deadlines for feeding and hydrating traveling athletes.

VII. FUNDAMENTAL AND ADVANCED FUELING TACTICS FOR TRAVEL

Table 11.1 offers an example of an "advanced" set of fueling tactics for eating on the road for a typical competition. These plans are sent out to hotels as part of a travel plan that not only outlines the nutrition requirements, but also covers other travel requirements.

The detail in this travel plan is what makes the plan "advanced" as much as the items themselves. Nothing is left to chance. The hotel does not need to wonder what the team's expectations are, which hotel management appreciates, as they often find themselves reacting to the needs of guests as opposed to having the needs outlined in advance. The applied sports nutritionist should develop this plan in great detail and send it to the hotel where the team will be staying. This also allows athletic departments to get a bid on the cost of meals long before the team arrives. The bid should include taxes, etc. so that the hotel and the applied sports nutritionist are able to sign a contract for nutrition services at that hotel.

Table 11.1 Advanced Fueling Tactics Plan

1. *Beverage Table for Strategic Planning Room*

Coaches and athletes will frequent this room throughout the stay at the hotel. The types of beverages and disposable serving containers and utensils that are to be available are detailed; bananas and red delicious apples also must be available. Most teams supply their own bottled water, Gatorade®, "energy" bars, and "recovery" bars, which will also be placed on the beverage table. However, these items must be stored by the hotel and served at appropriate temperatures. Some teams require a beverage table in several different rooms.

2. *Buffet Check List*

This details the manner in which the hotel should serve the players. Items described include color of table linen, meat-carving stations, types of seating tables and number of players per table, seating tables for coaches, portion control, and presentability and replacement of food on the buffet.

3. *Buffet Layout*

A typical pre-game dinner/breakfast layout is given in Figure 11.2. The players are to consume foods from specified tables first and these are to be arranged as specified by the applied sports nutritionist. This arrangement encourages the players to eat more of specific types of foods than other types.

4. *Dinner Buffet for the Evening Prior to the Game*

This is the dinner buffet for the athletes preceding the competition day. Food must be on the buffet line as specified by the applied sports nutritionist. The fruits, vegetables, nuts, and seeds should come first, followed by the starches, and then the protein items. Do not let the hotel staff decide on the arrangement. Most teams supply their own bottled water and Gatorade®, but the hotel must serve these beverages. The applied sports nutritionist needs to be sure the dining room is not so crowded that the quality of the dining experience is compromised.

Tables required for buffet:

- Two double-sided soup, salad, bread, and fruit tables
- two double-sided entree tables (use menu 1, 2, or 3 given below)
- one beverage table
- one condiment table
- one dessert table

Entree Menu 1: Asparagus spears, candied baby carrots, corn on the cob, baked potatoes, cheese sauce, spaghetti, meatless marinara sauce, beef spaghetti sauce (lean), baked cod fillets, char-grilled skinless barbecued chicken (100 g or 3 ounces), carved beef tenderloin *au jus*

Entree Menu 2: Broccoli spears, candied baby carrots, cheese sauce, mashed potatoes, beef gravy, rotini pasta, meatless marinara, beef spaghetti sauce (lean), meatless lasagna, char-grilled tuna or salmon steaks with lime butter, skinless shake-and-bake chicken (1/8 of chicken per serving), carved barbecue inside round of beef (visible fat removed before cooking and seasoning), *au jus*

Entree Menu 3: Whole green beans, candied baby carrots, twice-baked potatoes, cheese sauce, *mostaccoli* with meatless marinara, rice pilaf, baked orange roughy with bread crumbs, char-grilled skinless teriyaki chicken breast, carved prime rib (visible fat removed before cooking and seasoning), *au jus*

The experienced applied sports nutritionist could supply the hotel with estimates of the quantities of each of the items that are typically consumed. He or she should also taste certain foods for appropriate spice content and double-check food temperature and freshness before all meals consumed on the road. It is best to travel in advance of the team and check on hotel catering staff and be sure they are prepared for the team.

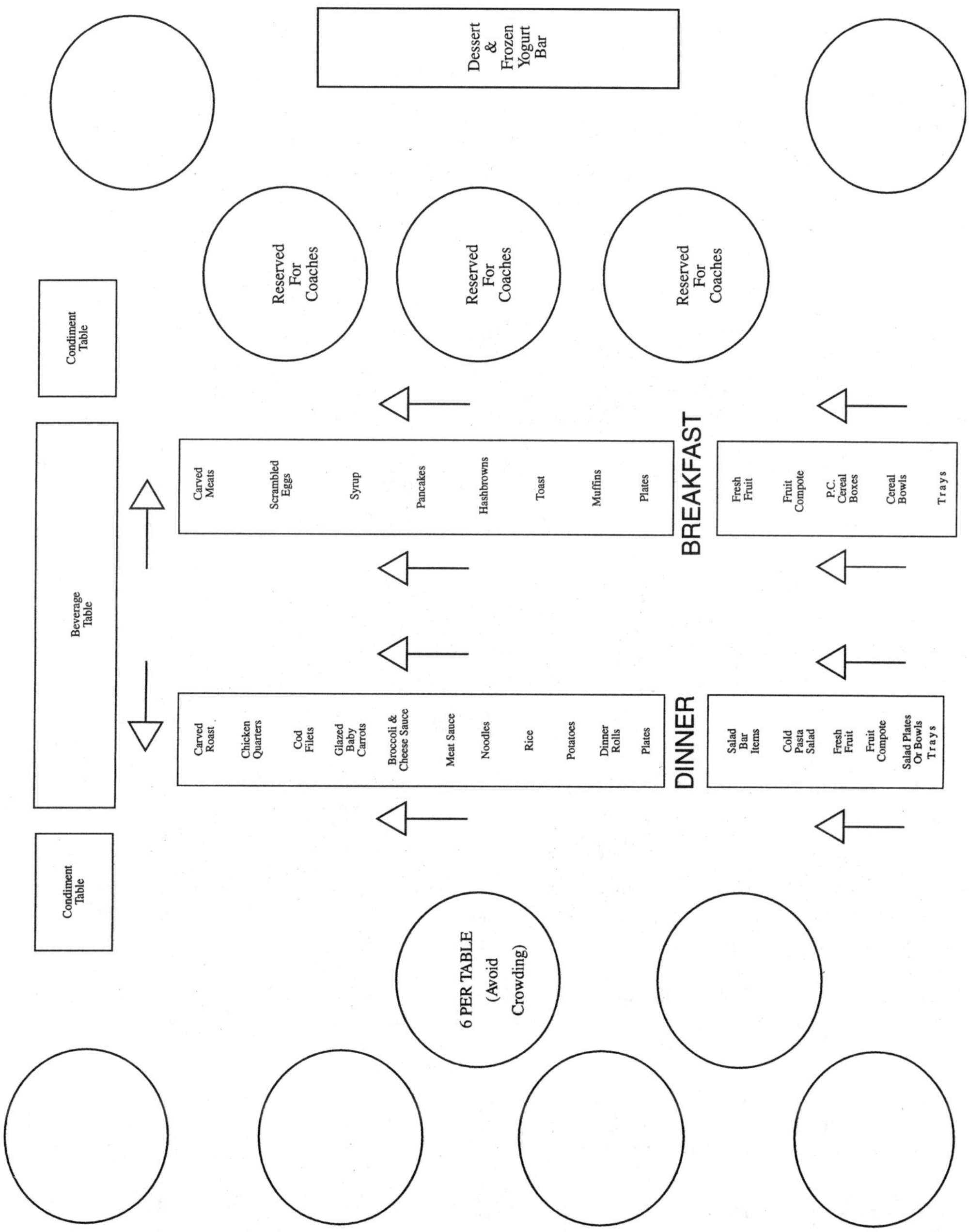

Figure 11.2 A typical pre-game dinner or breakfast layout.

5. Snack-Bag Buffet for the Night Prior to the Game

Two tables, double-sided, containing snack-bag buffet items are needed for the athletes from the first evening they arrive. They will obtain food from these tables at a specified time, take it to their hotel room, and eat it there. The foods should be arranged on the tables in a specified order. The applied sports nutritionist should limit players to a maximum amount of the various kinds of foods allowed. A typical menu is given below.

Items available:

- bags (plastic with handles preferred)
- ripe bananas and red delicious apples
- portion-controlled flavored yogurts, puddings (low-fat), and Jello®
- disposable spoons
- ~15 cm (6-inch) individually wrapped and labeled subs — turkey, roast beef, and ham (mix white and whole wheat buns), each containing ~135g (4 ounces) of shaved meat, no condiments added during preparation
- portion-controlled low-fat yellow and white cheese slices (individually wrapped)
- portion-controlled lettuce and tomato packets (individually wrapped)
- portion-controlled mustard, mayonnaise, and ketchup packets
- oatmeal cookies and chocolate chip cookies (individually wrapped)
- portion-controlled bags of potato chips and pretzels
- napkins
- Beverage table — same as for dinner

The experienced applied sports nutritionist could supply the hotel with estimates of the quantities of each of the items that are typically consumed. The athletes should understand that the snack is to be eaten immediately and not saved for later.

6. Pre-Game Breakfast Buffet

The hotel catering staff should follow the breakfast layout (Figure 11.2). Food items should be arranged as illustrated.

Tables for buffet

- two double-sided for cereal, muffins, and fruit
- two double-sided for entrees
- one beverage table
- one condiment table

Entree menu 1: White and whole wheat toast (lightly buttered), grits, hash browns (low oil), pancakes, waffles, maple and blueberry syrup, hot apple and strawberry topping, cheese omelets, carved smoked turkey breast, and mild low-fat beef sausage patties or links, or turkey-bacon strips

Entree menu 2: White and whole wheat toast (lightly buttered), grits, hash browns (low oil), pancakes, french toast, maple and blueberry syrup, hot apple and strawberry topping, scrambled eggs, mild low-fat turkey sausage patties or links, and carved Canadian bacon

Entree menu 3: White and whole wheat toast (lightly buttered), grits, hash browns (low oil), pancakes, maple and blueberry syrup, hot apple and strawberry topping, scrambled eggs, cheese quiche, baked breaded chicken strip, and low-fat pork sausage patties or links

The experienced applied sports nutritionist should supply the hotel with estimates of the quantities of each of the items that are typically consumed. Eggs should be well cooked. Turkey and Canadian bacon should be carved at the end of the buffet table.

7. Pre-Game for Night Game

This meal should be light in calories. The food should be arranged on the buffet as specified. The last meal should be served about 4 hours before the start of competition. When that is not feasible (early-morning or multiple-event sports), protein items in the meal that could slow digestion should be limited or eliminated.

Tables for buffet:

- two double-sided for soup, salad, bread, and fruit
- two doubled-sided entree tables
- beverage table
- condiment table

Entree menu: Baked potatoes, spaghetti, meatless marinara, lean-beef spaghetti sauce, kaiser buns, deli meat (turkey, roast beef, ham), breaded and baked cod fillet, lettuce, tomato (for sandwiches), white rice, beef, chicken, and vegetable (broccoli, carrots, pea pods) stir-fries

The experienced applied sports nutritionist should supply the hotel with estimates of the quantities of each of the items that are typically consumed. The stir-fries should not be spicy, but should be lightly seasoned with soy and thickened with cornstarch. The meat should be lean, not fried or breaded. The rice should be placed before the stir-fries in the buffet. Parmesan cheese and soy sauce can be on the condiment table. No pickles or onions should be served at this meal.

8. Cereal, Muffin, and Fruit Bar

This bar is served at breakfast. Either portion-controlled boxes or bulk cereal are acceptable. Hot water should be available for instant hot cereal. No poppy seed or chocolate items of any type should be on this bar. Regional and seasonal fruits may be offered with permission from the applied sports nutritionist.

Items available:

Cut fruit: sliced cantaloupe,peaches, banana, fresh blue berries or cherries, sliced strawberries, and raisins
Whole fruit: grapes, bananas, and apples
Cereal bar: bran flakes, corn flakes, granola cluster®, Honey Nut Cheerios®, hot cereal packets (flavored oatmeal and cream of wheat)
Breakfast rolls and muffins: bagels, fruit breads (peach or banana), and muffins

9. Soup, Salad, Bread, and Fruit Bar

This bar is served at lunch or dinner. The salad buffet should be refrigerated or iced and well lighted.

Items available:

Cut fruit: sliced cantaloupe, watermelon cubes, pineapple rings, sliced peaches, sliced pears, and fruit cocktail.
Whole fruit: grapes, bananas, apples, and seasonal options (must be approved by the applied sports nutritionist)
Salad bar: iceberg lettuce, romaine lettuce, grated carrots, sliced red cabbage, sliced green onion, sliced mushrooms, cherry tomatoes, sweet peppers, garbanzo beans, bean sprouts, croutons, sunflower seeds, imitation bacon bits, grated cheddar and mozzarella cheese, parmesan cheese, crumbled blue cheese, sliced ham, and sliced chicken breast
Salad dressings: ranch, french, creamy italian, thousand island, honey mustard, blue cheese, and vinegar and oil, all low-fat or fat-free, and labeled
Cold pasta salad: dressed with light oil, not mayonnaise
Bread: warm multi-grain dinner rolls or bread sticks, white bread, and wheat bread
Soup: chicken noodle, turkey rice, or vegetable beef

10. Beverage Table

Only portion-controlled beverages should be on the table. Disposable cups (473–591 mL or 16–20 ounce) and ice should also be available adjacent to the portion-controlled beverages. Local tap water will not be used for any beverages other than coffee. Bottled water, Gatorade®, and some special supplement beverages will be provided to the catering staff for serving to the team; these should be stored and chilled appropriately by the catering staff.

Items available:

Fruit juice: fruit punch (red), orange, grape, apple, and pineapple. (also, grapefruit and V-8® at breakfast only)
Other: Gatorade®, bottled water, milk (skim, 2% white, and 2% chocolate), coffee (regular and decaffeinated), hot water, assorted hot teas, instant hot chocolate packets, mini-marshmallows, sliced lemons, sugar, Nutra-Sweet®, non-dairy and dairy cream, styrofoam cups, cup lids, and stir straws

The catering staff should confirm dates on all beverages, especially dairy products, for freshness. The athletes should be provided with distilled water and supplement beverages that the applied sports nutritionist brings along with other team equipment.

11. Condiment Table

This table should have plenty of space for the athletes to set down their trays or plates. It should be close to the end of the buffet.

Items available:

- brown sugar, parmesan cheese, grated cheese (when no salad bar), pepper, and a variety of seasoning salts
- honey, soy sauce, barbecue sauce, salsa, Louisiana hot sauce, tabasco, worcestershire sauce, creamy horse radish, A1® and Hines 57® steak sauces (when serving red meat), Dijon mustard, yellow mustard, tartar sauce, cocktail sauce, lemon slices (when serving fish or seafood), and low-fat sour cream with chives (when serving baked potatoes)

Regional alternatives for condiments may be substituted with the permission of the applied sports nutritionist. The athletes will take the condiment bottles to a table, so supply several bottles of each condiment.

12. Dessert Table

Items available:

- warm brownies (no nuts)
- bananas and banana split boats
- low-fat, sweetened frozen yogurt (chocolate, vanilla, and strawberry) scooped into bowls that hold two to three scoops; also available should be sliced bananas, hot caramel, hot fudge, strawberry topping, pineapple topping, whipped cream, cherries, and sprinkles (should be served only the evening prior to the competition)

Catering staff should dispense the yogurt into bowls for the athletes. Disposable dishes and utensils should be used, as athletes frequently take dessert to their hotel rooms or to meetings.

13. Bid for Catering Services

The hotel should provide a detailed estimate of their costs for feeding the team. The applied sports nutritionists can help hotel catering staffs provide cost-effective meals. Often, the chef may have an inflated image of how much food to prepare for a group of athletes, which will increase food costs and waste. This bid should include taxes, gratuities, and other miscellaneous charges. The school may be tax-exempt, and, if so, the hotel catering administrator should be so informed. The applied sports nutritionist should inform athletic department administrators of the final costs for feeding the team.

VIII. HYDRATION AND REST

A fundamental fueling tactic is to encourage the athletes to use water and sports drinks in a liberal fashion in the 48 hours prior to competition. The cost-effective way to do this is to issue squeeze bottles to each athlete and have a cooler full of water and a cooler full of sports drinks in the bus, van, or plane for the athletes to utilize for drinking throughout the trip. If at all possible, use distilled water brought from the home training table at all times. If necessary, purchase bottled distilled water while on the road. The team cannot afford to have traveler's diarrhea from drinking the local tap water. Distilled water is the most practical product to use on the road and athletes do like the taste of distilled water. The only caffeinated beverages supplied on trips should be coffee for the coaches.

Athletes need to be rested prior to a competition. They should get adequate sleep, particularly for the 2 nights prior to the competitions. Sometimes, athletes may be given melatonin to help them sleep,[9] particularly those who are anxiety prone or just do not sleep well away from their own beds. Trips overseas that offer little time to adjust circadian rhythms may necessitate some efforts to change practice, meals, and rest patterns in the days prior to departure. This will decrease the amount of time needed to acclimate to the time change.

IX. SUMMARY

Much preplanning and work is needed for taking care of the nutritional needs of athletes on the road. These trips are exhausting for everyone involved. Difficulty for the applied sports nutritionist ranges, in order of demand, from the athletes practicing twice a day, to bowl games, to games on the road, to games played at home, with the latter being the easiest. Unfortunately, too few nutritionists have had the opportunity to travel along with a team and perform duties as an applied sports nutritionist. The sports community has yet to truly accept sports nutritionists, primarily due to financial issues. Doing what is best for the athletes' performance is not convenient or inexpensive, but it is the right thing to do. Feeding the athlete on the road is a fundamental fueling tactic that must be enhanced. Whether fueling tactics are at an advanced level of planning or just a fundamental effort to guide athletes to the best selections at their disposal, someone needs to be responsible. To have athletes board a van or bus without water, sports drinks, and snacks such as fresh fruit and breakfast bars, is inexcusable. It takes minimal effort to have some official on the trip make a couple of phone calls ahead of time to determine the best options for stopping for hot meals en route. Upon arrival, a trip to a local grocer can extend the supply of portion-controlled beverages and snacks that can be used incidental to practice, competition, and the trip home. A visit to a restaurant where athletes might be fed can be helpful to be sure that the meal options are appropriate and do not compromise performance (such as heavily spiced, smoked, or calorie-rich foods). The key to providing this is to allow someone in the travel party to plan ahead for the athletes. If athletes are going to eat at fast-food establishments, it should be after the competition.

Even the best-laid plans can go awry through miscommunication. For example, every morning in Tokyo the chef would serve french fries and hot dogs. Then the applied sports nutritionist talked with the chef about the difference between hashbrown potatoes and french fries and between breakfast sausage and hot dogs. Whoever is playing the role of the applied sports nutritionist will find that some degree of flexibility is required. Schedules change. Coaches change plans, weather changes plans, even the television changes the time that the competition starts. Planes and buses are late, hotel catering staffs make errors. The applied sports nutritionist must be alert and constantly checking on the agenda with the decision makers; the catering bill from the hotel should be obtained and checked to be sure that all the charges are correct. The applied sports nutritionist is an invaluable asset to athletic administrators and the team in that this person ensures that athletes are fed nutritious diets in a cost-effective manner.

REFERENCES

1. Driskell, J.A., *Sports Nutrition*, CRC Press, Boca Raton, FL, 2000.
2. Wolinsky, I. (Ed.), *Nutrition in Exercise and Sport*, Third Edition, CRC Press, Boca Raton, FL, 1998.
3. American Dietetic Association, Position of The American Dietetic Association: Nutrition for physical fitness and athletic performance for adults, *J. Am. Diet. Assoc.*, 87, 933-939, 1987.
4. Grandjean, A. Personal communication of January 10, 2000.
5. John Adams, Sports Editor, Vols catch up with Huskers, *Knoxville Sentinel* (Knoxville, TN newspaper), July 10, 1998.
6. Bujko J., Schreurs, V. V., Koopmanschap, P. E., Furstenberg, E., and Keller, J. S., Benefit of more but smaller meals at a fixed daily protein intake, *Z. Ernahrungswiss*, 36(4), 347-349, 1997.
7. National Collegiate Athletic Association, *1999-2000 NCAA Division I Manual*, p. 218, NCAA, Indianapolis, IN, 1999.
8. National Collegiate Athletic Association, Proposal #99-31, http:www.ncaa.org/databases/legislational/1999/99summary expenses.html.
9. Watson, R.R. (Ed.), *Melatonin in the Promotion of Health*, CRC Press, Boca Raton, FL, 1999.

CHAPTER 12

Eating Before, During, and After the Event

Robert E. Keith, Heather B. Holden, and Lisa S. McAnulty

CONTENTS

0-8493-8199-1/00/$0.00+$.50

I. INTRODUCTION

Food and beverages consumed in the hours prior to athletic performance, during an event, and immediately following an event can have a significant impact on an individual's ability to perform during the event and recover following performance. Many athletes have their own conceptions as to what foods they should consume before, during, and after an event. While some of these ideas may be good, many of the foods consumed by athletes in these time periods may be inappropriate or perhaps detrimental to performance and recovery. This chapter outlines the important concepts and reviews the literature concerning proper aspects of eating and drinking prior to, during, and following an athletic event.

II. EATING BEFORE ATHLETIC EVENTS

A. Related Physiology

Before discussing the aspects of a good pre-event eating pattern, a basic understanding of the physiological processes related to such eating is warranted. These physiological aspects include digestive processes, distribution of blood, and synthesis of liver glycogen.

1. Digestive Processes

Performance in an athletic event will be better if there is virtually no food in the stomach or small intestines at the time the event is being conducted. Food must be digested in the stomach and small intestines. This food then must be absorbed from the small intestines and enter the body's blood and lymph systems. The time needed for this process to be complete varies in relation to several factors.[1-3]

One of the factors that influences the time needed for food to clear the stomach and small intestines is the macronutrient composition of the meal. For example, carbohydrates are relatively easy to digest and absorb. Consumed carbohydrates generally clear the stomach and small intestines in 1 to 4 hours, depending on the type of carbohydrate. Complex carbohydrates, such as bread and pasta, may take 3 to 4 hours to clear. Simple carbohydrates, such as the sugars found in sports drinks, may clear in an hour or less. Fats and proteins generally take much longer to be digested and absorbed than carbohydrates. These macronutrients can take up to 7 hours to clear the gastrointestinal tract. Fats and proteins are digested slowly and remain in the intestinal system for a long time. Another problem with proteins and fats is that they tend to make the blood and tissues more acidic. This lowering of tissue pH may be counterproductive in high-intensity aerobic events.[1,2]

Another factor that influences the digestive rate is the size of the meal consumed. Large meals may require many hours to digest and absorb. Small meals and snacks can be digested and absorbed in 2 hours or less.[1-3]

Finally, nervousness that is often associated with athletic events also can impair the normal digestive and absorptive processes. This may allow food to linger in the gastrointestinal system when it normally would have been gone.[1-3]

2. Blood Supply

An average-size adult will have approximately 5 quarts of blood circulating throughout the body. Children will have less, depending on the size of the child. During times of rest and following ingestion of a meal, blood is diverted from body areas of low need to the stomach and small intestinal systems. This extra blood helps in the processes of digestion and absorption of the food that has been consumed. During light or moderate exercise, blood flow to the stomach and intestines is reduced to 60 – 70% of normal. This is still enough blood to allow for some digestion and absorption to take place (although at a slower rate). However, during strenuous exercise, blood flow to the gastrointestinal system is significantly reduced. Blood is diverted to the working muscles and skin for sweat production and cooling. Thus, digestion and absorption of food can be significantly impaired during strenuous exercise. Under these conditions, it would be advantageous for the athlete to have digestive and absorptive processes virtually complete by the time exercise starts. There should be little or no food in the stomach or intestines at the time of exercise.[1-4]

3. Liver Glycogen

The liver is capable of storing a small amount of glycogen (approximately 80–90 grams). This glycogen can undergo glycogenolysis during exercise with the resulting glucose being released to the blood to be used by working muscle and tissues of the central nervous system.

If the liver glycogen becomes depleted and blood glucose falls to hypoglycemic levels, working muscles and the brain can be deprived of adequate amounts of an important fuel source. This causes the working muscle and brain to function less than optimally and performance will suffer.[1,5,6]

The liver can store enough glycogen to supply the brain and resting muscles for 12 to 15 hours. However, working muscles will use the glucose produced from liver glycogen breakdown at a greatly accelerated rate. Thus, making sure that liver glycogen stores are maximized prior to strenuous activity is important for the athlete about to enter an event.[1,5,6]

B. Components of a Proper Pre-Event Meal

Certain components of a proper pre-event meal can be important to athletic performance. The meal should be structured so that the ingested food will clear the gastrointestinal tract by the start of the event. The meal also should be able to enhance the available liver glycogen stores, help support hydration for the athlete, and prevent sensations of hunger.[4,6,7]

Guidelines for proper pre-event meals have been developed. These are outlined in Table 12.1 and discussed in more detail in the following paragraphs.

Table 12.1 Important Components of a Proper Pre-Event Eating Plan

- Foods should be high in carbohydrate content and low in fat and protein.
- Liquid meals generally should be completed at least 1 hour prior to the event. Solid food pre-event meals should be consumed three to four hours prior to the event.
- Consumed foods should be somewhat bland, safe, and familiar to the athlete. Spicy, gas-producing, and other irritating foods should be avoided.
- Total caloric consumption in the hours prior to an event should be under 1000 kilocalories. Generally, kilocalorie consumption in the 300–500 range is considered appropriate.
- The dietary fiber content of foods consumed during the pre-event period should be minimized.
- Hypotonic drinks (water, sports beverages) should be consumed frequently to maintain pre-event hydration status.

1. *Timing of the Meal*

Because almost all food should be cleared from the stomach and small intestines by the start of exercise, timing of the meal becomes an important issue. In general, pre-event meals should be consumed 1 to 4 hours prior to competition or heavy training. Larger, mixed, or solid meals should be taken 3 to 4 hours prior to exercise, while smaller or liquid meals could be eaten 1 to 2 hours prior to competition.[4,6,7]

Consuming small amounts of food 30–60 minutes prior to exercise may or may not have adverse effects on performance. Some studies[8-12] reported decreased performance and/or hyperinsulinemia and hypoglycemia when meals or drinks high in glucose were consumed within an hour of exercise. However, other authors[5,13] have not seen significant hypoglycemia and/or a decrease in performance. Some athletes may be more sensitive to hypoglycemia and care probably should be taken in consuming high glucose foods and drinks 30–60 minutes prior to exercise.

2. *Composition of the Meal*

Several aspects related to the composition of the pre-event meal are important. These include the carbohydrate content, the type of food (bland versus spicy, etc.), the dietary-fiber content, and the level of fluid consumed.

As previously mentioned, carbohydrate foods are relatively easy to digest and absorb; typically clearing the gastrointestinal tract in 4 hours or less. Carbohydrates also would be the fuel of choice to maximize liver glycogen stores. Thus, pre-event meals should consist primarily of high-carbohydrate-type foods that contain small amounts of protein and fat. Some examples of high-carbohydrate pre-event foods can be found in Table 12.2. Neither the form of the carbohydrate (liquid versus solid) nor low versus high glycemic index value seem to make any clear differences as related to performance.[3,14-16] Thus, the athlete could choose a solid or liquid meal, pasta, potatoes, or cereal for their pre-event meal. The athlete can choose the high-carbohydrate meal that best meets their food preferences. Obviously, foods with high protein and fat content should be minimized. This would include the traditional "steak and eggs" meal previously used prior to football games, as well as foods such as hot dogs, nuts, hamburgers, bacon, and any food with a high butter or margarine content.

Table 12.2 Examples of High Carbohydrate Pre-Event Foods

Toast and jelly	Macaroni	Skim milk
Low fiber cereals	Baked potato	Applesauce
Apple juice	Spaghetti	Low fat yogurt
Pancakes	Bagels	Canned fruit
Bananas	Waffles	English muffins
Breads	Sherbert	Rice
Puddings	Cream of wheat	Oatmeal raisin cookies
Dried fruit	Saltine crackers	Graham crackers
Sports drinks	Cornbread	Tortillas

Foods eaten in the hours prior to exercise should be somewhat bland. They should not produce gas or cause gastrointestinal motility to increase. Spicy foods containing pepper or chili powder should be avoided. Foods such as onions, cabbage, broccoli, and various beans also should be avoided. These foods contain chemicals that may agitate the gastrointestinal system or be gas producing. While a small amount of a carbonated beverage may be acceptable in the hours prior to exercise, consumption of large quantities of these beverages need to be avoided due to possible gas production. The pre-event meal should consist of appropriate foods that are safe and familiar to the athlete. New or strange foods should be avoided during the pre-event period.[4,7,17,18]

While some athletes may use caffeine as a possible ergogenic aid, caffeine consumption in the hours prior to an event should be minimized. Caffeine will cause an increase in gastrointestinal motility. This may cause some distress to an already nervous athlete. Caffeine also has a diuretic action that can compromise an athlete's state of hydration in the pre-event period. Likewise, alcohol consumption needs to be avoided in the time prior to competition. Alcohol also exerts a diuretic action and may interfere with the athlete's ability to perform.[4,17]

The amount of dietary fiber is another important point to consider when developing a pre-event meal plan. Normally, diets should be high in fiber to promote good health. However, some types of dietary fiber can stimulate defecation. This may cause the urge to move the bowels during an athletic event, which would not be advantageous to performance. Therefore, the inclusion of high-fiber foods in the diet during the pre-event period should be minimized. This low-fiber period probably should include the day before the event. Foods high in dietary fiber include dried beans, various types of bran, nuts, raw vegetables, corn, and seeds.[4,7,17,18]

The consumption of ample quantities of fluid in the hours prior to an athletic event is an important component of a good pre-event eating plan. Ample fluid consumption will ensure that the athlete does not go into the event in a state of hypohydration. Beverages such as low-fat or skim milk or fruit juices can be consumed up to 2 hours before an event. Water and sports drinks should be consumed 2 hours or less before the start of the event. As previously mentioned, consumption of carbonated beverages as well as drinks containing caffeine and alcohol should be minimized or avoided during the pre-event time period.[4,7,17]

3. Meal Size

Large meals take a longer time, perhaps 6 to 8 hours, to be digested and absorbed than small meals. Therefore, the consumption of large meals on the day of competition is generally contraindicated. Large meals eaten the day before the event would be acceptable. Consumption of large pre-event meals virtually guarantees that food will still be in the stomach and small intestines at the time of competition. This can cause minor to serious discomfort for the athlete. General recommendations are that pre-event meals not exceed 1000 kcal. A meal this size should be consumed 3 to 4 hours prior to exercise. Meals of 300–400 kcal may be tolerated even 1 to 2 hours prior to exercise.[17] For example, a turkey sandwich made with white bread, mustard, and a small amount of lettuce and tomato contains approximately 350 kcal. Add a glass of apple juice (120 kcal) and a cup of flavored yogurt (220 kcal) and the total pre-event meal adds up to approximately 700 kcal. A breakfast of two 6-inch pancakes (200 kcal), two pats of butter (90 kcal), four ounces (103 ml) of syrup (100 kcal) and an eight ounce (206 ml) glass of orange juice (120 kcal) would provide just over 500 kcal total.

Research also has been reported on the amount of carbohydrate that should be consumed prior to exercise.[5,6] Sherman et al.[5,6] suggested that 1.0 to 4.5 grams of carbohydrate per kilogram of body weight be consumed 1 to 4 hours pre-event. The 4.5-gram amount should be consumed 3 to 4 hours prior to exercise while the 1.0 gram amount could be consumed up to 1 hour prior to an athletic event.

C. Adverse Effects of an Improper Pre-Event Meal

Improper pre-event nutrition can harm the athlete in several ways. These adverse effects are outlined in Table 12.3. Adverse effects can generally be classified as problems related to the gastrointestinal system, problems with blood glucose concentrations, and problems with hypohydration.

Most adverse effects of improper pre-event meals are associated with food still remaining in the stomach and intestines when physical activity begins. As mentioned, once exercise begins, blood flow to the gastrointestinal system is significantly impaired, which leads to reduced digestion, absorption, and movement of the food. This situation can result in various gastrointestinal disturbances ranging

Table 12.3 Adverse Symptoms Related to Improper Pre-event Eating

- Problems associated with the gastrointestinal system
  Nausea
  Intestinal cramping
  Belching
  Vomiting
  Flatulence
  Diarrhea or the urge to defecate
- Other problem areas and concerns
  Symptomatic hypoglycemia (weakness, anxiety, tremors)
  Hypohydration
  Sensations of hunger

from excess gas production to vomiting and diarrhea. All of these adverse effects will, more than likely, cause the athlete to perform less than optimally. Even if symptoms are not severe, the athlete's performance is still probably being compromised.[17]

A second problem area relates to the maintenance of normal blood glucose concentration. Symptomatic hypoglycemia may occur as a result of improper pre-event eating. Eating solely high-glycemic carbohydrate foods in a 30–60-minute time period prior to exercise will cause a rapid increase in blood glucose and insulin concentrations. The high insulin secretion will then cause a reduction in blood glucose. If this occurs in conjunction with intense exercise, symptomatic hypoglycemia could occur shortly after the initiation of exercise. While most studies in this area do report hypoglycemia upon exercise, not all report physical symptoms related to the hypoglycemia. In addition, the eating of some low-glycemic carbohydrates or small amounts of protein and fat along with the high-glycemic food will favorably modify the blood glucose response and prevent symptoms from occurring.[19]

Symptomatic hypoglycemia also may occur when an athlete enters a competition following a period of fasting. This can occur in early-morning events following a skipped pre-event meal, meaning that no food has been consumed for a period of 12–14 hours. This athlete would then enter the event with blood glucose concentrations in the low normal range. Upon exercise, glucose concentrations could continue to fall, resulting in symptoms later in the event. Eating some appropriate carbohydrate-containing foods prior to exercise would prevent this condition from occurring.[6]

Finally, suboptimal hydration in the pre-event period could adversely affect performance. Thus, the athlete needs to consume ample fluids prior to competition. The athlete should drink fluids in the pre-event period until urine volume is adequate and urine color is clear. Low urine volume and highly colored urine in the pre-event period are indications of hypohydration.[4]

D. Effects of the Pre-Event Meal on Performance

Several studies have documented increased performance in endurance events after consuming a pre-event meal. Sherman et al.[5] had subjects cycle at 70% of maximum for 90 minutes following ingestion of 1.1 to 2.2 grams of carbohydrate per kilogram of body weight 1 hour prior to exercise. Time trial performance was increased by 12.5% following the carbohydrate meal, as compared with a placebo meal. Sherman et al.[20] also reported increased cycling performance following a 312-gram carbohydrate meal (versus a placebo) given 4 hours prior to exercise. In another study, Schabort and colleagues[21] had subjects consume a carbohydrate breakfast (100 grams) 3 hours prior to exercise or had them enter exercise following an overnight fast. Cycling time to fatigue was significantly longer (136 minutes) when the subjects ate the breakfast meal versus the overnight fast (109 minutes). Finally, Anderson et al.[16] reported increased cycling time to fatigue in subjects following the consumption of oatmeal (84 minutes) versus when the subjects consumed a placebo

(66 minutes). In summary, it does appear that appropriate pre-event nutrition can significantly and positively impact endurance performance.

III. EATING DURING AN EVENT

Nutrition for optimal performance does not stop when an athlete heads for the starting line or competition field. What occurs during endurance events or day-long tournaments, regarding nutrition and hydration, could mean the difference between finishing or being carried off the playing field.

As previously mentioned, some planning for nutrition and hydration should occur before the actual event begins. The amount of planning will depend on various factors such as competition experience, type of event, etc. Other factors to consider include body composition, exercise intensity and duration, age, and gender. Another major factor is the weather. When training and competing in hot and humid or cold and windy conditions, special attention to proper hydration is warranted.

During exercise, many physiological processes are occurring concurrently. Heart rate increases, hormones are secreted, metabolic rate is increased, and body temperature is elevated.[22] There are several rate-limiting steps that affect the overall performance of the activity. One example is the increase in heat production which, in turn, causes an increase in body water and electrolyte losses. If this condition is not corrected, performance is hindered.

A. Nutrition During High Intensity, Short Duration, and Stop-and-Go Events

During an athletic event of short duration and high intensity (sprinting, high jumping, power weightlifting) the muscles are fueled by adenosine triphosphate (ATP) and creatine phosphate (CP).[17,23] ATP is further regenerated through chemical reactions from carbohydrates. This reaction is referred to as anaerobic glycolysis because the reaction can occur without oxygen. The anaerobic pathway will provide energy for events of high intensity lasting less than 1 minute. This system also provides energy for bursts of activity such as in tennis, soccer, basketball, and baseball.[17] The anaerobic system can produce only a limited amount of energy and is further hampered by the by-product of this pathway, lactic acid. The energy supply for anaerobic glycolysis comes from carbohydrates stored in limited amounts in the muscles. This storage accumulates from the foods eaten during the days prior to competition and, to a lesser degree, the pre-event meal. It is critical that all athletes try to consume adequate amounts of carbohydrate before a competition to have fuel for short bursts of energy (anaerobic work).

Athletes who participate in high-intensity stop-and-go sports such as basketball, football, soccer, wrestling, or hockey, could benefit by consuming carbohydrates during competition.[24] One study[24] conducted at the University of South Carolina looked at the ingestion of carbohydrates before and during high-intensity exercise. Men and women exercised on a stationary bike in 1-minute bursts of high-intensity exercise, followed by 3 minutes of rest. One group consumed an 18% carbohydrate drink before exercise, followed by a 6% solution every 20 minutes during exercise. A control group drank similar volumes of a placebo solution. The group that consumed carbohydrates maintained a high-intensity effort 28 minutes longer, on average, than the control group.

Several researchers have looked at carbohydrate and fluid requirements of soccer players.[25,26] Soccer involves high-intensity exercise intermingled with endurance. Intermittent, quick bursts of speed are needed to maneuver around a defender when handling the ball. A world-class soccer player averages approximately 5 miles during a 90–minute game, with numerous sprints interspersed in the match.[24] One review showed that carbohydrate supplementation during soccer matches resulted in a significant sparing of muscle glycogen.[25]

Recently, carbohydrate intake has been shown to improve weightlifting performance during a second workout.[27] A carbohydrate supplement (0.3 g/kg) or a placebo was given following an initial weightlifting session. After a 4-hour period of recovery, subjects performed a series of sets of squats until exhaustion. The total number of sets of squats, total repetitions, and total duration of the second workout were significantly improved following the carbohydrate supplement, as compared with the placebo.

Nutrition for intermittent day-long events or tournament competition provides some challenges. An example is a championship track and field meet where the athlete may have to compete in a sprint event at two different times — a preliminary trial and the finals. A swim meet is another example, where an athlete may have a time trial in the morning to qualify for the finals in the evening. Several factors must be considered. One is the amount of time between the events. Another factor is the psychological condition of the athlete. If the athlete is nervous, liquids may be tolerated better than solids. Liquid meals used during day-long events leave the stomach quicker than solid foods.[4,17] Fluid replacement also must be considered. Fluid replacement is discussed later in this section.

If, at least 1 hour exists prior to further competition, guidelines previously established for pre-event meals would apply. If there is less than an hour between events, the athlete should consume small amounts of carbohydrates (less than 300 kcal), either as a liquid (sports drinks) or as solid food such as a banana, bagel, low-fat crackers, or dried cereal.

Events that are high intensity and lasting 4 to 10 minutes and longer are classified as intermediate-duration events. Examples are wrestling matches, middle-distance swimming, and the mile run.[17] The major fuel source for these events is still muscle glycogen. In this situation, the glycogen can be metabolized by both anaerobic and aerobic pathways. An athlete competing in these events must have good muscle glycogen stores before the competition begins. The biochemical changes that are a result of training influence the amount of glycogen stored in the muscles.[4] Consequently, trained athletes have higher muscle glycogen storing capacities than untrained individuals.

Intermediate-duration events require the athlete to concentrate on consuming plenty of carbohydrates during training to ensure adequate muscle glycogen stores going into the competition. For competition lasting less than 60 minutes, the outcome of the event will hinge largely on nutrition and hydration practices that were followed prior to the event as well as the pre-event meal. Due to the intensity and length of the event, consuming carbohydrates during the event is extremely difficult. Proper hydration prior to the start of the event is also critical.

B. Nutrition During Prolonged-Activity Events

1. Carbohydrates

When you need energy during prolonged activity, your body will use a mix of glycogen and fat (free fatty acids) to fuel muscles. The body uses glycogen initially and then relies mostly on its fat stores for fuel. However, use of muscle glycogen and blood glucose as a fuel source for intense prolonged activity is still of major importance. Research has documented that muscle glycogen depletion is a major limiting factor to endurance exercise that exceeds 90–120 minutes.[17]

The central nervous system's sole source of energy is glucose. Liver glycogen and gluconeogenic processes maintain the blood glucose concentrations to provide glucose to the central nervous system. Furthermore, when muscle glycogen stores are low, glucose from the blood also will be used to provide glucose for the muscles. This, in turn, reduces liver glycogen. Blood glucose levels then drop, which impairs central nervous system and muscle function.[3]

Therefore, it is advantageous to consume carbohydrates during endurance events lasting longer than 60–90 minutes.[3,4,17] The consumption of carbohydrates during prolonged events helps support blood glucose and provides an important energy substrate for the central nervous system and the working muscles.

Several studies looking at cyclists and carbohydrate feedings indicated that carbohydrate feedings during exercise improved performance.[28-31] In one experiment, seven trained men were studied during prolonged cycling that alternated between 60% and 85% VO_{2max} every 15 minutes.

Carbohydrate feeding throughout exercise resulted in a 19% increase in the amount of work performed.[28] Another study[29] looked at no carbohydrate and carbohydrate feedings before and/or during endurance cycling at 70% VO_{2max}. Total work produced during exercise was 19–46% higher when carbohydrates were consumed. Performance was improved the most when carbohydrates were consumed before and during exercise. However, performance was improved when carbohydrates were consumed either before and/or during exercise.

Recommendations for carbohydrate intake include consuming approximately 100–300 calories of carbohydrates per hour after the first 60 to 90 minutes of exercise.[4] The carbohydrates can be in liquid or solid form, depending on the preference of the athlete. One study[31] observed the effects of liquid and solid carbohydrate (CHO) ingestion in cyclists exercising continuously for 190 minutes with intensity varying every 15 minutes between 45% and 75% VO_{2max}. Times to fatigue for solid CHO and liquid CHO treatments did not differ, but were significantly greater than the placebo treatment. Numerous carbohydrate-supplement products are currently available on the market. There are liquid carbohydrates, energy bars, carbohydrate gels, and sports drinks that contain carbohydrates and electrolytes.[4] Energy bars and carbohydrate gels should be consumed with plenty of fluid to avoid gastrointestinal distress. Any of these products, as well as various carbohydrate food sources, are capable of supplying sufficient carbohydrate to support optimal athletic performance.

Ultra-endurance events provide unique nutritional challenges because of the tremendous amount of time the athlete is in competition. The athlete has several options available to replenish carbohydrates during the competition. The options include sports drinks with carbohydrates and electrolytes, power bars, carbohydrate gels, solid foods, or any combination of these choices. The important factor to consider is what the athlete is able to tolerate without gastrointestinal distress.

A few studies have documented nutritional intakes during ultra-endurance races. One study[32] looked at the food and fluid intake of male ultra-endurance runners during a 1,005-km race completed over 9 days. Food and fluid intake occurred every 15 to 20 minutes and consisted of 62% of the energy from carbohydrate, 27% from fat and 11% from protein for a total of 25,000 kJ of energy each day. Another study[33] of male participants in a 100-km ultramarathon showed an energy intake of 4,233 kJ. This intake was 88.6% carbohydrate, 6.7% fat, and 4.7% protein, with a mean of 5.7 liters of fluid intake. A third study observed male cyclists during a 2,050-mile (3100-km) ride that occurred for 15–18 hours a day for 10 days.[34] The nutrient intake was 63% from carbohydrate, with 44% from simple sugars, cookies, sweetened drinks, and candy; 27% from fat, and 10% from protein. Total fluid intake averaged 10.5 liters per day (54% as water) with an average of 620 ml/hour of riding time. Athletes competing in ultra-endurance events need a variety of high-energy, high-carbohydrate foods and plenty of fluids during the event to maintain performance. It is important for the athlete to determine during training what methods will work best. Due to the jostling that runners experience, liquid carbohydrates are preferred over solid foods, while cyclists can usually tolerate solid foods. It is helpful to have a support team during ultra-endurance events to help remind the athlete to consume carbohydrates and fluids throughout the competition.

2. *Fluid Replacement*

Maintaining hydration is the most important nutritional concern during prolonged endurance activities. Water is a critical nutrient during prolonged exercise. During exercise, muscle contractions and metabolism generate heat. When the heat builds up, there is a subsequent increase in body temperature. Heat is removed primarily by sweating. Sweat evaporates from the skin to cool down the body. Approximately 600 kcal are eliminated by the cooling effect of evaporation of 1 liter of sweat.[35] Fluids lost through sweat must be replaced to avoid dehydration. The decision on how much fluid to ingest during exercise is based on avoiding or minimizing the effects of dehydration.

The body triggers certain responses to counterbalance dehydration. In sedentary individuals, these responses include stimulation of thirst by the hypothalamus in the brain. The hypothalamus/pituitary gland exerts hormonal control on the kidneys and renal tubules to reduce urine output and conserve sodium.[35] However, during exercise, the thirst mechanism is not sufficient to stimulate a large enough increase in fluid intake to counter the amount of fluid lost through sweating.[36] Dehydration then results unless that athlete has an adequate rehydration plan. Dehydration constituting as little as 1–2% of body weight impairs athletic performance and physiological responses. Weight losses of 5% of body weight or more may seriously impair the health of the athlete.[17,36-38] Every liter (2.2 lbs) of water loss will cause heart rate to increase approximately eight beats per minute and core temperature to rise by 0.3°C when exercising for prolonged periods of time in the heat.[39]

Several factors determine the amount of sweat produced and the amount of fluid lost during exercise. Factors that add to fluid needs include: high temperature, high humidity, solar radiation, improper clothing, and increased fluid losses from drinking caffeine or alcohol prior to competition.[38] Sweat losses of 1.5 liters per hour are typical during endurance sports, and under particularly hot conditions, sweat rates exceeding 2 to 3 liters per hour are not uncommon.[35]

Recommendations for fluid intake include consuming 300–500 ml (12–16 ounces) of fluid immediately prior to exercise followed by 120–240 ml (4–8 ounces) of fluid every 15–20 minutes.[17,37,38] Cool water (5 to 10°C; 40 to 50°F) is acceptable for events lasting 1 hour or less. Sports drinks should be consumed for events that last longer than 1 hour.[37,38,40] If the amount of sweat lost is not counterbalanced with fluid intake, dehydration is the end result. It is common for athletes to dehydrate by 2–6% of their body weight during exercise in the heat.[36,39] Runners generally drink only 300–500 ml of fluids per hour, which may be insufficient to maintain hydration.[39] Again, thirst would not be a good indicator of the level of dehydration, and the athlete should develop an adequate drinking plan prior to competition.

Continued heat exposure and dehydration can lead to heat cramps, heat exhaustion, and heat stroke. Heat cramps are the first signals that the body is having trouble with the heat. Heat cramps occur predominately in the legs and abdomen.[17,41] Treatment is as simple as resting in a cool place while drinking cool water or a sports drink. Massaging and stretching the affected muscles helps relieve the cramping. If the athlete continues exercising, heat exhaustion could occur, followed by heat stroke. Heat exhaustion symptoms include cool, moist, pale, or flushed skin, headache, nausea, dizziness, weakness, or exhaustion.[17,38,41] Heat stroke is a serious medical condition. The body systems are overwhelmed by the heat and begin to stop functioning. Symptoms include red, hot, dry skin; changes in consciousness; rapid, weak pulse or rapid shallow breathing.[41]

Most dehydration problems occur when competing in the heat, but dehydration can occur when competing in cold weather. When exercising in the cold, heat is lost by radiation and conduction (wind chill).[42] Cold air is usually dry air, which leads to an increase in respiratory water loss due to rapid breathing. Cold exposure also leads to an increase in vasoconstriction of skin blood vessels and shivering to conserve body heat and maintain core temperature.[42] Cold weather decreases the sense of thirst, therefore thirst is not a reliable indicator of the level of dehydration. In a cold, dry environment sweat can evaporate quickly and the athlete may not have a clear indication of how much fluid loss has occurred.[42] Loss of body fluids can cause the same problems as exercising in the heat.

For competitions lasting longer than 1 hour, sport scientists recommend that the athlete consume a carbohydrate, electrolyte-containing beverage. Recommendations include consuming 100–300 calories (25–75 g) of carbohydrate per hour as a replacement for depleted muscle glycogen stores.[4,17] The recommended glucose concentration is 6 to 8%, which is equivalent to 14–25 grams of carbohydrate per 8 ounces (240 ml).[4,17,36,38,40] Most commercial sports drinks contain carbohydrates at the recommended percentage. Table 12.4 gives a comparison of various sports drinks and other beverages. A higher carbohydrate concentration may delay gastric emptying time and could cause gastrointestinal distress. The presence of some carbohydrate and electrolytes in the beverage also may enhance the rate of fluid absorption.[4,17]

Table 12.4 Beverage Comparison Chart

Ingredient per 8 oz. (240 ml)	Gatorade®	Powerade®	AllSport®	Orange Juice	Coca-Cola®	Water	What to look for
Type of carbohydrate	Sucrose, Glucose, Fructose	Fructose, Glucose polymers, Maltodextrins	High Fructose corn syrup	Glucose, Fructose, Sucrose	High fructose corn syrup/ Sucrose	0	Sucrose, Glucose, Fructose, Mix of CHO
Carbohydrate content (%)	6%	8%	8–9%	10%	10–11%	0%	6–8% CHO
Carbohydrate (grams)	14 g	19 g	19 g	26 g	25 g	0 g	about 14g CHO
Sodium (milligrams)	110 mg	55 mg	55 mg	6 mg	28 mg	0 mg	At least 100 mg
Potassium (milligrams)	30 mg	30 mg	55 mg	436 mg	trace	0 mg	At least 28 mg
Carbonation	no	no	yes	no	yes	no	None

*Adapted from Gatorade Sports Science Institute[42]

A fluid containing electrolytes also is recommended for exercise lasting longer than 4 to 6 hours, because the electrolytes in the beverage may be needed to replace those lost during sweating.[36] This is important to prevent electrolyte disturbances and the condition of hyponatremia if only water is consumed during the prolonged event. Electrolytes such as sodium, potassium, and chloride help regulate muscle contraction, nerve impulse conduction, acid–base balance of the blood, blood clotting, and normal heart rhythm.[35] Sodium is found in the largest amounts in the extracellular fluid and is the primary electrolyte lost in sweat.

Special consideration regarding fluid intake should be given to children, adolescents, and older athletes. Unfortunately, little research has been carried out on the younger population due to ethical considerations of subjecting children to the rigors of heat exposure research. Children and adolescents must pay special attention to exercising in hot, humid weather as they have the potential to overheat at a greater rate than adults. The younger population often does not drink enough water because the beverage lacks taste appeal. One study looked at flavored drink consumption compared with water in 9–12-year-old boys performing three 3-hour intermittent exercise sessions.[43] Three different types of beverages were given. The beverages were: unflavored water, grape-flavored water, and grape-flavored water plus 6% carbohydrate and 18 mmol/l NaCl (sodium chloride). Drinking was allowed *ad libitum*. Consumption of the grape-flavored water with carbohydrate and NaCl resulted in over-hydration, whereas intake of the other two beverages resulted in underhydration.

Little nutritional information is available for the over-60 age group.[44] Older adult athletes pose special challenges for proper hydration due to decreased neural and renal function and heat tolerance.[44] Therefore, older athletes should be well hydrated before, during, and after exercise. Older athletes should pay special attention to the warning signs of dehydration.

IV. EATING AFTER ATHLETIC EVENTS

Adequate ingestion of carbohydrate, protein, and fluid post-exercise is crucial to replenishing glycogen stores, promoting net protein synthesis, and restoring fluid and electrolyte balance. Inadequate consumption of any of these nutrients following exercise would greatly compromise the ability to perform subsequent exercise. Therefore, this section of the chapter is devoted to a brief overview of glycogen resynthesis and a discussion of current recommendations for carbohydrate, protein, and fluid intake during recovery.

A. Recommendation for Carbohydrate Intake

1. *Glycogen Resynthesis*

Glycogen concentration in the liver is greater than that of skeletal muscle. However, the total amount of approximately 300–400 g stored in muscle exceeds the 80–90 g stored in the liver. The combined amount from these two tissues, in addition to the approximately 20 g of blood glucose, account for about 1800 kcal. This amount, however, is quickly diminished as muscle glycogen is increasingly utilized as a source of energy during prolonged intense exercise. Consequently, inadequate carbohydrate ingestion post exercise will prevent muscle glycogen from being adequately replenished between training bouts, and efforts to supercompensate muscle glycogen stores also will be unsuccessful.[3,4]

As discussed in a review by Ivy,[45] muscle glycogen resynthesis following exercise-induced depletion is biphasic. The first phase occurs immediately following exercise. With sufficient carbohydrate ingestion, a rapid resynthesis of muscle glycogen to near pre-exercise levels occurs within a 24-hour period. Factors influencing this rapid phase of glycogen resynthesis include increased glycogen synthase in the active form, increased muscle cell membrane permeability to glucose, and increased sensitivity of muscle to insulin. Conversely, an intermediate form of glycogen synthase that is highly sensitive to glucose-6-phosphate activation appears to regulate the slow phase of glycogen synthesis. Conversion of glycogen synthase to this form may be due to constant exposure of muscle tissue to elevated plasma insulin concentrations secondary to several days of high carbohydrate ingestion.

Usual glycogen stores for trained athletes, exercising daily and consuming a diet of 45–50% carbohydrate, are between 130–135 umol/g wet weight. It is possible, however, that abstinence from training for several days and consumption of a high-carbohydrate diet (70% carbohydrate) can result in glycogen levels greater than 210 umol/g wet wt.[45]

Because of the importance of glycogen as an energy substrate during prolonged intense exercise, extensive research has been conducted to elucidate the most effective method of rapidly replenishing muscle glycogen stores following exercise. Findings from several of these studies, with regard to amount, type, and timing of carbohydrate ingestion, are presented below.

2. *Amount*

Blom et al.[46] studied the rates of glycogen synthesis when varying amounts of glucose were ingested every 2 hours during the first 6 hours of recovery following exhaustive exercise. Glycogen storage averaged 5.7 umol/g wet weight/hour when carbohydrate supplements of 0.70 or 1.40 g glucose/kg body weight were given at 2-hour intervals. Reduction of carbohydrate to 0.35 g glucose/kg body weight at 2-hour intervals resulted in a subsequent decrease in rate of muscle glycogen resynthesis by 50%. Similar results were reported by Ivy et al.[47] The effects of ingesting carbohydrate supplements with varied concentrations (0, 1.5, or 3.0 g glucose/kg body weight) were examined during 4 hours of recovery from exercise. Although ingestion of either 1.5 or 3.0 g glucose/kg body weight resulted in significantly greater muscle glycogen storage compared with the basal rate, rates of glycogen storage were not different between the 1.5 and 3.0 g treatments during the first or second 2 hours of recovery. These results indicated that a carbohydrate supplement of 1.5 g/kg body weight provided at 2-hour intervals was able to maintain a relatively rapid rate of glycogen storage during the first 4 hours after exercise and that doubling the amount of the supplement did not provide any additional benefit with regard to glycogen resynthesis during the initial hours following exercise.

On a daily basis, an upper sufficient level of carbohydrate intake ranging from 500 to 600 g per day has been reported.[48] Ingestion of carbohydrate above this amount resulted in little additional

tion per unit body weight (g/kg/d).

As long as carbohydrate ingestion is sufficient, restoration of muscle glycogen appears to be unaffected by frequency of intake (i.e., total amount of carbohydrate fed as two meals or seven meals).[50]

3. Type

The effect of the type of dietary carbohydrate on muscle glycogen resynthesis was examined during a 48-hour period after strenuous running.[50] Feeding isocaloric diets containing either simple sugars (glucose, sucrose, fructose) or complex carbohydrates (starches) resulted in similar muscle glycogen levels 24 hours after exercise. However, the complex carbohydrate diet resulted in significantly greater muscle glycogen levels during the next 24 hours. The authors proposed that the increased muscle glycogen levels observed with the complex carbohydrate diet may have been due to sustained elevation of serum insulin during the second 24-hour period. This study, however, has received some criticism for categorizing carbohydrate foods on the basis of chemical composition rather than on the basis of their actual postprandial glycemic impact.

Recent studies have focused on the ingestion of low versus high glycemic index (GI) foods and rates of glycogen resynthesis. Kiens et al.[51] compared the effects of diets of 70% carbohydrate with either low or high GI for 44 hours following glycogen-depleting exercise. The rate of muscle glycogen resynthesis was reported to be twice as fast after 6 hours of post-exercise recovery with the high GI diet, but no difference in glycogen storage was observed by 22 hours following exercise. Burke et al.[52] fed five cyclists diets containing either low or high GI foods for 24 hours following a glycogen-depleting ride. Both diets provided 10 g/kg carbohydrate divided equally among four meals. Contrary to the findings of Kiens et al.,[51] results from the study by Burke et al.[52] showed that muscle glycogen stores, after 24 hours, were significantly greater on the high-GI diet than on the low-GI diet. The glycemic index of some representative foods can be seen in Table 12.5.

Rate of glycogen resynthesis does not appear to be influenced by carbohydrate feeding provided in solid or liquid form.[53] Following exhaustive exercise, provision of 3 g CHO/kg body weight in a solid or liquid form resulted in no differences in muscle glycogen storage rates during the 4-hour recovery period. Furthermore, the authors concluded that the rate of storage was not limited by the gastric emptying rate of the supplement.

Enhanced insulin response has been found when a carbohydrate supplement is provided in conjunction with protein.[54] Based on these findings, Zawadski et al.[55] studied the effects of a carbohydrate-protein supplement on muscle glycogen resynthesis following exercise. In addition to the synergistic insulin response observed in the previous study, the carbohydrate–protein supplement resulted in a lower blood glucose response and a faster rate of glycogen resynthesis than the carbohydrate supplement alone. The researchers proposed that the increased rate of muscle glycogen resynthesis was due to increased clearance of glucose by the muscle secondary to the increased blood insulin response. This same enhanced insulin response was not observed when a carbohydrate supplement was given with individual amino acids.[56] Although carbohydrate given with arginine resulted in a greater rate of glycogen resynthesis during the 4-hour recovery period, no difference was found in the blood glucose or blood lactate responses between the two treatments. These findings suggested that the increased glycogen resynthesis rate in the carbohydrate-protein treatment was due to a greater conversion of muscle glucose uptake to glycogen secondary to suppression of carbohydrate oxidation.

Table 12.5 Glycemic Indexes of Common Foods

High Glycemic Index (60–100)	Moderate Glycemic Index (40–59)	Low Glycemic Index (<39)
Breads and Grains	**Fruits**	**Dairy**
waffle - 76	watermelon - 72	ice cream - 61
doughnut - 76	pineapple - 66	yogurt, sweetened - 33
bagel - 72	raisins - 64	milk, high fat - 27
wheat bread, white - 70	banana - 53	milk, skim - 32
bread, whole wheat - 69	grapes - 52	
cornmeal - 68	orange - 43	**Snacks**
bran muffin - 60	pear - 36	jelly beans - 80
rice, white - 56	apple - 36	graham crackers - 74
rice, brown - 55		corn chips - 73
spaghetti - 41	**Starchy Vegetables**	angel food cake - 67
	potatoes, baked - 83	wheat crackers - 67
Cereals	potatoes, smashed - 73	popcorn - 55
Rice Krispies - 82	carrots - 71	oatmeal cookies - 55
Corn Flakes - 77	sweet potatoes - 54	potato chips - 54
Cheerios - 74	green peas - 48	peanuts - 14
shredded wheat - 69		
Grape Nuts - 67	**Legumes**	**Sugars**
oatmeal - 61	baked beans - 48	honey - 73
All Bran - 42	chick peas - 33	table sugar - 65
	kidney beans - 27	lactose - 46
Beverages	soy beans - 18	fructose - 23
soft drinks - 68		
orange juice - 57		
apple juice - 41		

4. Timing

The timing of carbohydrate supplementation between competition or a prolonged bout of exercise greatly impacts the rate of muscle glycogen resynthesis. In a study by Ivy et al.,[57] immediate post-exercise carbohydrate supplementation resulted in a glycogen resynthesis rate of approximately 6–7 umol/g wet weight/hour for approximately 2 hours. During the following 2 hours, however, this rate declined nearly 50% as a result of decreasing blood glucose and insulin concentrations.

In the same study by Ivy,[57] delaying carbohydrate supplementation for 2 hours following exercise caused a reduction in the glycogen resynthesis rate to 3–4 umol/g wet weight/hour for 2 hours after consumption. Although the rate of glycogen resynthesis increased during the following 2 hours, delayed ingestion of carbohydrate resulted in an overall reduced rate of glycogen storage compared with ingestion of carbohydrate immediately post-exercise. The decrease in glycogen resynthesis with delayed ingestion of carbohydrate may have been due to increased insulin resistance by the muscle. Parkin et al.,[58] however, found that delayed feeding of a high-GI meal by 2 hours produced no effect on the rate of muscle glycogen resynthesis at 8 and 24 hours post exercise, given adequate ingestion of carbohydrate during the recovery period.

The finding that rate of glycogen storage is most rapid immediately post exercise is of great importance to athletes who have only 4 to 8 hours of recovery between exercise sessions and desire to maximize glycogen storage. Ingestion of carbohydrate immediately post exercise, however, does not appear to be imperative for athletes who consume sufficient amounts of carbohydrate within 6 hours and are not required to exercise again within 8 hours. This also should be encouraging for those individuals who report diminished appetite immediately following and for up to 3 hours after strenuous exercise.

B. Recommendations For Protein Intake

1. Strength–Power Athletes

The exact mechanism by which muscle growth occurs with resistance training is poorly understood. Possible explanations for this phenomenon include muscle contraction-activated amino acid uptake and hormonal status following exercise. Hormones such as insulin, growth hormone, testosterone, and IGF-1 have been shown to influence protein synthesis. However, few studies have been conducted in the area of post-exercise protein supplementation of athletes. Chandler[59] studied the effects of carbohydrate, protein, or carbohydrate-protein supplements on the hormonal state of the body after weight-training exercise in nine healthy trained male weightlifters. Supplementation with carbohydrate and carbohydrate-protein immediately and 2 hours post exercise resulted in elevated plasma concentrations of insulin and growth hormone beyond that of the protein and control groups. Given the anabolic nature of these hormones, the authors concluded that carbohydrate and carbohydrate-protein supplementation following weight-training exercise may promote an environment more favorable for muscle growth.

2. Endurance Athletes

Although aerobic exercise has been shown to promote muscle protein catabolism, muscle mass is not significantly reduced because of enhanced protein synthesis during recovery. The rate of muscle protein synthesis was measured in six healthy subjects by direct determination of the rate of incorporation of labeled leucine into muscle at rest, at the end of 4 hours of aerobic exercise at 40% VO_{2max}, and after 4 hours of recovery.[60] Rate of muscle protein breakdown was assessed by 3-methylhistidine excretion and urinary nitrogen excretion. Findings from this study suggested that any increase in muscle protein breakdown during and after exercise was balanced to a large extent by an increase in muscle protein synthesis in recovery. Although no specific recommendations are available, it would appear reasonable that protein ingestion during recovery from prolonged aerobic exercise would enhance muscle protein synthesis during this period.

3. Individual Amino Acids

Protein synthesis is suppressed during exercise, while protein catabolism is increased. As a result, an increased pool of available free amino acids is created. This pool provides a source of energy for the exercising muscle through the oxidation of branched-chain amino acids and the use of alanine in gluconeogenesis. Additionally, increased availability of amino acids may enhance protein synthesis following exercise.[61]

Amino acid infusion following exercise has been successful in increasing availability of amino acids to the muscle and in regulating anabolic hormones.[62] Subsequently, protein synthesis is enhanced. However, current research has not provided strong evidence for the use of oral amino acid supplementation to obtain anabolic effects similar to those observed with amino acid infusion. Furthermore, amino acid supplementation at pharmacologic, rather than nutritional, dosages should raise concern for potential toxic effects of amino acid imbalance. One final point worth mentioning is that restrictive diets may limit intake of one or more amino acids, thereby decreasing intracellular availability of these amino acids for protein synthesis.

C. Fluid Requirements

As exercise intensity increases, body temperature also rises, unless the environmental temperature is low. Prolonged exercise, especially in a hot environment, results in substantial sweat losses with sweating rates possibly exceeding 2 liters per hour. The loss of both water and electrolytes raises a concern with regard to exercise performance and ability to thermoregulate. While ingestion of fluids helps minimize the negative effects on health and performance, the volume consumed usually fails to match the rate of sweat loss. Therefore, with the understanding that exercise is generally followed by some degree of fluid deficit, or dehydration, fluid replacement and restoration of energy substrate stores become crucial during recovery. Failure to achieve adequate rehydration would have negative repercussions on subsequent exercise. Figure 12.1 illustrates the cascade of events leading to decreased exercise capacity with dehydration.

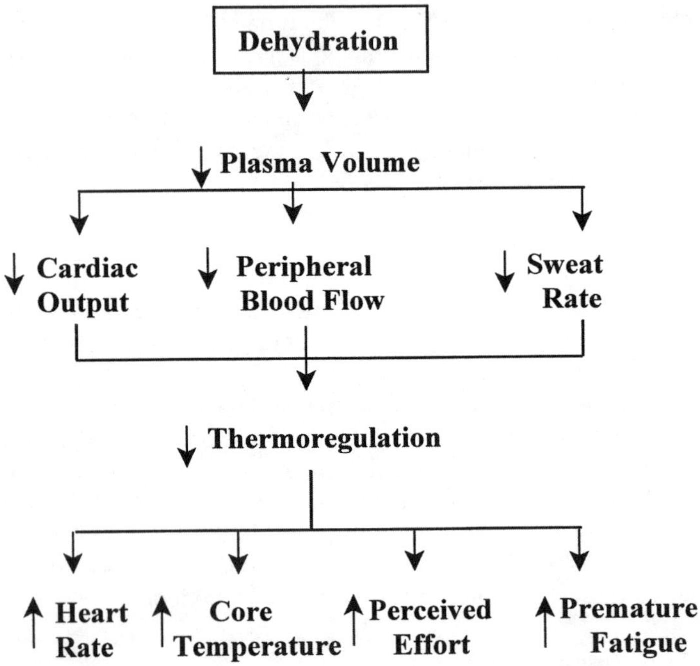

Figure 12.1 Physiological effects of dehydration.

1. Amount

Fluid ingestion equal to sweat loss has not been shown to be totally effective in rehydration based on urine losses.[63] This finding may indicate a necessity to revise the frequently used recommendation that the amount of fluid consumed following exercise should equal the body mass loss.

Recommendations for fluid intake greater than sweat loss were reported in a study by Shirreffs et al.[64] examining the effects of varying the volume of fluid ingested after exercise-induced dehydration as well as the concentration of sodium on the rehydration process. The drinks chosen included sodium concentrations of 23 mmol/l and 61 mmol/l, which correspond to the lower end and upper end of the ranges of normal values for the sodium content of sweat, respectively. Drink volumes consumed were equivalent to 50%, 100%, 150%, and 200% of body mass loss. Findings from this study suggest that a drink volume that exceeds sweat loss during exercise must be consumed to restore fluid balance. Additionally, sodium content of the beverage must be high enough to prevent increased urinary output.

2. Water Alone Versus Water/Electrolytes

Ingestion of plain water following exercise has been shown to result in a rapid decline in the plasma sodium concentration and in plasma osmolality.[65] The resulting effect is a reduced stimulus to drink (thirst) and increased urine output. Decreased fluid intake and increased urine loss would be detrimental to the rehydration process. In contrast, sodium chloride capsules ingested with water (77 mmol/l) have been shown to restore plasma volume within 20 minutes. Voluntary fluid intake also was observed to be higher and urine output was less than with ingestion of water alone.

Gonzalez-Alonso et al.[66] reported that a dilute carbohydrate-electrolyte solution (60 g/l carbohydrate, 20 mmol/l Na^+, 3 mmol/l K^+) was more effective in promoting rehydration after exercise than either plain water or a low-electrolyte diet cola. The difference between the drinks was primarily a result of differences in the volume of urine produced over the study period and appeared to be related to the electrolyte content. The primary electrolytes lost in sweat are sodium and chloride, the major ions of extracellular fluid, and, to a much lesser extent, potassium. Values for sweat sodium concentration are typically in the range of 20–80 mmol/l and for potassium 4-8 mmol/l. Normal plasma sodium concentration is approximately 140 mmol/l, compared with an intracellular concentration of about 10 mmol/l. Intracellular potassium concentration is about 150 mmol/l, and plasma potassium concentrations are generally 4–5 mmol/l. Because of the great differences in electrolyte loss that occur with different types of exercise under various conditions, it is difficult to develop a general recommendation for electrolyte replacement. Even in the absence of specific guidelines for electrolyte replacement, rehydration following exercise-induced dehydration in the heat has been shown to be more effectively achieved through the addition of electrolytes to the rehydration fluid. Furthermore, net fluid balance does not appear to be affected by the type of chloride salt used (e.g., sodium or potassium), nor does there appear to be an additive effect of including both salt forms in the rehydration beverage.[63]

Maughan and Leiper[67] examined the effects of different amounts of sodium rehydration fluids in subjects dehydrated 2% body mass by intermittent exercise of moderate intensity in the heat. Subjects ingested test drinks that contained 2, 26, 52, or 100 mmol/l Na^+ in addition to a flavoring. The amount of fluid consumed was based on degree of sweat loss. Urine output during the recovery period was inversely proportional to the sodium content of the test drinks. Subjects achieved positive sodium balance and remained in positive fluid balance only when the sodium content was greater than 50 mmol/l.

Ingestion of food plus fluid has been reported to reduce urine volume over a 6-hour period compared with drink alone.[68] The greater electrolyte content of the meal (e.g., higher sodium and potassium) may have been responsible for restoration of whole body water balance.

3. Caffeine and Alcohol Consumption

Beverages that induce a diuretic effect and facilitate water loss from the body are contraindicated for fluid replacement. Therefore, beverages containing alcohol or caffeine are not recommended for rehydration purposes following exercise. The effects of alcohol ingestion after sweat loss induced by exercise in a hot environment were investigated by Shirreffs and Maughan.[69] Once a 2% loss of body mass was reached while exercising in the heat, subjects then ingested a volume of fluid equivalent to 3% of the pre-exercise body mass. Test drinks were composed of alcohol-free beer and the addition of ethanol at a concentration of 0, 1%, 2%, or 4%. Urine volume increased over the next several hours as the alcohol concentration in the drinks increased, and a small but significant increase in urine output was observed with the highest alcohol concentration. While drinks containing low concentrations of alcohol were not found to greatly impair ability to rehydrate following exercise, alternative beverages that are better suited for fluid and electrolyte replacement as well as energy stores should be chosen.

V. SUMMARY

The food and beverages that are consumed before, during, and following strenuous exercise or a competition can influence the outcome of the event, and perhaps events that follow, within a short time span. Pre-event meals can have both a positive and negative effect on subsequent performance. Generally, pre-event meals should be high in carbohydrate, consumed 1 to 4 hours prior to the event, and should be composed of safe and somewhat bland foods. The total energy content of the meal should be under 1000 kcal. In addition, the fiber content of the meal should be low and adequate fluids must be consumed during the pre-event period.

Eating during high-intensity short-term events is impractical and probably not necessary. However, the consumption of adequate carbohydrate and fluids during more-prolonged events has been shown to improve performance during the event. Studies indicate that athletes performing in prolonged events should consume 25 to 75 grams of carbohydrate for each hour of the event. Thirst is not a good indicator of the level of dehydration during exercise. Therefore, athletes, on average, should consume fluids at the rate of 4 to 8 ounces (120–240 ml) every 15–20 minutes of an event. Water is acceptable for events lasting less than an hour. However, sports drinks should be the fluid replacement beverage for events lasting longer than 1 hour.

Consumption of adequate carbohydrate and replacement fluids is important following exercise. Research has shown that carbohydrates should be consumed almost immediately post exercise and this consumption should continue for 4 to 6 hours. Carbohydrate consumption should be around 1 gram per kilogram of body weight per hour. Fluids also need to be replaced in the post-exercise period. One liter or more of fluid should be consumed for each kilogram of lost body weight. Fluid consumption should continue until adequate urine volume is produced.

REFERENCES

1. Stamford, B., When to eat and exercise, *Phys. Sportsmed.*, 16, 184, 1988.
2. Clark, N., Eating before competing, *Phys. Sportsmed.*, 26, 73, 1998.
3. Coleman, E.J., Carbohydrate — the master fuel, in *Nutrition for Sport and Exercise*, 2nd ed., Berning, J.R. and Steen, S.N., Eds., Aspen Pub., Inc., Gaithersburg, MD., 1998, chap. 2.
4. Clark, N., *Sports Nutrition Guidebook*, 2nd ed., Human Kinetics, Champaign, IL., 1997.
5. Sherman, W.M., Peden, M.C., and Wright, D.A., Carbohydrate feedings 1 h before exercise improves cycling performance, *Am. J. Clin. Nutr.,* 54, 866, 1991.
6. Sherman, W.M., Pre-event nutrition, *Sports Sci. Exch.,* Gatorade Sports Sci. Inst., Barrington, IL 1(12), 1989.
7. Kanter, M., What to eat before and after exercise, in *Endurance Training for Performance,* Gatorade Performance Series, Gatorade Sport Sci. Inst., Barrington, IL., 1994, p. 13.
8. Costill, D.L., Coyle, E.F., Dalsky, G., Evans, W., Fink, W., and Hoopes, D., Effects of elevated plasma FFA and insulin on muscle glycogen usage during exercise, *J. Appl. Physiol.,* 43, 695, 1977.
9. Foster, C., Costill, D.L., and Fink, W.J., Effects of pre-exercise feedings on endurance performance, *Med. Sci. Sports,* 11, 1, 1979.
10. Keller, K. and Schwarzkopf, R., Pre-exercise snacks may decrease exercise performance, *Phys. Sportsmed.,* 12, 89, 1984.
11. Coggan, A.R. and Swanson, S.C., Nutritional manipulation before and during endurance exercise: effects on performance, *Med. Sci. Sports Exerc.,* 24, S331, 1992.
12. Koivisto, V.A., Karonen, S-L., and Nikkila, E.A., Carbohydrate ingestion before exercise: comparison of glucose, fructose, and sweet placebo, *J. Appl. Physiol.: Respirat. Environ. Exerc. Physiol.,* 51, 783, 1981.
13. Alberici, J.C., Farrell, P.A., and Kris-Etherton, P.M., Effects of pre-exercise candy bar ingestion on substrate utilization and performance in trained cyclists, *Med. Sci. Sports Exerc.,* 21, S47, 1989.
14. Thomas, D.E., Brotherhood, J.R., and Brand, J.C., Carbohydrate feeding before exercise: effect of glycemic index, *Int. J. Sports Med.,* 12, 180, 1991.

15. Thomas, D.E., Brotherhood, J.R., and Miller, J.B., Plasma glucose levels after prolonged strenuous exercise correlate inversely with glycemic response to food consumed before exercise, *Int. J. Sport Nutr.,* 4, 361, 1994.
16. Anderson, M., Bergman, E.A., and Nethery, V.M., Pre-exercise meal affects ride time to fatigue in trained cyclists, *J. Am. Diet. Assoc.,*94, 1152, 1994.
17. Coleman, E. and Steen, S.N., *The Ultimate Sports Nutrition Handbook,* Bull Pub. Co., Palo Alto, Ca., 1996.
18. Anderson, J.J.B. and McMurray, R.G., Overview: Nutrition in Exercise and Sport, in *Nutrition in Exercise and Sport,* 3rd ed., Wolinsky, I., Ed., CRC Press, Boca Raton, FL, 1998, 49.
19. Rankin, J.W., Glycemic index and exercise metabolism, *Sports Sci. Exchang.,* Gatorade Sports Sci. Inst., Barrington, IL, 10(1), No. 64, 1997.
20. Sherman, W.M., Brodowicz, G., Wright, D.A., Allen, W.K., Simonsen, J., and Dernbaugh, A., Effects of 4 h pre-exercise carbohydrate feedings on cycling performance, *Med. Sci. Sport Exerc.,*21, 598, 1989.
21. Schabort, E.J., Bosch, A.N., Weltan, S.M., and Noakes, T.D., The effect of a pre-exercise meal on time to fatigue during prolonged cycling exercise, *Med. Sci. Sport Exerc.,* 31, 464, 1999.
22. Brooks, G.A., and Fahey, T.D, *Exercise Physiology: Human Bioenergetics and its Applications*, John Wiley & Sons, New York, 1984, Chap. 5.
23. Borts, S., Schoonen, J.C., Kanter, M. Kosharek, S., and Benardot, D., Physiology of Anaerobic and Aerobic Exerice, in *Sports Nutrition: A Guide for the Professional Working with Active People*, 2 ed., Benardot, D., Eds., The American Dietetic Association, Chicago, 1993, Chap. 1.
24. Kanter, M., Refueling for stop-and-go sports, Gatorade Sports Sci. Inst., Coaches Corner, (www.gssiweb.com/), 1996, accessed, Sept. 1999.
25. Hawley, J.A., Dennis, S.C., and Noakes, T.D., Carbohydrate, fluid, and electrolyte requirements of the soccer player: a review, *Int. J. Sport Nutr.*, 4, 221, 1994.
26. Hargreaves, M., Carbohydrate and liquid requirements of soccer, *J. Sport Sci.*, 12, S13, 1994.
27. Haff, G.G., Stone, M.H., Warren, B.J., Keith, R.E., Johnson, R.L., Nieman, D.C., Williams, F., and Kirksey, K.B., The effect of carbohydrate supplementation on multiple sessions and bouts of resistance exercise, *J. Strength Cond. Res.,* 13, 111,1999.
28. Coggan, A.R. and Coyle, E.F., Effect of carbohydrate feedings during high-intensity exercise, *J. Appl. Physiol.*, 65, 1703, 1988.
29. Wright, D.A., Sherman, W.M., and Dernbach, A.R., Carbohydrate feedings before, during, or in combination improve cycling endurance performance, *J. Appl. Physiol.*, 71, 1082, 1991.
30. Jeukendrup, A., Brouns, F., Wagenmakers, A. J., and Saris, W. H., Carbohydrate-electrolyte feedings improve 1 hour time trial cycling performance, *Int. J. Sports Med.*, 18, 125, 1997.
31. Yaspelkis, B.B., Patterson, J.G., Anderla, P.A., Ding, Z., and Ivy, J.L., Carbohydrate supplementation spares muscle glycogen during variable-intensity exercise, *J. Appl. Physiol.*, 75, 1477, 1993.
32. Eden, B.D. and Abernathy, P.J., Nutritional intake during ultra-endurance running race, *Int. J. Sport Nutr.*, 4, 166, 1994.
33. Fallon, K.E., Broad, E., Thompson, M.W., and Reull, P.A., Nutritional and fluid intake in a 100–km ultramarathon, *Int. J. Sport Nutr.*, 8, 24, 1998.
34. Gabel, K.A., Aldous, A., and Edgington, C., Dietary intake of two elite male cyclists during 10-day, 2,050-mile ride, *Int. J. Sport Nutr.*, 5, 56, 1995.
35. Groff, J.L., Gropper, S.S., and Hunt, S.M., *Advanced Nutrition and Human Metabolism*, 2nd ed., West Publishing, St. Paul, 1995, Chap. 9.
36. American College of Sports Medicine, Position stand: exercise and fluid replacement, *Med. Sci. Sport Exerc.*, 28, i, 1996.
37. Lyle, B.J. and Forgac, T., Hydration and fluid replacement, in *Sports Nutrition for the 90s*, Berning, J.R., and Steen, S.N., Eds., Aspen Publishers, Gaithersburg, MD, 1991, Chap. 10.
38. Kleiner, S.M., Water: an essential but overlooked nutrient, *J. Am. Diet. Assoc.*, 99, 200, 1999.
39. Coyle, E.F., Fluid and carbohydrate replacement during exercise: how much and why?, *Sports Sci. Exchang.,* Gatorade Sports Sci. Instit., Barrington, IL, 7(3), No. 50, 1994.
40. Fike, S, Kanter, M., and Markley, E. Fluid and electrolyte requirements of exercise, in *Sports Nutrition A Guide for the Professional Working with Active People*, 2nd ed., Benardot, D., Eds., The American Dietetic Association, Chicago, 1993, 38-45.

41. American Red Cross, *Standard First Aid*, Mosby Lifeline, St. Louis, 1993, 218-221.
42. Gatorade Sports Sci. Instit., Fluids 2000: how do sports drinks work?, (www.gssiweb.com), Summer, 1998, accessed, Sept. 1999.
43. Wilk, B. and Bar-Or, O., Effect of drink flavor and NaCl on voluntary drinking and hydration in boys exercising in the heat, *J. Appl. Physiol.*, 80, 1112, 1996.
44. Mueller, C., Adult years, in *Sports Nutrition, A Guide for the Professional Working with Active People*, 2nd ed., Benardot, D., Eds., The American Dietetic Association, Chicago, 1993, 123-126.
45. Ivy, J.L., Muscle glycogen synthesis before and after exercise, *Sports Med.*, 11, 6, 1991.
46. Blom, C.S., Hostmark, A.T., Vaage, O., Kardel, K.R., and Maehlum, S., Effect of different post-exercise sugar diets on the rate of muscle glycogen synthesis, *Med. Sci. Sports Exerc.,* 19, 491, 1987.
47. Ivy, J.L., Lee, M.C., Brozinick, J.T., and Reed, M.J., Muscle glycogen storage after different amounts of carbohydrate ingestion, *J.Appl.Physiol.,* 65, 2018, 1988.
48. Lamb, D.R., Rinehardt, K.F., Bartels, R.L., Sherman, W.M., and Snook, J.T., Dietary carbohydrate and intensity of interval swim training, *Am.J.Clin.Nutr.,* 52,1058, 1990.
49. Wilkinson, J.G. and Liebman, M., Carbohydrate metabolism in sport and exercise, in *Nutrition in Exercise and Sport*, 3rd ed., Wolinsky, I. Ed., CRC Press, Boca Raton, FL. 1998, Chap. 3.
50. Costill, D.L., Sherman, W.M., Fink, W.J., Maresh, C., Witten, M., and Miller, J.M., The role of dietary carbohydrates in muscle glycogen resynthesis after strenuous running, *Am. J. Clin. Nutr.*, 34, 1831, 1981.
51. Kiens, B., Raben, A.B., Valeur, A.K., and Richter, E.A., Benefit of dietary simple carbohydrates on the early post-exercise muscle glycogen repletion in male athletes (abstract), *Med. Sci. Sports Exerc.,* 22, 1990.
52. Burke, L.M., Collier, G.R., and Hargreaves, M., Muscle glycogen storage after prolonged exercise: effect of the glycemic index of carbohydrate feedings, *J. Appl. Physiol.,* 75,1019, 1993.
53. Reed, M.J., Brozinick, J.T., Lee, M.C., and Ivy, J.L., Muscle glycogen storage postexercise: effect of mode of carbohydrate administration, *J. Appl. Physiol.,* 66, 720, 1989.
54. Spiller, G.A., Jensen, C.D., Pattison, T.S., Chuck, C.S., Whittam, J.H., and Scala, J., Effect of protein dose on serum glucose and insulin response to sugars, *Am. J. Clin. Nutr.,* 46, 474,1987.
55. Zawadski, K.M., Yaspelkis, B.B., and Ivy, J.L., Carbohydrate-protein complex increases the rate of muscle glycogen storage after exercise, *J. Appl. Physiol.,* 72, 1854, 1992.
56. Ivy, J.L., Glycogen resynthesis after exercise: effect of carbohydrate intake, *Int. J. Sports Med.,* 19, S142, 1998.
57. Ivy, J.L., Katz, A.L., Cutler, C.L., Sherman, W.M., and Coyle, E.F., Muscle glycogen synthesis after exercise: effect of time of carbohydrate ingestion, *J. Appl. Physiol.*, 64,1480, 1988.
58. Parkin, J.M., Carey, M.F., Martin, I.K., Stojanovska, L., and Febbraio, M.A., Muscle glycogen storage following prolonged exercise: effect of timing of ingestion of high glycemic index food, *Med. Sci. Sports Exerc.*, 29, 220, 1997.
59. Chandler, R.M., Byrne, H.K., Patterson, J.G., and Ivy, J.L., Dietary supplements affect the anabolic hormones after weight-training exercise, *J. Appl. Physiol.*, 76, 839, 1994.
60. Carraro, F., Hartl, W.H., Stuart, C.A., Layman, D.K., Jahoor, F., and Wolfe, R.R., Whole body and plasma protein synthesis in exercise and recovery in human subjects, *Am. J. Physiol.,* 258, E821,1990.
61. DiPasquale, M.G., *Amino Acids and Proteins for the Athlete*, CRC Press, Boca Raton, FL., 1997, Chap. 4.
62. Biolo, G., Maggi, S.P., Williams, B.D., Tipton, K.D., and Wolfe, R.R., Increased rates of muscle protein turnover and amino acid transport after resistance exercise in humans, *Am. J. Physiol.*, 268, E514, 1995.
63. Maughan, R.J., Owen, J.H., Shirreffs, S.M., and Leiper, J.B., Post-exercise rehydration in man: effects of electrolyte addition to ingested fluids, *Eur. J. Appl. Physiol.,* 69, 209, 1994.
64. Shirreffs, S.M., Taylor, A.J., Leiper, J.B., and Maughan, R.J., Post-exercise rehydration in man: effects of volume consumed and drink sodium content, *Med. Sci. Sports Exerc.*, 28, 1260, 1996.
65. Nose, H., Mack, G.W., Shi, X., and Nadel, E.R., Shift in body fluid compartments after dehydration in humans, *J. Appl. Physiol.,* 65, 318, 1988.
66. Gonzalez-Alonso, J., Heaps, C.L., and Coyle, E.F., Rehydration after exercise with common beverages and water, *Int. J. Sports Med.,* 13, 399, 1992.

67. Maughan, R.J. and Leiper, J.B., Sodium intake and post-exercise rehydration in man, *Eur. J. Appl. Physiol.*, 71, 319, 1995.
68. Maughan, R.J., Leiper, J.B., and Shirreffs, S.M., Restoration of fluid balance after exercise-induced dehydration: effects of food and fluid intake, *Eur. J. Appl. Physiol.*, 73, 317, 1996.
69. Shirreffs, S.M. and Maughan, R.J., Restoration of fluid balance after exercise-induced dehydration: effects of alcohol consumption, *J. Appl. Physiol.*, 83, 1152, 1997.

Part IV

Eating and Addictive Disorders/Conditions

CHAPTER 13

Nutritional Implications of Eating Disorders Among Athletes

Jaime S. Ruud

CONTENTS

I. INTRODUCTION

Today there is enormous pressure on young athletes to be successful and to achieve an ideal body weight. Franseen and McCann[1] write: "The level of competition for elite athletes puts demands on them that most people never experience. Expressions like "no pain, no gain" or "some is good, more is better" suggest that athletes must push beyond a healthy limit. This attitude can cause serious injuries, overtraining or weight loss that is unhealthy and dangerous."

0-8493-8199-1/00/$0.00+$.50

This is especially true for athletes who must maintain a low body weight for their sport. Athletes in "thin-build" sports (gymnastics, figure skating, ballet) report greater body dissatisfaction and more persistent dieting than athletes in normal-build sports (e.g. basketball, volleyball, field hockey).[2]

The inability to control weight and body shape can lead to frustration, guilt, and even despair. Athletes with a history of low self-esteem and difficulty with problem solving and handling stress may turn to food as a coping mechanism. What begins as a casual diet to shed a few pounds to please the coach or improve performance can end in a lifelong battle with food.

Many cases of eating disorders go unnoticed, especially in the athletic world, because there is such a fine line between healthy and unhealthy eating. Successful athletes are disciplined and determined. They often set very high goals and train at the limit of their physical ability. It's not uncommon for athletes to skip meals, have pre-game rituals, and work out several hours a day.

Healthy eating means consuming balanced meals and snacks at regular times; taking in enough calories to maintain a healthy weight; and eating for health and performance. When the athlete eats for reasons other than nourishment and pleasure, the function or purpose of eating can become disordered.

Disordered eating can be defined as eating or not eating in response to an external cue rather than an internal one.[3] An external cue might be "willpower," "a planned diet," or emotional reasons such as loneliness, anxiety, or anger. Internal cues are feelings of hunger, satiety, and fullness.

Almost everyone experiences disordered eating at some time in his or her life. It is when the time spent in external eating is greater than the time spent eating in response to internal hunger cues that the situation can develop into an eating disorder.[3] Athletes, coaches, trainers, team physicians, and sport nutritionists need to be aware of athletes with weight concerns and help them achieve a body weight that promotes optimal health and performance. This chapter presents an overview of eating disorders in athletes, including definition and diagnostic criteria, risk factors, effects on health and performance, and the role of the sports nutritionist in treatment.

II. DEFINITION AND DIAGNOSTIC CRITERIA

According to the fourth edition of the *Diagnostic and Statistical Manual of Mental Disorders* (DMS –IV), eating disorders are characterized by severe disturbances in eating behaviors.[4] The term eating disorder typically refers to anorexia nervosa, bulimia nervosa, or binge-eating disorder. However, eating disorders can range from anorexia nervosa to obesity (Figure 13.1). Within this continuum one can find a number of categories for disorders that do not meet specific DSM–IV criteria, including concerns about weight and shape, excessive dieting, bingeing behaviors, and anorexia athletica.

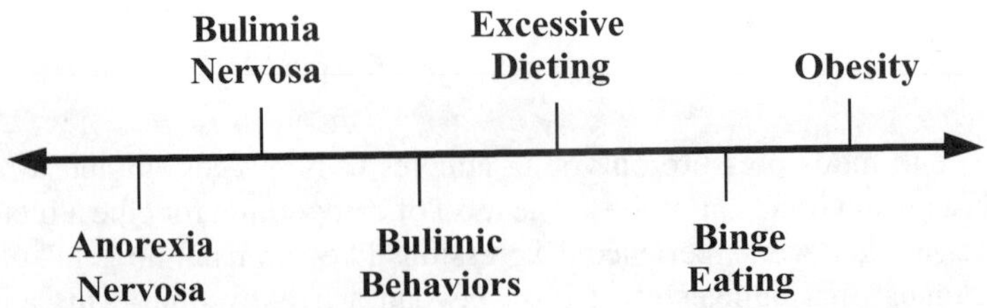

Figure 13.1 The range of eating disorders.

A. Eating Disorders Not Otherwise Specified

Many young women and men can experience a preoccupation with food and weight, but don't suffer from severe malnutrition or the emotional and psychological behaviors associated with eating disorders such as depression, anxiety, obsessive-compulsive behaviors, and low self esteem. The DSM–IV refers to disorders that do not meet the criteria for anorexia, bulimia, or binge eating, as eating disorders not otherwise specified (NOS).[4]

The term sub-clinical eating disorder has also been used to identify individuals who display some but not all of the signs of an eating disorder. These individuals may restrict food intake significantly but not enough to be diagnosed as anorexic.[5] They may also binge and purge, but only occasionally. Regardless of the situation, serious eating problems and health consequences can develop if the proper education and support are not provided.

Within sub-clinical eating disorders is a growing problem, seen among athletes, known as anorexia athletica.[6] According to Ledin,[7] individuals classified as having anorexia athletica not only have an intense fear of being fat, but also use compulsive exercise as a means of controlling their weight. The diagnostic criteria for anorexia athletica include:

- An intense fear of gaining weight or becoming fat even though an individual is already underweight (< 5% of body weight)
- Restrictive energy intake below that required to maintain the energy requirement of high-volume training
- Compulsive exercise
- Occasional bingeing or purging (once a week or once every 3 months)

It is important to differentiate between the athlete with a clinical eating disorder and one who manifests a sub-clinical eating disorder because intervention at this point may prevent progression to more-serious symptoms such as anorexia nervosa, bulimia nervosa, or binge-eating disorder. Table 13.1 presents a complete list of criteria for identifying the athlete with a sub-clinical eating disorder.[5]

Table 13.1 Proposed Diagnostic Criteria for Anorexia Athletica [5]

- Preoccupation with food, calories, body shape, and weight, as evidenced by a score of 20 on the Eating Attitudes Test (EAT-26)
- Distorted body image, as evidenced by a score of ≥ 14 on the Body Image Dissatisfaction scale of the Eating Disorder Inventory (EDI)
- Intense fear of gaining weight or becoming fat even though moderately or extremely underweight (5 to15% below normal weight for height) or extremely low body fat
- Over at least a 1-year period, the athlete maintains a body weight below "normal" (5 to 15%) for age and height using one or a combination of the following:
    - restricting energy intake (energy intake ≥ 80% of energy expenditure)
    - severely limiting food choices or food groups, as evidenced by food frequency, a 7- to 14-day diet record, or both
    - excessive exercise (i.e., more than necessary for success in sport or as compared to athletes of similar fitness levels
    - absence of medical illness or affective disorder explaining the weight loss or maintenance of low body weight
- Gastrointestinal complaints
- Menstrual dysfunction (i.e., primary or secondary amenorrhea or oligomenorrhea)
- Frequent use of purging methods (i.e., self-induced vomiting, or use of laxatives or diuretics for at least 1 month)
- Bingeing (≤ eight episodes per month for at least 3 months).

B. Anorexia Nervosa

Anorexia nervosa is a disorder in which anxiety, compulsive tendencies, and preoccupation with food and dieting lead to excessive weight loss. Anorexics have an intense fear of gaining weight, and, as a result, issues related to food become highly emotional. Despite an emaciated body, anorexics see themselves as fat when they look in the mirror.

Anorexia is characterized by four primary factors:

1. Body weight less than 85% of expected weight (or Body Mass Index (BMI 17.5)
2. Intense fear of weight gain
3. Inaccurate perception of own body size, weight, or shape
4. Amenorrhea

The classic anorexic is intelligent, high achieving, and willing to please. The individual may have been slightly overweight as an adolescent, and, on the subtle suggestion of family or coach, begins to diet. The person achieves a very low body weight by restricting food, and in the process becomes involved in daily rituals, including frequent weigh-ins, skipping meals, counting fat grams, and exercising to burn calories. While the most apparent physical characteristic of anorexia is extreme weight loss, there are other distinguishing features, including lanugo, (a fine, downy hair on arms, legs, and face), bloating or constipation, and dry skin and hair.

Anorexia is a potentially life-threatening disorder. It has the highest mortality rate of all psychiatric diagnoses and a suicide rate equivalent to that of schizophrenia. Although many people undergo a single episode of anorexia and fully recover, if treatment is not successful, death can occur from starvation, suicide, or complications in electrolyte imbalance.[8] The course of anorexia is often cyclical, exacerbating under stress and improving in times when life events feel under control. Treatment is important, as evidence is emerging suggesting that brain tissue is lost with chronic caloric restriction, increasing the likelihood of permanent disability and impaired functioning in the untreated individual. From 0.5 to 1% of adolescent and young women have anorexia nervosa.

C. Bulimia Nervosa

Bulimia nervosa occurs in roughly 2 to 5% of the population. It is described as reoccurring episodes of binge eating, usually followed by purging. To meet the criteria, the binge eating and purging must occur, on average, at least twice a week for 3 months.[4] Purging is defined as dietary restriction, self-induced vomiting, misuse of laxatives or diuretics, or excessive exercise.

Bulimia is characterized by four primary factors:

1. Recurrent binge eating
2. Recurrent purging, excessive exercise, or fasting
3. Excessive concern about body weight or shape
4. Absence of anorexia nervosa

The typical bulimic is an 18- to 25-year-old Caucasian female who is concerned about her appearance although she is usually of normal weight or slightly overweight. To control her weight, the bulimic becomes entrapped in a vicious cycle: diet, starve, binge, and purge. The binge–purge behavior occurs in an effort to relieve guilt and shame.

Bulimics, by their nature, are very secretive and inconspicuous, which is why this disorder is often difficult to diagnose. Unlike anorexia, where extreme weight loss is apparent, many physical features of bulimia do not appear until late in the course of the illness. Common signs of binge–purge behavior include swollen parotid glands (cheeks), calluses on the back of hands, and dental erosion.

D. Binge Eating Disorder

Binge eating disorder is a serious and prevalent problem among the overweight population.[9] It is characterized by recurrent overeating episodes when an individual consumes a large amount of food while feeling a loss of control over eating behaviors.[4] This disorder differs from bulimia nervosa in that compensatory behaviors, such as purging, fasting, and compulsive exercise are not present. To meet criteria for the diagnosis, a person must engage in binge eating at least 2 days per week for 6 months, and report marked distress about their symptoms.[4]

Binge eating disorder is characterized by the following criteria:[4]

1. Recurrent episodes of binge eating (eating, within any 2-hour period, a large amount food, being unable to control overeating during the episode)
2. Eating until uncomfortably full
3. Eating large amounts of food, even when not physically hungry
4. Eating alone out of embarrassment
5. Feelings of disgust, depression, low self esteem, lack of willpower
6. Occurs, on average, at least 2 days a week for at least 6 months
7. Not associated with the regular use of inappropriate compensatory behaviors (i.e., purging, fasting, excessive exercise)

Binge-eating disorder is frequently associated with a history of depression, low self-esteem, and personality disturbances. A distorted body image and preoccupation with food are also prevalent. Although binge-eating disorder is not usually an issue with athletes, it is likely to manifest in the case of a serious injury.

E. Muscle Dysmorphia

Muscle dysmorphia is a relatively new term used to describe individuals who are pathologically preoccupied with being fit and muscular. It is a form of body dysmorphic disorder (BDD), which is an obsession with a defect in visual appearance, usually involving the face, skin, hair, or nose.[10] Muscle dysmorphia is not considered an eating disorder but rather a psychiatric disturbance involving body image.

Muscle dsymorphia affects both men and women, although it may be more common in men. Sufferers have extreme body dissatisfaction coupled with low self esteem and depression. Despite being large and muscular, they perceive themselves as small and weak.[10] To achieve their desired body image, they become totally consumed by weightlifting and dieting and become extremely anxious if something interferes with their daily rituals. The individual frequently gives up important social, occupational, or recreational activities to maintain the rigorous workout and diet regimen. Abuse of anabolic steroids and other substances is common.[11] Muscle dysmorphia parallels obsessive-complusive disorder in that the person has obsessive thoughts and behaviors, such as checking, comparing, reassurance seeking, and excessive exercise.

Characteristics associated with muscle dysmorphia include[10]

1. Preoccupation with body size
2. Long hours of lifting weights
3. Excessive attention to diet
4. The individual gives up important social, occupational, or recreational activities to maintain workout and diet schedule
5. The individual avoids situations where his/her body is exposed to others
6. Preoccupation with body size causes clinically significant distress or impairment
7. Fear of being too small or not muscular
8. The individual continues to work out, diet, or use ergogenic substances despite knowledge of adverse physical and mental consequences

III. PREVALENCE OF EATING DISORDERS IN ATHLETES

Athletes have followed bizarre diets and rigorous training schedules since ancient times. But not until the last 20 years have researchers really looked at actual numbers of athletes afflicted by these behaviors and the impact they can have on health and performance.

Early studies on the prevalence of eating disorders in athletes focused more on pathogenic weight control behaviors than clinical symptoms.[12] More-recent data have used self-reported questionnaires including the Eating Attitudes Test (EAT)[13] or the Eating Disorder Inventory (EDI)[14] to measure dieting behaviors and attitudes associated with eating disorders. The EAT is a 40-item assessment. A cut-off score of 30 is used to classify individuals at risk for eating disorders. The EDI is a 64-item, multi-scale measure designed to assess a wide range of psychological and behavioral traits common in individuals with eating disorders.[14]

Sundgot-Borgen[15] evaluated the prevalence of eating disorders in 522 Norwegian elite female athletes representing 35 different sports. In her study, the EDI was used as a screening instrument. Athletes were interviewed and then clinically examined. According to Sundgot-Borgen, both personal interviews (survey data) and clinical examinations are necessary to obtain reliable data on the prevalence of ED in athletes.

Results showed that 18% of the total population met the criteria for an eating disorder. When data were compared between sport groups, notable differences were observed. Eating disorders were significantly higher among athletes in aesthetic (34%) and weight-dependent (27%) sports than in endurance (20%), technical (13%), and team sports (11%). Further analysis revealed differences within sport groups. For example, within the endurance-sport group, the prevalence was significantly higher in cross-country skiers (33%) than orienteers (0%). In another large study involving 363 athletes (173 females and 190 males) representing 21 different sports, Fogelholm and Hiilloskorpi[16] reported that the prevalence of weight and diet concerns was highest among athletes in weight-class sports (judo, wrestling, boxing, and karate) and aesthetic sports (ballet, gymnastics, and figure skating).

IV. RISK FACTORS

Many sociocultural, familial and psychological factors have been implicated in the development of eating disorders (Table 13.2).[17] Females are at greater risk because society places greater demands on women to achieve and maintain an ideal body shape. Studies show that even young girls who are underweight for their height are dieting to combat their fears of being overweight and not being accepted in society.[18] For many girls, weight and dieting concerns emerge as early as age 8.[19]

Table 2. Risk Factors for Eating Disorders

Biological Factors:	Psychological Factors:	Behavioral Factors:	Sociol-environmental Factors:	Cultural Norms:
Body weight	Body dissatisfaction	Excess dieting	Peer pressure to be thin	Society's glamorization of thinness
Early maturation	Low self-esteem	Bingeing	Negative parental attitudes toward weight control	
Pubertal development				

Adapted from: Taylor et al. Factors associated with weight concerns in adolescent girls. *Int. J. Eating Disorders* 24, 31, 1998.

Dieting at an early age appears to be a major predictor of an eating disorder.[19,20] A 3-year study involving adolescents concluded that females who dieted (severely restricted food intake) were 18 times more likely to develop an eating disorder than those who did not diet.[20] Even subjects who dieted at a moderate level were five times more likely to develop an eating disorder than those who did not.

For many athletes, weight concerns and, subsequently, dieting becomes the focal point of their athletic existence.[5] Athletes who are strongly committed to their sport are at greatest risk of dieting to improve appearance and chances of success. As noted by Smith,[21] "Hunger pains become gratifying signals of accomplishment and food becomes 'the opponent' in a contest the athlete is determined to win."

Another factor implicated in the development of eating disorders in athletes relates to the sport. Two large-scale studies involving athletes from a variety of sport groups concluded that aesthetic (e.g., ballet, gymnastics, figure skating) and weight-dependent (e.g., wrestling, boxing, judo, and karate) sports have a higher percentage of athletes with eating disorders.[6,16] In sports where athletes are judged on appearance, presentation, and performance, there is enormous pressure to achieve an ideal body shape. Many athletes fall victim to eating disorders in a desperate attempt to be thin to please coaches and judges. Gymnastics is one sport where body size has changed dramatically over the years. In 1976, the average gymnast was 5'3" and weighed 105 lbs (47.7 kg). In 1992, the average gymnast was 4'9" weighing 88 lbs (40 kg).[22]

Some athletes do not have the genetic makeup to attain the "ideal body" for their particular sport.[23] There are three basic body types: ectomorph, mesomorph, and endomorph. Athletes generally exhibit a predominance of one body type with aspects of the other two.[24] Ectomorphs typically are lean and slightly muscular. Mesomorphs are naturally muscular and strong. Endomorphs exhibit a stocky build; they have a wide chest and hips and short bones. For the endormoph, weight gain is easy and fat loss is difficult.

Do athletics cause an eating disorder? When comparing disordered eating in female athletes and college women, Ashley et al.[25] concluded that it is not athletics per se that predisposes one to develop an eating disorder but a particular psychopathology. Personality characteristics (high self-expectation, perfectionism, competitiveness) and pressures from coaches and parents to meet certain weight expectations may increase the likelihood. One study found that athletes at risk for an eating disorder are those who are experiencing considerable distress achieving self-identity, who are conflictually dependent on their parents, and who engage in destructive forms of self-restraint.[26]

Former world-class gymnast Cathy Rigby who suffered from an eating disorder for 12 years, does not blame her coach or her sport, but something inside her. "What started it for me," she said, "was the fact that my disposition is very competitive and somewhat obsessive-compulsive. I think I was born that way. So the very things that gave me the need to be good at what I did, to work harder than everybody else, that's what led to it."[27]

A. Warning Signs

Detection of eating disorders among athletes can be very difficult because many pathogenic weight control behaviors are secretive in nature.[12] Athletes may avoid treatment or under-report disordered eating behaviors for fear of being discovered and losing their position on the team.[15] Preoccupation with weight and dieting do not automatically signal an eating disorder. Some athletes may show signs of disordered eating during season but resume normal eating habits when the season is over.[28] Coaches and trainers must recognize when healthy training routines become an obsession and when an athlete is using pathogenic weight control behaviors to become thin. An assessment is warranted if the athlete displays any of the following warning signs:

- Negative comments about food
- Omission of entire food groups such as meat or dairy

- Dramatic decrease in performance
- Excessive concern about weight
- Dramatic weight loss
- Mood Swings
- Depression
- Wearing baggy and layered clothing
- Social withdrawal from teammates
- Visits to the bathroom following meals

V. EFFECTS ON HEALTH AND PERFORMANCE

Athletes with eating disorders are at greater risk for injury and illness. They already place a lot of stress on their bodies as a result of strenuous exercise. Add to that chronic energy restriction and the combination of the two will eventually take its toll on health and performance.

The medical signs and complications of eating disorders have been described and discussed at length elsewhere.[29] This section will briefly review the nutrition- and performance-related issues affecting athletes with eating disorders.

A. Nutritional Status

Researchers [30,31] have examined the energy intake and nutritional status of athletes with sub-clinical eating disorders. Beals and Manore[30] studied 48 female athletes between the ages of 16 and 36 who trained at least 6 hours a week. Subjects were screened for sub-clinical eating disorders using a health and diet history questionnaire, the EDI, and the Body Shape Questionnaire. Twenty four athletes met the criteria for sub-clinical eating disorder; 24 athletes served as the control group. Energy and nutrient intakes and energy expenditure were determined by weighed food records and 7-day activity logs. Results showed that energy intakes of athletes with sub-clinical eating disorders were significantly lower than in the control athletes, 1989 kcal/d vs. 2293 kcal/d, respectively. The athletes with sub-clinical eating disorders also consumed significantly less fat (43 g/d or 19% of total calories) than the control athletes (61 g/d or 23% of total calories).

In another study that assessed the nutrient intake of female athletes with eating disorders, Sundgot-Borgen[31] reported diets low in energy and essential vitamins and minerals, particularly, calcium, vitamin D, and iron. Mean carbohydrate intakes were significantly lower than the 8 to 10 g/kg bw/d recommended for optimal performance.[32] The anorexics averaged 1.7 g/kg bw/d with a range of 1.0 to 2.3 g/kg.

Chronic energy deprivation coupled with high levels of physical activity can lead to serious health consequences including chronic fatigue, compromised immune function, poor or delayed healing, electrolyte imbalances, cardiovascular alterations, and reduced bone density.[30] Roemmich and Sinning[33] assessed the influence of energy restriction on growth, maturation, body composition, protein nutrition, and muscular strength in adolescent wrestlers and a control group. Subjects were evaluated before, at the end (late season), and 3 to 4 months after a wrestling season. Wrestlers consumed a high-carbohydrate, low-fat diet during the season but did not consume adequate energy or protein intake. Although dietary restriction and wrestling training had little effect on growth or maturation, it did produce significant reductions in protein nutritional status, body protein and fat stores, and muscular strength and power.

B. Female Athlete Triad

Female athletes with eating disorders are at risk of developing amenorrhea and premature osteoporosis, two components of the Female Athlete Triad.[34] The triad includes eating disorders, amenorrhea, and osteoporosis, and each component of this triad increases the chance of morbidity and mortality.

Some groups of female athletes, such as runners, gymnasts, and dancers, exercise and diet to the point where they develop eating problems and menstrual irregularities. Amenorrhea is the absence of menstrual cycles and is characterized by low levels of circulating estrogen. There are two major categories of amenorrhea: primary and secondary. Primary amenorrhea is the absence of menstrual periods by age 16. Secondary amenorrhea is the absence of 3 to 6 consecutive menstrual periods after normal menses have begun.

Many nutritional and physiological factors have been associated with amenorrhea. Frequently cited are weight loss, low body-fat levels, excessive exercise, and nutritional inadequacy.[35] Research has failed to consistently show that one single factor causes amenorrhea; in all likelihood, it results from a combination of factors.

The prevalence of amenorrhea in athletes varies between and within sport groups. In a study of 226 elite female athletes, gymnasts had the highest incidence of amenorrhea (71%), followed by lightweight rowers (46%) and runners (45%).[36] Among ballet dancers, the reported incidence of amenorrhea ranges from 27% to 47%.[36,37]

A primary concern of amenorrheic athletes is reduced bone mineral density.[23,12] Compared with regularly menstruating athletes, amenorrheic athletes have significantly lower bone mineral density and this can occur at multiple skeletal sites including the femoral neck, lumbar spine, and lower leg.[38,39] Goebel et al.[40] found that low bone mineral density was significantly correlated to present and past minimum weights in patients with eating disorders.

The primary cause of reduced bone mineral density in amenorrheic athletes is low circulating levels of estrogen. The major health consequences of decreased bone mineral density are higher chances of stress fractures and premature osteoporosis.

In managing athletic amenorrhea, treatment goals include:[41]

- reestablish normal weight and menstrual cycles
- reduce training level
- increase caloric intake

Although an increase in bone density may occur before the return of normal menses, this increase may still be significantly below the normal range for optimal bone health.[42] If female athletes are not willing to change their training routine or diet, estrogen replacement therapy and calcium supplementation may be necessary to preserve and protect bone mass.[35,43,44]

VI. IDENTIFICATION

If an athlete is suspected of having an eating disorder, it is important to intervene. Many colleges and universities have developed policies and procedures addressing the identification, intervention, and treatment of eating disorders. A multidisciplinary team of professionals who have knowledge in the different areas of recovery offers the best approach. The team includes a physician, psychologist, psychiatrist, nutrition therapist, and coach or athletic trainer.

Members of the treatment team work closely together so that messages communicated to the athlete are consistent.[45] The team should have experience working with athletes and have an appreciation for the particular sport. Athletes can be afraid to talk about eating disorders because they are fearful of losing a financial scholarship or their place on the team.

If an athlete's eating disorder puts them at risk for medical complications and they are not willing to comply, a written contract signed by the coach, treatment team, and the athlete may be necessary. To stay on the team, the athlete is required to show up for counseling and medical appointments.

VII. THE ROLE OF THE SPORTS NUTRITIONIST IN TREATING EATING DISORDERS

The sports nutritionist is often the person in an athlete's life with the ability to identify and intervene when a potential eating disorder exists. It is not uncommon for an athlete to arrive at a consultation with complaints of fatigue, poor performance, the inability to gain weight with strength training, feeling cold, and extreme mood changes. In the early stages of an eating disorder, the athlete may present with a strong sense of denial. The goal is to establish a trusting relationship so that the athlete will return for further counseling. Assessment will not occur in a single session, but will evolve as rapport strengthens between the athlete and the sports nutritionist.[46]

The role of the sports nutritionist is to assist with the normalization of the athlete's weight and eating behavior. The responsibilities of the sports nutritionist include;[47]

- Evaluate the athlete's current food intake
- Estimate and determine the athlete's appropriate weight goal
- Support athletes as they try new eating behaviors
- Educate the athlete about normal and abnormal food intake patterns
- Help the athlete understand weight and performance issues
- Dispel myths and misconceptions about diet, health, and exercise (i.e., eating meat will make you fat; eating after 8 p.m. will result in weight gain)
- Teach principles of good nutrition and planning
- Work with the multidisciplinary team in treating the athlete

The initial assessment involves a detailed weight and height history, exercise history, menstrual history, three-day dietary analysis, and body composition measurements, using arm circumference and triceps skinfold for lean muscle mass, and three-site skinfold (triceps, suprailiac, and thigh) for estimate of percent body fat.[48] To obtain a more complete evaluation of nutritional status, ask about supplements, laxatives, diuretics, and other medications. The EAT-40 can be used to assess preoccupation with food, calories, body shape, and weight.[13] A score >30 is indicative of a subclinical eating disorder.

When counseling the athlete with an eating disorder, remember that each athlete's recovery process is unique and treatment plans and goals should be individualized.[49] For the underweight athlete, the most important goal is to establish 95% of normal body weight. Weight gain is a priority because many of the existing symptoms of an eating disorder are secondary to starvation.[45] A weight gain of 0.5 kg (1lb) per week is advised until the athlete achieves the desired goal weight.[50]

Case studies reveal the intense emotional anxiety that eating-disordered athletes have about food and the fear of getting fat during the first few weeks of treatment.[50,51,52] Visualization techniques, food and mood diaries, and journals are tools often used to help athletes verbalize their feelings related to food and body image.[50] The goal is to reverse the athlete's distorted thinking about food, weight, and body image, while promoting self esteem and positive feelings about body size.

VIII. PREVENTION

Physicians, trainers, coaches, and athletes should be informed about eating disorders and what to do if a problem is suspected. Early detection and intervention are important to the athlete's health and performance. The pre-participation exam provides an opportunity to screen for disordered-eating behaviors. Athletes should be questioned about weight and performance goals. If the athlete displays any of the warning signs of a possible eating disorder, nutrition counseling should be provided.

Emphasizing the role of good nutrition and weight control in optimizing athletic performance can reduce the risk of triggering an eating disorder. If an athlete's performance is declining, it is important not to suggest weight loss to improve speed, strength, or appearance, without ruling out other factors. Many times, it's not a body fat or body weight issue, and the attempt to lose weight by dieting or purging only predisposes the athlete to, or exacerbates, the depression that was the root of the problem to begin with.

Education is a primary tool for reducing the risk of eating disorders in athletes. Because coaches, trainers, and parents have the ability to negatively or positively influence the athlete, it is essential that these individuals be included in educational programs regarding healthy weight, body image, and performance. Results of a recent study found that less than half of 258 NCAA Division coaches from five universities (44.5%) reported ever having attended an educational program about eating disorders.[53] This is a surprise, considering that, in 1989, the NCAA provided NCAA schools with educational videos and materials on eating disorders.[53] Furthermore, a number of colleges and universities have implemented prevention, education, and intervention programs. Perhaps these programs are sponsored by campus recreation centers instead of athletic departments, making resources more available to students than athletes and coaches.

Programs aimed at reducing the cultural obsession with thinness and society's distorted meaning of gender identity are needed. Eating Disorders Awareness and Prevention, Inc. (EDAP) is a national, nonprofit organization dedicated to prevention of eating disorders. It provides information to health-care professionals, educators, families, friends, and sufferers. One of the programs sponsored by EDAP is *Eating Disorders Awareness Week (EDAW).* During a week in February, volunteer coordinators — health professionals and educators — organize educational outreach programs and presentations in schools and communities. EDAP also provides videos, curricula, a newsletter, conferences, workshops, and a national speaker's bureau.

IX. SUMMARY

Athletes need to be provided with realistic expectations about body weight, body image and athletic performance. They must also be cognizant of the influence coaches, parents, peers, and the media can have on their decision-making processes. Athletes need help developing greater self-acceptance and belief in their own personal effectiveness, to look beyond the purely physical aspects of their being, and to see themselves as total individuals who have both personal and social worth.[54]

REFERENCES

1. Franseen, L. and McCann, S. Causes of eating disorders in elite female athletes. *Olympic Coach.* Spring, 15, 1996.
2. Davis, C. and Cowles, M. A comparison of weight and diet concerns and personality factors among female athletes and non-athletes. *J. Psychoso. Res.* 33, 527, 1989.
3. Woolsey, M. When food becomes a cry for help. *J. Am. Diet. Assoc.*, 98, 395, 1998.
4. American Psychiatric Association. *Diagnostic and Statistical Manual of Mental Disorders* 4th ed., American Psychiatric Association, Washington D.C.., 1994, 539.
5. Beals, K.A. and Manore, M.M. The prevalence and consequences of sub-clinical eating disorders in female athletes. *Int. J. Sport Nutr.* 4, 175, 1994.
6. Sundgot-Borgen J. Risk and trigger factors for the development of eating disorders in female elite athletes. *Med. Sci. Sports Exerc.* 26, 414, 1994.
7. Ledlin, R. Anorexia Athletica. http://www.cewl.com/cewl/cewlol/articles/70001.htm. Accessed June 28, 1999.
8. Sullivan, P.F. Mortality in anorexia nervosa. *Am. J. Psychiatry,* 152, 1073, 1995.
9. Bruce, B. and Wilfley, D. Binge eating among the overweight population: A serious and prevalent problem. *J. Am. Diet. Assoc.* 96, 58, 1996.

10. Pope H.G., Gruber A.J., Choi P., Olivardia B.A. Phillips KA. Muscle dysmorphia. An underrecognized form of body dysmorphic disorder. *Psychosomatics* 38, 548, 1997.
11. Wroblewska, A.M. Androgenic–anabolic steroids and body dysmorphia in young men. *J. Psychosom. Res.* 42, 225, 1997..
12. Garner, D. M., Rosen, L.W., and Barry, D. Eating disorders among athletes: Research and recommendations. Child and Adolescent Psychiatric Clinics of North America. 7, 839, 1998.
13. Garner, D.M. and Garfinkel, P.E. The eating attitudes test: an index of the symptoms of anorexia nervosa. *Psych. Med.* 9, 273, 1979.
14. Garner, D.M., Olmstead, M. P., and Polivy, J. Development and validation of a multidimensional eating disorder inventory for anorexia nervosa and bulimia. *Int. J. Eating Disorders* 2, 15, 1983.
15. Sundgot-Borgen J. Prevalence of eating disorders in elite female athletes. *Int. J. Sport Nutr.*3, 29, 1993.
16. Fogelholm, M. and Hiilloskorpi, H. Weight and diet concerns in Finnish female and male athletes. *Med. Sci. Sports Exerc.* 31, 229, 1999.
17. Taylor, C.B., Sharpe, T., Shisslak, C., Bryson, S., Estes, L.S., Gray, N., McKnight, K.M., Crago, M., Kraemer, H.C., and Killen, J.D. Factors associated with weight concerns in adolescent girls. *Int. J. Eating Disorders* 24, 31, 1998.
18. Koff, E. and Rierdan, J., Perceptions of weight and attitudes toward eating in early adolescent girls. *J. Adolesc. Health* 12, 307, 1991.
19. Shapiro, S., Newcomb, M., and Loeb, T. B. Fear of fat, disregulated-restrained eating, and body esteem: prevalence and gender differences among 8- to 10-year-old children. *J. Clin. Child Psychol.* 26, 358, 1997.
20. Patton, G.C., Selzer, R., Coffey, C., Carlin, J. B., and Wolfe, R. Onset of adolescent eating disorders: population based cohort study over 3 years. *Brit. Med. J.* 18, 765, 1999.
21. Smith, N. Excessive weight loss and food aversion in athletes simulating anorexia nervosa. *Pediatrics.* 66, 139, 1980.
22. "Dying to win," *Sports Illustrated.* 81, 52, 1994.
23. West, R.V. The female athlete: The triad of disordered eating, amenorrhea, and osteoporosis. *Sports Med.* 26, 63, 1998.
24. Fleck, S. J. Weight training and body build, *Nat. Strength and Conditioning J.*, October, 61, 1994.
25. Ashley, C.D., Smith, J. F., Robinson, J. B., and Richardson, M.T. Disordered eating in female collegiate athletes and collegiate females in an advanced program of study: a preliminary investigation. *Int. J. Sport Nutr.* 6, 391, 1996.
26. Skowron E.A. and Friedlander M.L. Psychological separation, self-control, and weight preoccupation among elite women athletes. *J. Counsel. and Devel.* 72, 310. 1994.
27. Kenny, C., Rigby Beat "Insidious" Eating Disorders. *Omaha World Herald.* Sunday, March 14, 1999.
28. Leon, GR. Eating disorders in female athletes. *Sports Med.* 12, 219, 1991.
29. Becker, A. E., Grinspoon, S. K., Klibanski, A. and Herzog, D. B. Eating disorders. *N. Engl. J. Med.* 340, 1092, 1999.
30. Beals, K.A. and Manore, M.M. Nutritional status of female athletes with sub-clinical eating disorders. *J. Am. Diet. Assoc.* 98, 419, 1998.
31. Sundgot-Borgen J. Nutrient intake of female elite athletes suffering from eating disorders. *Int. J. Sport Nutr.* 3, 431, 1993.
32. Jacobs, K.A. and Sherman, W.M. The efficacy of carbohydrate supplementation and chronic high-carbohydrate diets for improving endurance performance. *Int. J. Sports Nutr.* 9, 92, 1999.
33. Roemmich, J. N. and Sinning, W. E. Weight loss and wrestling training: effects on nutrition, growth, maturation, body composition, and strength. *J. Appl. Physiol.* 82, 1751, 1997.
34. American College of Sports Medicine. The Female Athlete Triad. *Med. Sci. Sports Exerc.* 29, i, 1997.
35. Benson, J.E., Engelbert-Fenton, K.A., and Eisenman, P.A., Nutritional aspects of amenorrhea in the female athlete triad. *Int. J. Sport Nutr.* 6, 134, 1996.
36. Wolman, R.L. and Harries, M.G. Menstrual abnormalities in elite athletes. *Clin. Sports Med.* 1, 95, 1989.
37. Benson, J. E., Gieger, C. J., Eiserman, P.A., and Wardlaw, G. M. Relationship between nutrient intake, body mass index, menstrual function, and ballet injury. *J. Am. Diet. Assoc.* 89, 58, 1989.

38. Tomten, S.E., Falch, J.A., Birkeland, K.I., Hemmersbach, P. and Hostmark, A.T. Bone mineral density and menstrual irregularities. A comparative study on cortical and trabecular bone structures in runners with alleged normal eating behavior. *Int. J. Sports Med.* 19, 92, 1998.
39. Pettersson, U., Stalnacke, B., Ahlenius, G., Henriksson-Larson, K., and Lorentzon, R. Low bone mass density at multiple skeletal sites, including the appendicular skeleton in amenorrheic runners, *Calcif. Tissue Int.* 64, 117, 1999.
40. Goebel, G., Schweiger, U., Kruger, R. and Fichter, M. M. Predictors of bone mineral density in patients with eating disorders. *Int. J. Eating Disorders* 25, 143, 1999.
41. Dueck, C.A., Matt, K.S., Manore, M.M., and Skinner, J. S. Treatment of athletic amenorrhea with a diet and training intervention program. *Int. J. Sport Nutr.* 6, 24, 1996.
42. Jonnavithula, S., Warren, M.P., Fox, R.P., and Lazaro, M.I. Bone density is compromised in amenorrheic women despite return of menses: a 2-year study. *Obstet. Gynecol.* 81, 669, 1993.
43. Constantini, N.W. Clinical consequences of athletic amenorrhoea. *Sports Med.* 17, 213, 1994.
44. Drinkwater, B.L., Nilson, K., Chestnut, C. H., Bremner,W. J., Shainholtz, S., and Southworth, M. B. Bone mineral content of amenorrheic and eumenorrheic athletes. *N. Engl. J. Med.*, 311, 277, 1984.
45. Grandjean, A.C., Woscyna, G.R., and Ruud, J.S. Eating disorders in athletes. In: Mellion, M.B., (Ed). *Office Sports Medicine.* 2nd ed. Hanley & Belfus, Philadelphia; 1996, 113.
46. Stellefson, E.J., *Winning the War Within. Nutrition Therapy for Clients with Anorexia or Bulimia Nervosa.* Helm Publishing, Lake Dallas, Texas, 1999.
47. Reiff DW, Reiff KKL. *Eating Disorders: Nutrition Therapy in the Recovery Process.* Life Enterprise, Mercer Island, WA, 1997.
48. Vinci, D.M. Effective nutrition support programs for college athletes. *Int. J. Sport Nutr.* 8, 308, 1998.
49. Position of the American Dietetic Association: Nutrition intervention in the treatment of anorexia nervosa, bulimia nervosa, and binge eating. *J. Am. Diet. Assoc.* 94, 902, 1994.
50. Clark, N. Counseling the athlete with an eating disorder:a case study. *J. Am. Diet. Assoc.* 94, 656, 1994.
51. Clark, N. How to help the athlete with bulimia: practical tips and a case study. *Int. J. Sport Nutr.* 3, 450, 1993.
52. Thompson, R.A. and Sherman, R.T. *Helping Athletes With Eating Disorders.* Human Kinetics Publishers, Champaign, 1993.
53. Turk, J. C., Prentice, W. E., Chappell, S., and Shields, E. W. Collegiate coaches' knowledge of eating disorders. *J. Athl. Tr.* 34, 19, 1999.
54. Nagel, K.L. and Jones, K.H. Eating disorders: prevention through education. *J. Home Econ.* Spring, 53, 1993.

CHAPTER 14

Nutritional and Performance Implications of Use of Addictive Substances Among Athletes

Robert J. Moffatt, Samuel N. Cheuvront, and John B. Shea

CONTENTS

0-8493-8199-1/00/$0.00+$.50

I. INTRODUCTION

Sports participation is commonly believed to correlate with sound nutritional practices and a healthy lifestyle. It has become convincingly clear, however, that athletes are not as different from nonathletes as was once believed. Grandjean[1] has reported that, despite the growing knowledge of sports nutrition, athlete diets around the world do not differ considerably from their respective cultural norms. This observation is in agreement with direct comparisons between U.S. athletes and the general U.S. population published in 1989.[2] Nutrient intake data from 1991–1995 indicate that the median macro nutrient distributions among Americans are approximately 49% carbohydrate, 17% protein, and 33% fat.[3] In a recent review of the nutritional practices of a wide array of male and female athletes, average intakes of 48% carbohydrate, 17% protein, and 35% fat were estimated,[4] which again suggests little difference between athletes and a normally active population. Not only do these values represent intakes well below (carbohydrate) and above (fat) athlete recommendations,[5] they even fall shy of general dietary guidelines.[6]

Per capita caffeinated beverage consumption constitutes almost 50% of daily fluid intake in the United States.[7] Americans consume an average of 200 mg of caffeine daily in the form of coffee (52%), tea (29%), and soft drinks (59%),[8] but as many as 30% are estimated to consume up to 600 mg/d and another 10% as much as 1000 mg/d.[9] Unfortunately, very little data exist concerning the actual caffeine consumption of athletes in particular. Given the similarity between the diets of athletes and nonathletes, it is reasonable to speculate that average American caffeine intakes are representative of athlete intakes also. One available survey of women in competitive sports reported that almost 40% were habitual coffee and tea drinkers.[10] Interestingly, their pattern of caffeine intakes did not change whether subjects were "in training" or not. Although caffeine is considered the most commonly used psychoactive substance in the world,[11] ample evidence abounds that suggests that the social behaviors of athletes also include recreational drug use and high-risk activities previously thought to pervade only the sedentary community.

II. PREVALENCE OF DRUG USE IN SPORTS

The occurrence of recreational drug use among athletes appears to be similar or even greater than nonathletes in high school, college, and professional sports. Studies of high school students[12,13] show that the use of smokeless tobacco, alcohol, marijuana, and the occurrence of binge drinking are all more likely in athletic youth than sedentary youth. Numerous collegiate sport surveys[14–16] have also been conducted to ascertain whether this trend persists at the college level. Analysis of 3-day food records from one comprehensive North American study spanning 4 years and including 13 different collegiate sports reported mean alcohol intakes ranging from 0–47 g/day.[14] The majority of responses were, however, below the intakes of adult Americans in general (12–24 g/d) which is also within the definition of moderation.[3,6,17] This information must be interpreted cautiously, however, as alcohol intakes are commonly under reported in food records.[17] Anderson et al.[15] surveyed more than 2,000 varsity athletes representing five men's and women's sports at 11 universities on their recreational use of alcohol, marijuana, and cocaine. When compared with data for nonathletes, cocaine and marijuana use were lower but alcohol intake was the same. In absolute terms, about 5% of athletes used cocaine, 30% marijuana, 30% smokeless tobacco, and 90% alcohol. However, since the questions were based on use in the previous 12 months, speculation on abusive behavior is not detailed. When more than 17,000 college athletes in 140 different universities were questioned using various time frames ranging from 2 weeks to lifetime, the conclusion was that substantially more men and women student-athletes (50–61%) binge drink than their non-athlete (36–43%) counterparts.[16] Men were also more likely to use smokeless tobacco, but less likely to use marijuana and cigarettes. Student-athletes may therefore be more susceptible to recreational drug abuse, especially alcohol and tobacco.

Advertising in professional sports like auto racing and American football are evidence that tobacco and alcohol, respectively, are an integrated part of sport and society. However, data on alcohol intake among elite and professional athletes is scant. Gutgesell et al.[18] have suggested that serious runners (30 miles or 48km/wk) consume almost three times more alcohol per week (~24 g/d) than sedentary controls (~9 g/d) matched for age, gender, and marital status. While this may at first seem surprising, runner intakes remained within general intake guidelines. Professional soccer players[19] and Olympic caliber athletes[20] also consume only small amounts of alcohol (3–19 g/d). In contrast, tobacco use in sport appears more pervasive. Data collected in 1987–88 showed that between 35 and 45% of major league baseball players surveyed use smokeless tobacco and many (19%) felt that it was a natural part of the game.[21,22] An additional 15% of baseball players smoked 10 or more cigarettes per day. This usage is not limited to baseball, however, as 36% of soccer players in the 1993–94 French championships also reported smoking and half of this number smoked five or more cigarettes per day. [23] Athletes, like nonathletes, are clearly susceptible to recreational drug use. The premature deaths of Babe Ruth from oropharyngeal cancer and Len Bias from cocaine overdose are reminders that although sports participation provides numerous health and fitness advantages, it cannot protect against the potential hazards of chronic substance use or abuse.

III. PSYCHOSOCIAL ASPECTS OF ATHLETE DRUG USE

The use of drugs by athletes can be described by three motives. These motives are enhancement, coping, and social.[24] There has been little research concerning these motives and athletic performance. However, it can be assumed that coping motives are focused on the time interval just preceding an event, enhancement motives are focused on performance during the event, and social motives are focused on the time interval just following an event. Coping motives are directed toward relaxing and coping with the pre-event anxiety, while enhancement motives are directed toward improving the performance itself. Social motives come into play during the period following competition, perhaps to celebrate a win or mourn a loss. This three-factor model can be useful in understanding the role of sports performance in the use of nicotine, caffeine, cocaine, amphetamines, marijuana, and alcohol. In addition to the addictive potential of these drugs at a physiological level, each can be used as a learned response to environmental stimuli. Thus, an athlete may be introduced to nicotine, caffeine, cocaine, and, to a lesser extent, alcohol, as instrumental for performance enhancement. All these drugs have been associated with an increase in arousal and so they may be used for performance enhancement. Interestingly, all of these drugs cause withdrawal symptoms that include irritability and lack of concentration. Abstinence from nicotine, for example, has been demonstrated to result in as much as a 15% decrement in performance on certain skill performance tasks.[25, 26] This great a decrement at the highest levels of performance would be very damaging to an athlete's success in competition. In this case, performance becomes the reinforcement for continued drug use. In fact, enhanced performance as a result of nicotine use is confined to abstinent smokers and can be attributed to the release from the withdrawal symptoms associated with smoking cessation. Nicotine has little effect on the performance of non-smokers. The instrumental reinforcement of performance on addiction has received little attention, and it would seem to provide an important avenue for investigation in sports research. Alcohol in low dosages has been associated with greater levels of activation during performance, but it may be used in greater dosages for pre-event relaxation, as well as for post-event celebration. Because of its depressant effects on the central nervous system, alcohol may also be used to relax following a loss. Cocaine, and, to a much lesser extent, caffeine, are associated with increased arousal levels. They may be first encountered as a means to enhance performance. However, social motives may also play a role in cocaine use. This is a highly addictive drug and continued use of it may be associated with its physiological addictive characteristics. However, some addiction to cocaine has been associated with the attempt of athletes to reinstate the emotional "high" experienced during competition. Thus, performance enhancement in addition to social motives might play an important role in the use of cocaine.

Finally, marijuana is a drug associated with social, and, to a lesser extent, coping, motives. An athlete might choose to use marijuana the night before a competition to cope with anxiety and stress, but then use it as part of a celebration following competition. It is doubtful that marijuana would provide any use in meeting performance motives.

It can be ascertained from the three-factor model for drug addiction that athletes may become exposed to drug use for social, coping, and performance motives. This use of drugs as well as the effects of these drugs on performance and physiological strata has been documented by various investigators. However, the implications of drug use in athletics for the development of a drug dependence or addiction have received less attention. According to the discussion offered here, drug use may at first occur as an instrumental behavior related to athletic competition. It may therefore become a learned response that is generalized to other performance-related experiences. This would especially be the case where an ex-athlete associates former athletic behaviors with current job performance. In this case, it might be expected that such individuals would engage in drug-related behaviors learned during their years in professional work as athletes. This topic has received little attention by sports researchers.

IV. IMPLICATIONS OF DRUG USE ON PERFORMANCE

Several pharmacological agents have purported ergogenic properties and have been used extensively by athletes. This class of ergogenics has severe limitations, however, because of what constitutes legal usage. The pharmacological drugs presented in this chapter are alcohol, amphetamines, caffeine, cocaine, diuretics, marijuana and nicotine, and several (alcohol, caffeine) are banned at certain levels and by certain sports, while drugs such as amphetamines, cocaine, and marijuana are illegal. It is imperative that athletes, trainers, coaches, and team physicians know and understand the legality of drug use for ergogenic purposes (whether prescription drugs or not) and at what levels the so-called legal drugs are permissible (e.g., caffeine, alcohol). An updated list of banned substances can be accessed through the United States Olympic Committee's Web site (www.olympic-usa.org).

The following section will examine each of these drugs, exploring how they may work to help or hinder performance. The final section will examine the impact of these drugs on the athlete's nutritional status, with special attention to how these pharmacological agents impact dehydration, body weight, and micronutrient status.

A. Alcohol

The alcohol produced for consumption and found in many common beverages is ethyl alcohol. Alcohol is classified as a drug because of its depressant effect on the central nervous system (CNS). Alcohol can also be classified as a food since it is a source of calories.

Alcohol is probably considered for consumption by the athlete for several reasons. Some view it as a way to enhance energy production during competition or to reduce muscle tremor. Many use alcohol for its psychological effects, because it is believed to reduce anxiety, improve confidence, and reduce inhibitions while enhancing alertness. Athletes also use alcohol for social reasons.

Several laboratory studies have been conducted to examine the potential ergogenic benefits of alcohol use. Although alcohol contains a relatively large number of calories (7 kcal/g), its contribution to energy production during exercise is minor. Likewise, alcohol is a poor source of carbohydrates and, in fact, may interfere with glucose metabolism during high-intensity aerobic exercise.[27] Acute alcohol ingestion has been shown to have no beneficial affects on strength, power, speed, or cardiovascular endurance.

As an aid to psychomotor functions, acute ingestion of alcohol has been found to impair athletes' coordination, reaction time, accuracy, and balance even though they may feel more alert and self-confident.

Very little information is available regarding the effect of social drinking on physical performance. The ingestion of alcohol the night before an aerobic fitness test resulted in a decreased aerobic capacity.[28] Heavy drinking the day prior to athletic competition may exert what has been referred to as the "hangover effect,"[28] complications of which might be dehydration from excessive urinary water loss. This, of course, can have serious consequences to performance, particularly during competition in hot environments.

B. Amphetamines

Amphetamines, often called "pep pills," exert a strong pharmacological effect on the CNS. Amphetamines act to mimic the effect of catecholamines, causing an aroused level of sympathetic function — increased heart rate, blood pressure, cardiac output, respiratory rate, metabolism, and glycolysis. Amphetamines also affect blood flow redistribution, in that more blood is delivered to the skeletal muscle and less to the skin and splanchnic region. Aside from the drugs' increased sympathetic influence, amphetamines are reported to increase alertness, a perception of increased energy and self-confidence, and a decreased sense of muscle fatigue.

Scientific reports of the drugs' effectiveness are mixed. However, more-recent laboratory studies have shown that strength, power, maximal heart rate, and peak lactate response were all increased with amphetamine use.[29,30] Chandler and Blair[30] also reported an increased time to exhaustion despite no improvement in aerobic power. It is this finding that is of concern and suggests that the perception of fatigue may be delayed, thus extending work beyond what would be normal. This could be especially problematic during exercise in hot, humid environments where body temperature balance could be compromised.

Regardless of the benefits, real or otherwise, amphetamines are a controlled substance whose continued use could lead to either physiological or psychological addiction. General side effects include nervousness, acute anxiety, confusion, weight loss, aggressive behavior, and insomnia, all of which may act negatively on performance. Further, drugs like amphetamines that alter perception to fatigue, pain, and heat stress might severely compromise the athletes' health and safety.

C. Caffeine

Caffeine is one of the most widely consumed drugs by non-athletes and athletes alike. This drug is commonly found in coffee, tea, soft drinks, chocolate, and a wide variety of other foods, and is also common in some over-the-counter medications. Caffeine is a CNS stimulant that has been reported to exhibit ergogenic properties. As such, users report enhanced reaction time, improved concentration and alertness, increased fatty acid mobilization, and increased muscle triglyceride usage.

The potential of caffeine as an aid to performance is exerted through its effects on the CNS and mobilization of fuels for muscular work. As a CNS stimulant, caffeine is reported to decrease the perception of fatigue.[31] The primary means through which caffeine is believed to exert its effects are in lipid mobilization during exercise. Although considerable controversy exists, several studies have demonstrated marked improvement in endurance performance for recreational and competitive cyclists and highly trained distance runners,[31–35] whereas others have not.[36–38] If an ergogenic effect does exist, it is most likely related to the role of caffeine on mobilizing fatty acids during exercise. Fatty acid mobilization has been shown to rapidly increase at rest as a result of caffeine ingestion and remain elevated for several hours.[39] Caffeine's influence on fatty acid mobilization during exercise is not as clear, however, since some report significant elevations[40,41] in plasma free fatty acids, while others report no effect.[32,42] Additionally, fat utilization as indicated by respiratory exchange ratios may[33,42] or may not[32,41] be reduced during submaximal exercise.

For those unaccustomed to caffeine or for those who consume high doses, caffeine might produce undesirable side effects such as anxiety, insomnia, tremors, diarrhea, and diuresis. The diuretic effect could place the athlete at risk for dehydration, especially when competing in hot environments.

D. Cocaine

Cocaine, a powerful CNS stimulant, can be characterized as a sympathio-mimetic drug. Cocaine is commonly taken by snorting or smoking, or intravenously. In all likelihood, cocaine use by athletes is intended for recreational purposes. The drug creates a sense of euphoria and is thought to increase physical power, self-confidence, and motivation, and some athletes believe it has ergogenic properties. Much like amphetamines, cocaine makes the athlete feel energetic and more alert, while masking pain and fatigue.

Available research regarding cocaine's potential on human physical performance is scant, but it is clear that no ergogenic benefits are derived from its use.[43-46] In fact, available evidence demonstrates detrimental effects on endurance performance.[44,47,48]

Cocaine is highly addictive, and habitual use potentiates psychological problems (i.e., anxiety, agitation, and paranoia) as well as physiological effects (arrhythmia, hypertension, death).

E. Diuretics

Diuretics are often used in the control of blood pressure. This effect is brought about through reducing body water levels, which acts to decrease blood volume, thereby lowering blood pressure. Certain athletes routinely use diuretics for reasons other than control of blood pressure. Although these drugs are not necessarily addictive, they nevertheless have the potential to exert detrimental affects on physical performance.

Diuretics are frequently used by athletes (e.g., wrestlers, rowers) when there is concern about "making weight," a term used to indicate the need to be at, or less than, a certain weight to participate. Diuretics may lead to a significant weight loss (through a loss of body water), but there is no evidence that other ergogenic benefits are derived. In fact, the opposite effect is quite possible in that excessive body water loss results from reduced plasma and extracellular fluid volumes. This, of course, has implications for athletes participating in activities dependent on optimal aerobic endurance. Reductions in plasma volume lower maximal cardiac output and therefore aerobic capacity.

Performance studies, particularly those of long duration, generally show diminished exercise tolerance proportionate to the level of dehydration induced.[49,50] Additionally, this partial dehydration caused by a reduced plasma volume impairs temperature regulation during competition and also may encourage electrolyte imbalance.

It may be worth noting that some athletes who take banned drugs may also use diuretics. This is done not for performance enhancement, but simply in an attempt to mask drug detection by increasing urine volume and thereby diluting the concentration of illegal drugs measured in urine.

F. Marijuana

Marijuna exerts its influence on the CNS either as a stimulant or depressant. Although not considered an ergogenic aid, its use is reportedly common among athletes. Its use appears to be for its recreational value; however, since its effect on performance is generally ergolytic, it is presented here.

Marijuana has been proven to depress motor- and eye–hand coordination, reaction time, and tracking.[46] In addition, users frequently report a relaxed feeling to the point of general apathy and loss of ambition and impaired judgment.

G. Nicotine

Nicotine is a stimulant that is ingested either by smoking or in the smokeless form such as chewing tobacco, snuff, and tobacco plugs. Smokeless tobacco use appears to be increasing in popularity among athletes where they can be observed using it on the playing fields and promoting its sales through commercials and advertisements.

Owing to its purported ergogenic effect, some athletes turn to nicotine. Many become addicted and use nicotine on a daily basis. Many athletes believe that nicotine makes them more alert and better able to concentrate while at the same time, calming them. Nicotine can simultaneously increase sympathetic, parasympathetic, and CNS activity. Nicotine from cigarettes or smokeless tobacco causes increased heart rate and blood pressure and autonomic activity as well as vasoconstriction, decreased peripheral circulation, increased anti-diuretic hormone, catecholamines, insulin, and glucagon. There is evidence that both resting metabolic rate[51,52] and cardiovascular responses to light exercise[53] are increased after nicotine use.

Smokers have been observed to have increases in the work of breathing,[54] delays in the time needed for consumption of oxygen to attain submaximal exercise,[55] and lower maximal aerobic capacities than non-smokers.[56] This effect is due, in large part, to a reduced oxygen transport carrying capacity resulting from increased carbon monoxide binding to hemoglobin. Nicotine has generally been found to be of little, if any, value to athletic performance. It must be mentioned however, that nicotine users may incur as much as a 15% decrement in skill performance.[25,26] This might explain, in part, why many professional baseball players continue to use nicotine products (i.e., smokeless tobacco) during play.

There are serious long-term health effects resulting from this highly addictive drug. Tobacco uses are linked to several cancers, most notably to mouth, pharynx, larynx, and lungs. Smoking leads to respiratory infections and emphysema. Smoking has also been reported to negatively alter lipoprotein profiles[57,58] and promote atherosclerosis.

V. IMPACT OF DRUG USE ON NUTRITION

A. Dehydration

Water is an essential nutrient that accounts for more than two-thirds of an athlete's body weight. Although wide variability exists, insensible perspiration, urinary, fecal, and respiratory water losses approximate 2.5–3 L/day. Sweat (1–2 L/hr) and respiratory water losses that accompany the added metabolic heat load and ventilatory exchange of exercise can add significantly to fluid requirements. In addition to the recommended water intake of 1–1.5 mL/kcal of energy expenditure suggested for normal living,[7] supplemental fluid intakes[59] have been designed to help offset exercise losses and maintain fluid homeostasis. However, voluntary fluid replacement rarely exceeds 50% of losses during exercise,[60] which is explained, in part, by a delayed thirst response. Preventing dehydration with sound food and fluid consumption is therefore a behavioral issue. Because even low levels (1–2%) of dehydration can significantly impair performance and the capacity to adequately regulate body temperature,[61] the chronic or mistimed consumption of a diuretic could potentially undermine the training and competitive status of any athlete and complicate the occurrence of heat illness.

1. Caffeine

The potential ergogenic allure of caffeine as an endurance-enhancing substance has made its use banned by the International Olympic Committee (IOC) in quantities exceeding 12 μg/mL of urine. However, this level of excretion represents an intake approaching 800 mg of caffeine (eight 6-oz. cups or ~1500 ml of coffee) and is evidence that a generous tolerance for caffeine intakes is recognized even at the Olympic Games. Caffeine has a stimulant effect on the kidney attributed to increased renal blood flow and elevated glomeruli filtration.[62] The diuretic potential of caffeine in quantities below the IOC limit has recently been shown. Following abstinence from caffeine for 5 days, casual coffee drinkers were given 900 ml of coffee (~650mg caffeine) while 24-hour urine samples were collected. A negative fluid balance equal to a 2.8% reduction in body water and 1% reduction in body weight was observed.[63] Just as in exercise-induced dehydration, subjects also admitted no thirst sensation despite their notable fluid losses. Urine output increased 41% compared with outputs from identical volumes of water intake. Since the natural physiological response of the kidney is to reduce urine output in times of dehydration, added urinary losses resulting from caffeine consumption could further exacerbate a negative fluid balance. Several investigators dismiss the acute diuretic potential of caffeine to cause dehydration or impair thermoregulation when taken in smaller doses (~350 mg),[64,65] but the chronic use of caffeine in large, but realistic, quantities and its potential impact on hydration status from day to day has not been evaluated.

2. Alcohol

The strong inhibitory effect of alcohol on antidiuretic hormone (ADH) make beer and other alcoholic beverages unacceptable choices for achieving positive hydration. In addition, alcohol acts as a vasodilator, thus increasing heat loss and the potential for hypothermia during cold-weather exercise.[66] Despite the obvious contraindications, the use of alcohol in sport has a long history dating back to the Greek Olympiads, when wine was enjoyed as the beverage of choice among athletes. Modern convictions for alcohol use in sport suggest that beer is an alternative source of carbohydrate, or "liquid bread." The actual quantity of carbohydrate in beer varies widely from 1–13 g per 12 oz (~360 ml) serving, making the mass consumption of beer as a carbohydrate source of far greater potential harm than good. The anti-tremor effect of alcohol is considered a potential advantage in precision sports such as archery, but alcohol use is currently banned only in the modern pentathlon.[67] This limited tether of control is also testimony to the popularity and acceptance of alcohol as a social drug. Because it is not clear when athletes consume alcoholic beverages or choose to binge drink, it is difficult to know how harmful current practices might actually be to overall health and performance.

3. Diuretics

Clinical diuretic use commonly reserved for the treatment of hypertension and edema is also practiced by many athletes despite its banned status. Although weight loss is achieved without thermal or exercise stress, the hypohydration produced by clinical diuretics has been shown to invoke a greater magnitude of plasma volume loss than other methods of diuresis and lead to an exaggerated impairment in thermoregulation.[68] It is therefore clear that the use of either dietary or clinical diuretics only serves to make the challenge of preventing dehydration more formidable.

B. Weight Control

Body weight and body image are important components of weight class and judged sports. The use and abuse of many recreational drugs can significantly compound the difficulty many athletes will encounter in achieving or maintaining a desired body weight.

1. Alcohol and Caffeine

Because, at 7 kcal/g, ethanol is an energy-dense chemical, the effect of its consumption in addition to the carbohydrate calories of beer and various mixed drinks is known to produce weight gain when added to an otherwise normal diet.[69] Caffeine, on the other hand, is known to raise basal metabolic rate for several hours in a dose-dependent manner. This has raised the question of whether the thermogenic effects of caffeine might be useful for weight control.[62,70,71] However, significant elevations require continual dosing (100 mg/2 hrs × 6),[71] which may be impractical. The direct side effect of dehydration and the indirect displacement of other nutrient-rich beverages probably offset this minor thermogenic benefit.

2. Nicotine and Marijuana

Athletes who smoke find quitting difficult due to the addictive nature of nicotine. Both athletes and the sedentary ex-smoker may also complain of weight gain with abstinence from smoking. Weight gain that accompanies smoking cessation is believed to be the result of nicotine's direct effect on the satiety center of the brain.[72] In this manner, smoking becomes the impetus for weight control. When body weight and body image are a high priority, the difficulty of quitting becomes compounded. In contrast to tobacco, anecdotal reports of extreme appetite ("munchies") following the use of marijuana may in fact have opposite weight control ramifications. Evidence for the selective clinical use of the active ingredient in marijuana (delta-9-tetrahydrocannabinol, or THC) in stimulating appetite and reducing the nausea associated with chemotherapy suggests that this is a real phenomenon[73] and may represent a new approach for encouraging drug abstinence.

C. Micronutrient Status and Health

Although the micronutrient intakes of athletes usually exceed both the scientific guidelines and non-athlete population intakes due to greater calorie intakes,[3,74] many female athletes fall short on calcium. Reasons for milk avoidance are numerous, but population data suggest that displacement of milk by other more popular beverage choices, including coffee, tea, and soft drinks, is one participating factor.[75]

1. Caffeine and Alcohol

More than half of dancers (ballet, jazz, modern dance) consume fewer than two servings of dairy products/day, yet 91% drink caffeinated beverages (2–4 beverages/day) and almost 75% consume alcohol (mean = 5 drinks/wk).[76] Across a myriad of women's sports, high school,[77,78] college,[14,79,80] and elite adult females[81,82] consume only about 75% of the current Dietary Reference Intake (DRI) for calcium (1000–1300 mg/d)[83] with the lowest intakes reported for adolescent female gymnasts, runners, and ballet dancers. Since lifetime milk and calcium intakes are well associated with bone mineral density (BMD),[84-86] the displacement of milk by caffeinated and alcoholic beverages may act to reduce BMD. Because peak bone mass is achieved for females between the ages of 18–30,[87,88] the long-term consequence of milk displacement by caffeinated beverages may be one contributing factor in the higher incidence of fracture and osteoporosis over the female lifespan. Alcohol may also potentiate this effect, as it is known to directly inhibit human osteoblastic cell activity.[89] The lower BMD commonly seen in dancers and other female athletes is undoubtedly a partial reflection of nutritional and lifestyle influences.

Additional micronutrient losses associated with ethanol intakes include the obligatory coenzyme utilization of thiamin, riboflavin, and niacin in alcohol metabolism. Its consumption also reduces the absorption of these vitamins while increasing the renal excretion rates of many minerals.

Although alcoholism and binge-drinking are well documented to have these effects,[90] whether moderate, but chronic, alcohol consumption results in altered micronutrient status is not known.

2. Diuretics and Smoking

The use of some clinical and over-the-counter drugs also have the potential to negatively impact both short- and long-term nutritional status. Almost all clinical diuretics produce significant losses of potassium, sodium, magnesium, chloride, and calcium. It is important to recognize that these losses are dose dependent and that hypokalemia, in particular, can be fatal. The harmful free radical species resulting from the oxidative stress imposed by cigarette smoke reduce plasma ascorbic acid levels,[91,92] thus raising the physiological need for vitamin C. Plasma concentrations of other important antioxidants (vitamin A, vitamin E) are also known to be lower in smokers even when the dietary intakes of these vitamins are similar to non-smokers.[93]

VI. SUMMARY

Although athletes commonly express dietary concerns related to performance, it is well documented that their actual eating practices approach those of the general population. Similarly, the lifestyle habits of many high school, college, and professional athletes are not consistent with the traditionally held role model stereotype. Parents, coaches, trainers, and athletes themselves should be aware that sports participation does not exclude athletes from the societal influences and pressures which often lead to substance use and abuse. Alcohol and tobacco use are especially prevalent at all levels of sport. Documentation of less pervasive athlete drug use, although evident, supports only tentative conclusions.

Many of the substances outlined in this chapter can be highly addictive (alcohol, amphetamines, cocaine, marijuana, nicotine) and many are illegal (amphetamines, cocaine, marijuana). Additionally, some (alcohol, caffeine, diuretics) are banned substances at many levels of athletic competition. The largely ergolytic consequences to performance and the negative nutritional impact these substances have with respect to hydration, weight control, and micronutrient balance make their use a logical contraindication for optimal athletic achievement.

REFERENCES

1. Grandjean, A. C., Diets of elite athletes: Has the discipline of sports nutrition made an impact?, *J. Nutr.*, 127, 874S, 1997.
2. Grandjean, A. C., Macronutrient intake of U.S. athletes compared with the general population and recommendations made for athletes, *Am. J. Clin. Nutr.*, 49, 1070, 1989.
3. Millen, B. E., Quatromoni, P. A., Franz, M. M., Epstein, B. E., Cupples, L. A., and Copenhafer, D.L. Population nutrient intake approaches dietary recommendations: 1991-1995 Framingham nutrition studies, *J. Am. Diet. Assoc.*, 97, 742, 1997.
4. Hawley, J. A., Dennis, S. C., Lindsay, F. H., and Noakes, T. D., Nutritional practices of athletes: Are they suboptimal?, *J. Sports Sci.*, 13, S75, 1995.
5. American Dietetic Association, Position of the American Dietetic Association: Nutrition for physical fitness and athletic performance in adults, *J. Am. Diet. Assoc.*, 87, 933, 1987.
6. United States Department of Agriculture, *Nutrition and Your Health: Dietary Guidelines for Americans*, 4th ed., Washington, D.C., United States Department of Agriculture and Health and Human Services, 1995.
7. Food and Nutrition Board, *Recommended Dietary Allowances*, 10th ed., Washington, D.C., National Academy Press, 1989, 249.

8. Lecos, C., *Caffeine Jitters: Some Safety Questions Remain*, Rockville, MD, Department of Health and Human Services, 4, 1988.
9. Greden, J. F., Coffee, tea and you, *Science*, 19, 6, 1979.
10. Werblow, J. A., Fox, H. M., and Henneman, A., Nutritional knowledge, attitudes, and food patterns of women athletes, *J. Am. Diet. Assoc.*, 73, 242, 1978.
11. Witters, W., Venturelli, P., and Hanson, G., *Drugs and Society*, Boston, Jones & Bartlett, 1992, 274.
12. Ewing, B. T., High school athletes and marijuana use, *J. Drug Educ.*, 28, 147, 1998.
13. Rainey, C. J., McKeown, R. E., Sarget, R. G., and Valois, R. F., Patterns of tobacco and alcohol use among sedentary, exercising, non-athletic, and athletic youth, *J. Sch. Health*, 66, 27, 1996.
14. Short, S. H. and Short, W. R. Four-year study of university athletes' dietary intake, *J. Am. Diet. Assoc.*, 82, 632, 1983.
15. Anderson, W. A., Albrecht, R. R., McKeag, D. B., Hough, D. O., and McGrew, C. A., A national survey of alcohol and drug use by college athletes, *Phys. Sportsmed.,* 19, 91, 1991.
16. Wechsler, H., Davenport, A. E., Dowdall, G. W., Grossman, S. J., and Zanakos, S. I., Binge drinking, tobacco, and illicit drug use and involvement in college athletics: A survey of students at 140 American Colleges, *J. Am. Coll. Health*, 45, 195, 1997.
17. Briefel, R. R., Sempos, C. T., McDowell, M. A., Chien, S., and Alaimo, K., Dietary methods research in the third National Health and Nutrition Examination Survey: under reporting of energy intake, *Am. J. Clin. Nutr.*, 65,1203S, 1997.
18. Gutgesell, M. E., Timmerman, M., and Keller, A., Reported alcohol use and behavior in long-distance runners, *Med. Sci. Sports Exercise*, 28, 1063, 1996.
19. Maughan, R. J., Energy and macronutrient intakes in professional football (soccer) players, *Br. J. Sports Med.*, 31, 45, 1997.
20. VanErp-Baart, A. M., Saris, W. H. M., Binkhorst, R. A., Vos, J. A., and Elvers, J. W. H., Nationwide survey on the nutritional habits in elite athletes. Part I. Energy, carbohydrate, protein, and fat intake, *Int. J. Sports Med.*, 10, S3, 1989.
21. Ernster, V. L., Grady, D., and Greene, J. C., Smokeless tobacco use and health effects among baseball players, *J. Am. Med. Assoc.*, 264, 218, 1990.
22. Connolly, G. N., Orleans, C. T., and Kogan, M., Use of smokeless tobacco in major league baseball, *NEJM*, 318, 1281, 1988.
23. Bouillard, J. and Branger, B., Smoking and professional soccer players in France, *Rev. Mal. Respir.*, 15, 753, 1998.
24. Cooper, M.L., Russell, M., Skinner, J.B., and Windle, M., Development and validation of a three-dimensional measure of drinking motives, *Psych. Ass.*, 4, 123, 1992.
25. Shea, J.B., Marzilli, T.S., and Fairbrother, J.T. The effects of smokeless tobacco on college baseball players' movement regulation. *Proc. Soc. Res. Nicotine and Tobacco*, 4, 48, 1999.
26. Shea, J.B., Marzilli, T.S., Fairbrother, J.T., and Lujan, R., Attention allocation and task difficulty: The effects of smoking deprivation on attention allocation and task difficulty, *Proc. Soc. Res. Nicotine and Tobacco*, 3, 27, 1998.
27. Kendrick, Z., Effect of ethanol on metabolic responses to treadmill running in well trained men, *J. Clin. Pharmacol.*, 33, 136, 1993.
28. O'Brien, C., Alcohol and Sport, *Sports Med.*, 15, 71, 1993.
29. Ivy, J.L., Amphetamines. *Ergogenic Aids in Sport*, Williams, M. H., ed., Human Kinetics, Champaign, IL, 1983, 101.
30. Chandler, J. V. and Blair, S. N., The effect of amphetamines on selected physiological components related to athletic success, *Med. Sci. Sports Exerc.*, 12, 65, 1980.
31. Costill, D. L., Dalsky, G., and Fink, W. J., Effects of caffeine ingestion on metabolism and exercise performance, *Med. Sci. Sports*, 10, 155, 1978.
32. Graham, T. E. and Spriet, L. L., Performance and metabolic responses to a high caffeine dose during prolonged exercise, *J. Appl. Physiol.*, 71, 2292, 1991.
33. Ivy, J. L., Costill, D. L., Fink, W. J., and Lower, R. W., Influence of caffeine and carbohydrate feeding on endurance performance, *Med. Sci. Sports*, 11, 6, 1979.
34. Spriet, L. L., MacLean, D. A., Dyck, D. J., Hultman, E., Cederblad, G,. and Graham, T. E., Caffeine ingestion and muscle metabolism during prolonged exercise in humans, *Am. J. Physiol.*, 262, E891, 1992.

35. Sasaki, H., Maeda, J., Usui, S., and Ishiko, T., Effects of sucrose and caffeine ingestion on performance of prolonged strenuous running, *Int. J. Sports Med.*, 8, 203, 1987.
36. Bond, U., Adams, R., Balkissoon, B., McRae, J., and Tearny, R. J., Effects of caffeine on cardiorespiratory function and glucose metabolism during rest and graded exercise, *J. Sports Med. Phys. Fit.*, 20, 135, 1987.
37. Powers, S. K., Dodd, S., Woodyared, J., and Magnum, M., Caffeine alters ventilatory and gas exchange kinetics during exercise. *Med. Sci. Sports Exerc.*, 18, 101, 1986.
38. Sasaki, H., Takaoka, I., and Ishiko, T., Effects of sucrose and caffeine ingestion on running performance and biochemical responses to endurance running, *Int. J. Sports Med.*, 8, 203, 1987.
39. Van Handel, P., Caffeine, *Ergogenic Aids in Sports*, Williams, M. H., ed., Human Kinetics, Champaign, IL, 1983, 128.
40. Dodd, S. L., Brooks, E., Powers, S. K., and Tulley, R., The effect of caffeine on graded exercise performance in caffeine naive versus habituated subjects, *Eur. J. Appl. Physiol.*, 62, 424, 1991.
41. Tarnopolsky, M., Atkinson, S., MacDougall, I., Sale, D., and Sutton, J. R., Physiological responses to caffeine during endurance running in habitual caffeine users, *Med. Sci. Sports Exerc.*, 21, 418, 1989.
42. Essig, D., Costill, D. L., and Van Handel, P., Effect of caffeine ingestion on utilization of muscle glycogen and lipid during leg ergometer cycling, *Int. J. Sports Med.*, 1, 86, 1980.
43. Cantwell, J. D. and Rose, F. D., Cocaine and cardiovascular events, *Phys. Sportsmed.*, 14, 77, 1986.
44. Conlee, R. K., Amphetamine, caffeine and cocaine, *Ergogenics — Enhancement of Performance in Exercise and Sport*, Lamb, D.R. and Williams, M.H., eds., Brown and Benchmark, Dubuque, IA, 1991, 285.
45. Lombardo, J., Stimulants and athletic performance: Cocaine and nicotine, *Phys. Sportsmed.,* 14, 85, 1986.
46. Wadler, G. and Hainline, B., *Drugs and the Athlete*, F. A. Davis, Philadelphia, PA, 1989,
47. Bracken, M. E., Bracken, D. R., Nelson, A. R., and Conlee, R. K., Effect of cocaine on exercise endurance and glycogen use in rats, *J. Appl. Physiol.*, 64, 884, 1988.
48. Marques-Magallanes, J. A., Koyal, S. N., Cooper, C. B., Kleerup, E. C., and Tashkin, D .P., Impact of habitual cocaine smoking on the physiological response to maximal exercise, *Chest*, 112, 1008, 1997.
49. Armstrong, L.E., Costill, D.L., and Funk, W.J. Influence of diuretic induced dehydration on competitive running performance, *Med. Sci. Sports Exerc.*, 17, 456, 1985.
50. Caldwell, J.E. Diuretic therapy and exercise performance, *Sports Med.*, 4: 290, 1987.
51. Moffatt, R. J. and Owens, S., Cessation from smoking: Effect on body fat, metabolism and caloric intake, *Metabolism*, 40, 465, 1991.
52. Marks, B. L. and Perkins, K., The effects of nicotine on metabolic rate, *Sports Med.*, 10, 277, 1990.
53. Perkins, K. A., Sexton, J. E., Solberg-Kassel, R. D., and Epstein, L. H., Effects of nicotine on perceived exertion during low intensity exercise, *Med. Sci. Sports Exerc.*, 23, 1283, 1991.
54. Rode, A. and Shepard, R. J., The influence of cigarette smoking on the oxygen cost of breathing in near maximal exercise, *Med. Sci. Sports*, 3, 51, 1971.
55. Biggerstaff, K.D. and Moffatt, R.J. Impact of smoking low nicotine cigarettes on steady state exercise responses. *Proc. Southeast Amer. Coll. Sports Med.*, 26, 22, 1998.
56. McDonough, P. and Moffatt, R. J., Smoking-induced elevations in blood carboxy-hemoglobin levels: Effect on maximal oxygen uptake, *Sports Med.*, 27, 275, 1999.
57. Moffatt, R. J., The effects of cessation from smoking on serum lipids and high density lipoproteins cholesterol, *Atherosclerosis*, 74, 85, 1988.
58. Moffatt, R. J., Stamford, B. A., Owens, S., and Chitwood, L., The time course for changes of HDL subfractions following cessation from cigarette smoking, *J. Smoking Rel. Dis.*, 3, 11, 1992.
59. American College of Sports Medicine, Position stand on exercising and fluid replacement. *Med. Sci. Sports Exerc.*, 28, i, 1996.
60. Broad, E., Burke, L. M., Cox, G. R., Heely, P., and Riley, M., Body weight changes and voluntary fluid intakes during training and competition sessions in team sports, *Int. J. Sport Nutr.*, 6, 307, 1996.
61. Sawka, M. N., Physiological consequences of hypohydration: exercise performance and thermoregulation, *Med. Sci. Sports Exercise*, 24, 657, 1992.
62. Arnaud, M., The pharmacology of caffeine, *Prog. Drug Res.*, 31, 273, 1987.

63. Neuhauser-Berthold, M., Beine, S., Verwied, S. C., and Luhrmann, P. M., Coffee consumption and total body water homeostasis as measured by fluid balance and bioelectrical impedance analysis, *Ann. Nutr. Metab.*, 41, 29, 1997.
64. Falk, B., Zylber-Katz, E., and Bashan, N., Effects of caffeine ingestion on body fluid balance and thermoregulation during exercise, *Can. J. Physiol. Pharm.*, 68, 889, 1990.
65. Gordon, N. F., Myburgh, J. L., Kruger, P. E., Kempff. P. G., Cilliers, J. F., Moolman, J., and Grobler, H. C., Effects of caffeine ingestion on thermoregulatory and myocardial function during endurance performance, *S. Afr. Med. J.*, 62, 644, 1982.
66. Haight, J. and Keatinge, W., Failure of thermoregulation in the cold during hypoglycemia induced by exercise and ethanol, *J. Physiol.*, 229, 87, 1973.
67. Catlin, D. H. and Murray, T. H., Performance-enhancing drugs, fair competition, and Olympic sport, *J. Am. Med. Assoc.*, 276, 231, 1996.
68. Claremont, A. D., Costill, D. L., Fink, W., and Van Handel, P., Heat tolerance following diuretic induced dehydration, *Med. Sci. Sports*, 8, 239, 1976.
69. Gruchow, H. W., Sobocinski, K. A., Barboriak, J. J., and Scheller, J. G., Alcohol consumption, nutrient intake and relative body weight among U.S. adults, *Am. J. Clin. Nutr.,* 42, 289, 1985.
70. Astrup, A., Toubro, S., Cannon, S., Hein, P., Breum, L., and Madsen, J., Caffeine: A double-blind, placebo-controlled study of its thermogenic, metabolic, and cardiovascular effects in healthy volunteers, *Am. J. Clin. Nutr.*, 51, 759, 1990.
71. Dulloo, A., Geissler, C., Horton, T., Collins, A. and Miller, D., Normal caffeine consumption: Influence on thermogenesis and daily energy expenditures in lean and post-obese human volunteers, *Am. J. Clin. Nutr.*, 49, 44, 1989.
72. Meyers, F. H., Jawetz, E., and Goldfein, A., *Review of Medical Pharmacology*, 6th ed., Los Altos, CA, Lange Medical Publications, 1979, 79, 294.
73. Voth, E. A. and Schwartz, R. H., Medicinal applications of delta-9-tetrahydrocannabinol and marijuana, *Ann. Intern. Med.*, 126, 791, 1997.
74. VanErp-Baart, A. M., Saris, W. H. M., Binkhorst, R. A., Vos, J. A., and Elvers, J. W. H., Nationwide survey on the nutritional habits in elite athletes. Part II. Mineral and vitamin intake, *Int. J. Sports Med.*, 10, S11, 1989.
75. United States Department of Agriculture, Nationwide Food Consumption Survey, Nutrient Intakes: Individuals in 48 States, Year 1977-78, Hyattsville, MD, Consumer Nutrition Division, Human Nutrition Information Service, United States Department of Agriculture, 1984.
76. Stensland, S. H. and Sobal, J., Dietary practices of ballet, jazz, and modern dancers, *J. Am. Diet. Assoc.*, 92, 319, 1992.
77. Moffatt, R. J., Dietary status of elite female high school gymnasts, *J. Am. Diet. Assoc.*, 84, 1361, 1984.
78. Benson, J., Gillien, D. M., Bourdet, K., and Loosli, A. R., Inadequate nutrition and chronic calorie restriction in adolescent ballerinas, *Phys. Sportsmed.*, 13, 79, 1985.
79. Kirchner, E. M., Lewis, R. D., and O'Connor, P. J., Bone mineral density and dietary intake of female college gymnasts, *Med. Sci. Sports Exerc.*, 27, 543, 1995.
80. Risser, W., Lee, E., LeBlanc, A., Poindexter, H. B., Risser, J. M., and Schneider, V., Bone density in eumenorrheic female college athletes, *Med. Sci. Sports Exerc.*, 22, 570, 1990.
81. Deuster, P. A., Kyle, S. B., Moser, P. B., Vigersky, R. A., Singh, A., and Schoomaker, E. B., Nutritional survey of highly trained women runners, *Am. J. Clin. Nutr.*, 45, 954, 1986.
82. Ellsworth, N. M., Hewitt, B. F., and Haskell, W. L., Nutrient intake of elite male and female Nordic skiers, *Phys. Sportsmed.*, 13, 78, 1985.
83. Yates, A. A., Schlicker, S. A., and Suitor, C. W., Dietary Reference Intakes: The new basis for recommendations for calcium and related nutrients, B vitamins, and choline, *J. Am. Diet. Assoc.*, 98, 699, 1998.
84. Fehily, A. M., Coles, R. J., Evans, W. D., and Elwood, P. C., Factors affecting bone density in young adults, *Am. J. Clin. Nutr.*, 56, 579, 1992.
85. Halioua, L. and Anderson, J. B., Lifetime calcium intake and physical activity habits: independent and combined effects on the radial bone of healthy premenopausal Caucasian women, *Am. J. Clin. Nutr.*, 49, 534, 1989.

86. Sandler, R. B., Slemeda, C. W., Laporte, R. E., Canley, J. A., Schramm, M. M., Barresi, M. L., and Kriska, A. M., Postmenopausal bone density and milk consumption in childhood and adolescence, *Am. J. Clin. Nutr.*, 42, 270, 1985.
87. Matkovic, V., Jelic, T., Wardlaw, G. M., Llich, J. Z., Goel, P. K., Wright, J. K., Andon, M. B., Smith, K. T., and Heaney, R. P., Timing of peak bone mass in Caucasian females and its implication for the prevention of osteoporosis, *J. Clin. Invest.*, 93, 799, 1994.
88. Recker, R. R., Davies, K. M., Hinders, S. M., Heaney, R. P., Stegman, M. R., and Kimmel, D. B., Bone gain in young adult women, *J. Am. Med. Assoc.*, 268, 2403, 1992.
89. Klein, R. F., Pausti, K. A., and Carlos, A. S., Ethanol inhibits human osteoblastic cell proliferation, *Alcohol. Clin. Exp. Res.*, 20, 572, 1996.
90. Halsted, C. H., Alcohol: Medical and nutritional effects, *Present Knowledge in Nutrition*, 7th ed., ILSI Press, Washington D.C., 1996, 547.
91. Lykkesfeldt, J., Loft, S., Nielsen, J. B., and Poulsen, H. E., Ascorbic acid and dehydroascorbic acid as biomarkers of oxidative stress caused by smoking, *Am. J.Clin. Nutr.*, 65, 959, 1997.
92. Giraud, D.W., Martin, H.D., and Driskell, J.A. Plasma and dietary vitamin C and E levels of tobacco chewers, smokers, and nonusers, *J. Am. Diet. Assoc.*, 95, 798, 1995.
93. Driskell, J.A., Giraud, D.W., Sun, J., and Martin, H.D,. Plasma concentrations of carotenoids and tocopherols in male long-term tobacco chewers, smokers, and non-users, *Int. J. Vitam. Nutr. Res.*, 66, 203, 1996.

CHAPTER 15

Nutritional Implications of Exercise Dependence Among Athletes

Nancy M. Betts

CONTENTS

I. INTRODUCTION

In the last 2 decades we have seen a growing awareness of the importance of exercise to health and well-being. But, at the same time, we have observed some people indulging in excessive exercise to the point of injury, even death. Perhaps this is inevitable in cultures where the attitude "if a little is good, a lot must be better" prevails. While there is no standard definition of "excessive exercise," this term is included in the diagnostic criteria for the eating disorders of anorexia nervosa and bulimia.[1] As in these eating disorders, excessive exercise may be practiced as a means to control body weight. However, unlike the eating disorders, excessive exercise is often viewed positively. Certainly, a regular program of moderate exercise is a positive action to improve or maintain health.

0-8493-8199-1/00/$0.00+$.50

However, while habitual exercise in and of itself does not necessarily constitute disordered behavior, there are habitual exercise patterns that do appear dysfunctional. These disordered exercise patterns have been given various labels, but the term "exercise dependence" currently seems the most popular descriptor.

II. EXERCISE DEPENDENCE DEFINED

The running craze of the early 1970s was lauded by many physicians and health professionals as one of the best ways to relieve stress, control weight, and improve cardiovascular health. Morgan[2] saw a different side, however, and was one of the first to describe recreational running as a "negative addiction." Crippling injuries among the individuals who pursued this activity most aggressively were the cause of concern. Morgan suggested that some individuals were either physically intolerant to long-distance running or unable to maintain a perspective of moderation in their running efforts. Running "addiction," in his terms, was present if people believed that they required exercise daily and if they showed signs of withdrawal when deprived of the opportunity to exercise for any reason. The "exercise addict" was described as a person who would become "depressed, anxious, and extremely irritable" if unable to run. These withdrawal effects could become sufficiently severe to promote continued exercise even when it was medically unadvisable, interfered with the addict's work, or caused serious social conflicts. Others also noted this growing behavioral syndrome and gave it a variety of terms, from "fitness fanaticism" to "athletic neurosis" to "obligatory running."[3] However, De Coverley Veale[4] made a strong case that the syndrome seemed most closely related to a dependence syndrome and coined the term "exercise dependence."

As described in the literature, De Coverley Veale[4] found similarities among the profiles of exercisers displaying compulsive exercise behaviors. One of the most consistent features is a mood disorder brought on when the exercisers, particularly runners, are unable to exercise. This mood disorder manifests itself as depression, irritability, impaired concentration, and sleep disturbance, all of which define a withdrawal state. The withdrawal symptoms are relieved by exercise, but as exercise continues, a tolerance level is reached and the exerciser feels he must increase the amount of exercise to relieve or avoid withdrawal. Relief from or avoidance of withdrawal becomes the highest priority in the exerciser's life and exercise is continued during sickness or injury and at the expense of work, social, and family life. These behaviors were sufficiently consistent for De Coverley Veale to propose a set of diagnostic criteria for exercise dependence that included:

- a rigid, stereotyped pattern of exercise performed at least once each day
- prioritizing exercise over other activities
- developing a tolerance to the level of exercise
- experiencing withdrawal symptoms in the form of mood alterations when unable to exercise
- avoiding withdrawal or relieving it by exercising
- exercising against the advice of a health professional
- continuing the exercise pattern even though it causes work, family, or social difficulties
- weight loss to enhance exercise performance
- awareness of their compulsion to exercise.

Although case studies and anecdotal evidence of exercisers who fit the criteria provide a compelling argument, there is still no agreement that exercise dependence is a primary behavioral disorder. Some researchers suggest that the most substantial symptomology indicating exercise dependence relates to mood alteration.[2-4,7,10] However, the tension-relieving effects of exercise have long been known and physicians often prescribe physical exercises to reduce feelings of stress.[3,7] Additional psychological benefits of exercise have been noted, including reductions in clinical mental depression, heightened cognitive functioning, improved occupational performance, and enhanced sleep patterns. These benefits are not only supported by subjective evidence but also by objective, physiological evidence. It is therefore accepted that all exercisers will likely experience some type of mood-altering effect from exercise. However, simply participating in a regular exercise program to relieve tension cannot be considered symptomatic of exercise dependence, even when the exercise appears excessive to others.

Perhaps the most profound example of mood alteration in exercise is the "runner's high"described by some endurance exercisers.[3-7] As many as 78% of runners in some studies have been reported as stating that they had experienced this euphoric state.[3] Nevertheless, attempts to study this phenomenon by examining neurotransmitters, corticosteroids, and plasma endorphins have largely met with failure.[3-7] Occurrence of the runner's high varies both among and within respondents, and descriptions of the euphoria appear to be highly subjective. The subjective nature, the unreliable occurrence, and the lack of physiological markers of the runner's high suggest that, rather than being an extreme mood alteration, runner's high may be the normal relaxation response to exercise as experienced by individuals who are not stressed, anxious, or depressed. Regardless of its nature, however, the runner's high does seem to provide additional incentive for habitual exercise in some cases.

As with the runner's high, the greatest difficulty in defining exercise dependence is the lack of physiological or biochemical markers. Attempts have been made to measure changes in plasma or urinary catecholamines, corticosteroids, and endorphins, but these measurements lack sensitivity and specificity.[3-7] Empirical evidence for the existence of the syndrome has been based on measurements of sleep disturbance and mood alterations resulting from voluntary or involuntary abstinence from exercise. These measurements are largely subjective. Perhaps the best "marker" to distinguish between non-abusive habitual exercise and exercise dependence is refusal to discontinue exercise in the face of medical, occupational, social, or familial contraindications. A similar definition for excessive exercise was reported as running or working out 2 to 3 hours per day despite injury and pain.[7] Such definitions suggest that the disorder may be a form of obsessive-compulsive behavior.[3, 6-8]

It is of interest that obsessive-compulsive behaviors are relatively common in the eating disorders anorexia nervosa and bulimia nervosa.[1,9] Excessive exercise is also a common feature for both disorders,[1] and this has sparked speculation that exercise dependence might be a variant of anorexia nervosa. Yates et al.[10] were the first to draw parallels between exercise dependence (called "obligatory running") and anorexia nervosa, and, while the case studies presented by the authors were later found to be fictitious, their publication began a continuing debate about the origin of both eating and exercise disorders. Eisler and le Grange[8] have summarized the debate by presenting four models:

1. Eating disorders and exercise dependence are separate syndromes.
2. Exercise dependence overlaps with and leads to eating disorders.
3. Both eating disorders and exercise dependence are aspects of another disorder.
4. Exercise dependence is a variant of eating disorders.

A. Separate Syndromes

De Coverly Veale,[4] in his paper proposing a diagnostic criterion for exercise dependence, separates primary exercise dependence from exercise dependence that is secondary to an eating disorder. He felt that "a diagnosis of primary exercise dependence can be differentiated from an eating disorder by clarifying the ultimate aim of the exercise." When performance of the exercise itself is the end point, with dieting and weight loss used as a means to improve performance, then the behavior should be classified as primary exercise dependence. In anorexia nervosa, the aim of excessive exercise is for achieving weight loss or preventing fatness, making the exercise a secondary behavior.

Owens and Slade[11] made a somewhat finer distinction between exercise dependence and eating disorders. They compared 35 female marathon runners with an unspecified number of anorexic and bulimic patients in terms of "Perfectionism" and "Satisfaction" using a questionnaire called SCANS. The runners and the patients scored similarly in terms of perfectionism but differed markedly in terms of satisfaction, with the marathon runners having high satisfaction scores and the patients having low satisfaction scores. The authors interpreted these findings as evidence for separate disorders. They believed the high perfectionism scores indicated high standards among the runners and, because the runners were not dissatisfied, running was likely used as a healthy means for maintaining their high standards. While this study is one of the few that compares female runners with female anorexics and bulimics, it was limited in terms of subject numbers and in terms of comparison measurements. A larger sample (n = 191) of both male and female exercisers responded to the Eating Disorders Inventory along with the Reasons for Exercising Inventory, both of which are considered valid and reliable.[12] This study found differences between the males and females, suggesting that females may use exercise for controlling their body weight while males use exercise to improve their fitness. In fact, there was a negative correlation for the males with respect to scores on the bulimia subscale and the fitness subscale. As the males in this study scored higher on exercising for fitness, they scored lower on the eating disorder subscale. The males who exercised for fitness reasons also scored higher on a self-esteem scale. The authors suggest that female exercisers who specifically cite weight control, muscle tone, or attractiveness as reasons for exercising should be examined for eating disorders but that excessive exercising in males is not related to disordered eating. These findings also suggest that exercise dependence may be a secondary disorder for females but a primary disorder for males.

In contrast, a well-designed study of females showed that obligatory exercisers did not demonstrate disordered eating tendencies compared with symptomatic bulimics and controls.[13] Unfortunately, bulimics who exhibited excessive exercise were excluded from this study and the groups, while equal, were small (n = 25 in each). The researchers used a number of reliable, valid instruments to measure disordered eating behaviors, one being the 26-item Eating Attitudes Test.[14] A score of 20 or higher on this scale is indicative of disordered eating. While the obligatory exercisers in this study had significantly lower scores than the bulimics, the mean score was 24 with a relatively large standard deviation (± 11.8). The authors expressed concern that some of the obligatory exercisers in this sample may show signs of disordered eating, or may have had a prior history of eating disorder. However, the subscale scores and the scores on the remaining scales did not indicate an overlap of exercise dependence and eating disorders.

B. Exercise Dependence Leads to Eating Disorders

In this model, exercise would begin in a normal, healthy manner but would progress to an excessive pattern, accompanied by diet manipulation leading to the development of an eating disorder.[8] De Coverley Veale[4] presents a very fine distinction between exercise dependence and anorexia nervosa by stating that the aim of the exercise differentiates the two. However, as Dewsnap[15] points out, "exercise aims" are abstractions and anorexic individuals may not provide an honest answer to their aims. Likewise, an exercise addict who says that the aim of his exercise is to develop higher levels of fitness may be equating fitness with lower levels of body fat. Thus, while in theory "exercise aim" may be the distinguishing feature between eating and exercise disorders, making the distinction may not be possible in practice.

Because excessive exercise is a diagnostic criterion for anorexia nervosa, bulimia, and bulimia nervosa,[1] several researchers have studied the role that exercise plays in these disorders. Richert and Hummers[16] found that, among the 345 college students participating in their survey, duration of jogging related to higher scores on the Eating Attitudes Test (EAT). The authors felt that hours of jogging among college students could be a predictor for eating disorders. However, the correlation coefficient, while statistically significant, was small (r = 0.20), data from males and females were not analyzed separately, and the "at risk" comparison group consisted of 29 students who scored higher than 30 on the EAT. In a more comprehensive study, 60 female college students were recruited with an equal number of distance runners who had lost at least 4.5 kg without diet manipulation, bulimia nervosa patients, and non-dieter-non-exerciser controls. A battery of reliable, valid measures of depression, bulimic symptoms, and body image disturbance were used to compare the three groups. No differences were found between the runners and controls on any of the inventories; however, the bulimics had significantly higher scores on all measures. The mean scores for the bulimic patients were all indicative of disorder. The authors stated that their findings could not support the notion that distance runners are at risk for eating disorders.

Contrary to the previous study, Kennedy et al.[17] found that excessive exercise preceded the onset of eating disorders. Forty-five patients admitted to an in-patient unit for eating disorders participated in a retrospective study of their exercise habits. A validated physical activity scale was used, along with a semi-structured interview and a symptom checklist. Over 50% of the patients were found to have engaged in regular exercise prior to beginning diet manipulation and were more physically active than controls, with exercise beginning in their early teens. The authors concluded that excessive exercise is an integral part of the development and maintenance of eating disorders. Brewerton et al.[18] found excessive exercise to be more common among anorexic patients than bulimic patients, but nearly 33% of their sample were compulsive exercisers. These researchers suggested that coaches and family members need to be alert to excessive exercising as an indicator of anorexia nervosa.

C. Another Disorder Underlies Both

While there is little data to support this model, some researchers and clinicians have suggested that both eating disorders and exercise dependence are manifestations of another psychiatric disorder.[8] De Coverley Veale[4] likened exercise dependence to a compulsive behavior and stated that the proposed diagnostic criteria were based on "the core features of a dependence syndrome." Morgan[2] also defined exercise dependence as an addictive behavior. Kennedy et al.[18] report literature describing anorexia nervosa as a starvation addiction. But, the most common root disorder suggested as underlying both eating disorders and exercise dependence is obsessive-compulsive behavior. Kaye et al.[9] found strong evidence of obsessive-compulsive behaviors that were beyond those related to the disorder itself among patients suffering from anorexia nervosa. Davis et al.[19] found that for males, but not for females, excessive exercise was significantly related to obsessive-compulsive tendencies. These researchers also stated that "there is general agreement that obsessive-compulsive characteristics are one of the common personality features associated with eating disorders." However, after conducting an in-depth review of the literature, Hauck and Blumenthal[7] were unable to agree that exercise dependence has its foundation in another underlying disorder. They cite small subject samples, lack of distinction between types of exercise, poor sampling methods, inconsistent measurement methods, and inattention to possible confounding variables as a few of the problems in the research to date that render a conclusion impossible. Standardized methods and a clearer definition of exercise dependence is needed before this model can be tested.

D. Exercise Dependence is a Variant of Eating Disorders

This is perhaps the most difficult model in terms of evaluation and acceptance.[8] This model suggests that the etiological factors leading to the development of an eating disorder in a woman are the same factors that lead to exercise dependence in a man. In other words, the process of developing either disorder is the same, but the expression of the disorders differs. Yates et al.[10] were the first to suggest this, based on their findings from 60 case histories. They determined that male obligatory runners and anorectic women share common personality characteristics, including introversion, depression, compliance, social anxiety, low self esteem, and inhibition of anger. They also state that the different cultural ideals for men and women contribute to the direction that the disorder takes. For men, the ideal is athletic prowess, which leads to exercise dependence, and for women, it is thinness, which leads to anorexia nervosa. The previously cited study by Mcdonald and Thompson[12] lends some support for this by finding that males exercised for fitness and showed few signs of eating disorders, while females exercised for weight control and showed more signs of eating disorders. An interesting study by Szymanski and Chrisler[20] compared 66 female athletes and 20 non-athletic, non-exercising women on a femininity–masculinity scale and on several other scales, including the Eating Disorders Inventory. Subjects who scored high on the feminine subscale scored significantly higher on bulimia and perfectionism subscales. They scored numerically higher on drive for thinness, ineffectiveness, and interpersonal distrust subscales. While the findings give some insight into gender traits related to eating disorders, the authors did not measure amount of exercise, and thus did not compare the feminine–masculine traits in relation to exercise habits. Such a study might lend some support to exercise dependence as a variant of eating disorders. However, Hauck and Blumenthal[7] rather emphatically state that available data do not support a relationship between eating disorders and exercise dependence. They also allege that the case studies of Yates et al.[10] were fictitious and that available evidence indicates eating disorders and exercise dependence are independent.

The previous discussion indicates that there is acceptance of exercise dependence as a syndrome. Unfortunately, few studies to date have been able to clearly identify the nature of exercise dependence. Unstandardized and inconsistent methods providing inconclusive results have thus far failed to identify exercise dependence as a primary disorder, or one secondary to eating disorders. Furthermore, exercise dependence cannot be ruled out as a syndrome overlapping with eating disorders or as a variant of eating disorders. There is also some suggestion that both exercise dependence and eating disorders are offshoots of another root disorder, most notably obsessive-compulsive disorder. One of the biggest difficulties in studying exercise dependence is in measuring it. There are as yet no clear markers for this syndrome, and there are no validated instruments for its measurement. Until a valid, reliable measurement for exercise dependence is developed, the nature of the syndrome will remain unresolved

III. MEASURING EXERCISE DEPENDENCE

In their comprehensive review of questionnaires used to identify compulsive exercisers, Hauck and Blumenthal[7] point out that the scales lack validation and their testing has not been conducted with clearly addicted exercisers. Kirkby and Adams[21] concur. After studying two of the most widely used questionnaires, they determined that the two instruments were measuring different qualities, suggesting that comparisons of exercise dependence across studies using different methods should be made cautiously. Along with the lack of measuring tools, the lack of physiological markers and the possible relationship with eating disorders complicates the identification of primary exercise dependence.

This section describes a series of studies that were conducted in an attempt to develop and validate a questionnaire for measuring exercise dependence. The process began by comparing five not yet validated questionnaires[19,22-25] to the De Coverley Veale[4] proposed diagnostic criteria. Each of the questionnaires had aspects of the diagnostic criteria but none included all of the criteria, and most of the response formats were dichotomous and thus limited in terms of statistical treatment. An Exercise Habits Inventory was constructed to reflect all of the diagnostic criteria and to provide a response format that would be somewhat more continuous in nature.

A. Study 1: Development and Initial Validation

Wanetka[26] drafted the two-part Exercise Habits Inventory (EHI). Part one consisted of demographic information and a series of questions concerning the respondent's exercise history. Part two consisted of 40 items reflecting themes related to exercise dependence as defined in the literature and constructed using a Likert-scale format. The questionnaire was completed by runners who were competing in a 10-kilometer race. Of the 261 runners, 185 were males and 76 were females ranging in age from 19 to 76 years with a mean age of 38.7 years. Weekly hours of exercise were computed and total weekly hours of exercise were calculated. The response to each item was scored and the item scores were added to produce a total score. Reliability was 0.92 using Coefficient Alpha. The high reliability score indicated that the items reflected the intent of the questionnaire.

Validity was examined using a principal components factor analysis with a varimax rotation. Factor loadings of 0.4 or higher were considered significant. An 11-component solution resulted for the total sample and, as seen in Table 15.1, the items grouped in a manner reflective of the literature descriptions of the proposed syndrome.

The factor analysis for the male respondents was similar to that seen in Table 15.1 but included a factor that suggested they experienced social pressure to be athletic and physically fit. For the females, this factor category was not seen. Instead, a 10-factor solution was found for the females, with items constituting "increased tolerance to exercise" either not loading significantly or loading with other factor components. There were some differences in item groupings that combined body weight concerns with continued exercise during illness, concerns about injury, and lowered self-esteem. The females also had a stronger factor relating to the priority given to exercise that included choosing to exercise over social activities, planning the day around exercise, exercising more than once per day, and having family or friends who had made negative comments about the respondent's exercise. Thus, for this sample, there are indications that males and females have somewhat different perceptions about exercise.

For the total sample, as number of hours of exercise per week increased, the scores on the EHI became more indicative of exercise dependence. Also, hours of weekly exercise were divided into quartiles, and, as the quartiles increased, the EHI scores were either numerically or statistically more indicative of exercise dependence.

Based on the results from this initial study, it was felt that the EHI showed promise. As total hours of exercise increased, so did the score on the EHI. There seemed to be some differences between the ways males and females responded and between the types of exercises performed. For example, the combination of aerobic exercise, running, and weight lifting, particularly among the females, was more highly related to EHI score than any of the three singly or than other types of exercise. Also, responses suggested that several of the items were interpreted differently from their intended meaning by some of the respondents.

B. Study 2: Comparison to the Eating Attitudes Test

Brown's[27] examination of the literature led to the belief that exercise dependence and eating disorders are in some way related. She attempted to examine this using a mail survey of a nationwide probability sample of adults who had indicated they were exercisers. To address scoring issues and to make response as simple as possible, the EHI was revised to more closely resemble the Eating Attitudes Test[14] and both questionnaires were mailed with postpaid business-reply envelopes. The response rate was 29%, with a total return of 427 questionnaires. Of these 427 responses, 102 reported that they did not exercise and were excluded from the analysis, leaving a total of 325 responses. The response rate in this study was low and might have been increased with multiple mailings and incentives; however, the resources available were insufficient to allow for this.

There were 165 male respondents and 160 female respondents, ranging in age from 19 to 83 years. The mean age at 53 years was higher than in Wanetka's[26] study. The literature indicates that exercise-dependent individuals are aware of their compulsion to exercise[4] and, because of this, Brown asked if the respondents felt a compulsive need to exercise. In the total sample, 41% responded "yes" and 55% responded "no" (the remainder provided no response). Also, only running, walking, and aerobics were included as exercise choices in this study due to the limited number

Table 15.1 Factor Loadings For The 40-Item Exercise Habit Inventory[26]

		Factor Loading
Mood[a]		
(25)[b]	Exercise makes me feel in control emotionally	0.787
(32)	I am more attentive, alert or focused after I exercise	0.713
(29)	There is a difference in my mood before and after exercise	0.703
(23)	Exercise helps me feel more confident	0.701
(24)	I experience a "high" after I exercise	0.649
(28)	When I don't work out, I feel sluggish	0.585
(3)	I feel mentally relieved after I exercise	0.585
(21)	When unable to exercise, I find myself worrying more about personal problems	0.499
Withdrawal/relief from withdrawal		
(36)	If I miss a workout, I constantly think about exercise	0.718
(16)	I get anxious and frustrated when upcoming events may interfere with my workout	0.667
(33)	If I feel I haven't "put everything" into my workouts, I feel depressed or frustrated	0.600
(27)	If I missed a planned workout, I would exercise twice as hard the next day	0.560
(5)	I feel guilty when I don't exercise	0.553
(9)	When I miss a scheduled workout time, I feel tense, irritable, or depressed.	0.526
(13)	I find myself thinking about exercise throughout the day	0.521
(17)	I need to work out longer and/or more frequently than others to be satisfied with my level of fitness	0.490
(26)	I feel more self-conscious about myself and have a lower self-esteem when I can't exercise	0.440
(34)	If I felt an injury developing, I would worry about the consequences of not being able to exercise	0.431
(6)	I increase my workout intensity or workout time to increase my desired level of fitness	0.414
Exercise despite injury, illness, medical advice		
(31)	I would, or have, continued to workout despite a physical condition that is aggravated by exercise	0.776
(8)	I exercise despite an injury or pain in my body	0.751
(20)	I have continued to exercise against the advice of a health professional	0.664
(2)	I have exercised when I had a cold (common cold, flu, etc.) or a long-term illness	0.617
Exercise despite interference with work, family, or social life		
(37)	I would consider refusing a new job, promotion, or any additional responsibilities that would possibly interfere with my exercise routine	0.802
(30)	I would consider terminating a relationship or job if it interfered too much with my exercise	0.746
(14)	I would miss a day of exercise if something unexpected came up	0.479
Exercise given high priority		
(7)	I plan the day's activities around my workout times	0.656
(1)	I have chosen to engage in my regular exercise routine over social activities with family and friends	0.513
Body weight and performance		
(10)	I feel that an increase in my body weight will inhibit my athletic performance	0.777
(4)	I lose weight to improve my athletic performance	0.719
(11)	Some days I feel the need to exercise more than once per day	0.465
Increased tolerance to exercise		
(40)	I follow the saying "No pain, no gain" when I exercise	0.749
(39)	If I accomplish an exercise-related goal, I strive for a harder goal the next time	0.676

Table 15.1 Factor Loadings For The 40-Item Exercise Habit Inventory[26] (Continued)

		Factor Loading
Difficulties with family or friends		
(35)	I have difficulties with my family, friends, or job in regard to my exercise routine	0.789
(19)	My family members or friends have made some negative comments about my exercise habits	0.666
Exercise in isolation		
(12)	I exercise alone rather than with a partner	0.769
(22)	I have taken substances (steroids, caffeine, supplements, etc.) to increase my athletic ability	0.481
Weight loss to improve athletic performance		
(18)	I use various weight control techniques such as laxatives, vomiting, fasting or diet pills to increase my athletic performance	0.775
Stereotyped exercise pattern		
(38)	I exercise at approximately the same time of day each day I exercise	0.837
(15)	I exercise regardless of the weather conditions such as high heat, rainstorms, and extreme cold	0.427

[a] The factor labels were arbitrarily assigned based on the items included in the factor.
[b] Numbers in parentheses indicate the item number on the questionnaire.

of people reporting that they engaged in other activities, the limited amount of time those who performed them reported, and the lack of relationship between those activities and EHI scores in Wanetka's[26] study. Instead, a category of "other" was included to account for the excluded activities.

As with Wanetka's study, this one found a reliability coefficient of 0.92 for the EHI with all but one item contributing to the overall reliability. Brown also examined the Coefficient Alpha of the Eating Attitudes Test (EAT) and found a coefficient of 0.78 for the test as a whole, 0.77 for the dieting subscale, 0.65 for the bulimia subscale, and 0.49 for the oral control subscale. Because the test as a whole showed the highest reliability, it was decided that the subscales would not be further examined.

Factor analysis provided a 10-item solution similar to Wanetka's. The major difference was that items in two categories dealing with exercise as a high priority and stereotyped exercise pattern were combined in this study. Interestingly, several items did not load at the 0.40 cut-off level. These items included choosing exercise over social activities, belief that increased body weight inhibits athletic performance, exercising regardless of the weather conditions, and exercising harder the day following a missed session. Brown felt that the differences might be explained by the generally higher age and the different sampling method in this study.

Surprisingly, score on the EHI was not correlated with total hours of exercise.[3-7] This was true for individual activities as well. However, further analysis showed that as age increased among this sample EHI score decreased, suggesting that younger individuals were more likely to show symptoms of exercise dependence. The older respondents in this study were found to have higher weekly hours of exercise than the younger respondents, but this was due to the nature of their exercise. The older respondents reported walking more often, while the younger respondents reported running and aerobics more frequently. Similar results were seen with the EAT scores and hours of exercise. Total EHI and total EAT scores were significantly related at $p \leq 0.01$, although the correlation coefficient was low at $r = 0.35$.

When examining the relationship between the EHI score and the EAT score by type of exercise a strong correlation was found for runners ($r = 0.62$; $p \leq 0.01$), a moderate one for walkers ($r = 0.46$;

p ≤0.01), and a moderate one for aerobic exercisers (r = 0.49; NS). The lack of statistical significance for the latter was due to the small number (n = 18) reporting aerobics as the sole activity. Brown felt that these findings showed support for exercise dependence and eating disorders as overlapping syndromes.

Brown examined predictors of exercise by age and gender using regression analysis. For the older women in the sample, EHI and EAT items relating to reducing body fat and controlling body weight seemed to be the greatest motivators for exercise. For the runners, exercise appeared to be seen as a way to relieve mental stress. Overall, the results suggested that for older adults, walking as an exercise requires a time commitment and that "exercise dependence" for the older exercisers was more a matter of trying to maintain good health and mobility.

C. Non-Exercisers

Berggren[28] had an interest in why individuals did not adopt an exercise program given the proven effects of exercise for health promotion and stress reduction. She felt that an instrument for measuring exercise dependence should be valid and reliable when used with non-exercisers, and that scores on the instrument should be indicative of an absence of exercise dependence. The same should hold true for eating disorders. To test the validity of both the EHI and EAT, a nationwide mail survey was conducted using names and addresses of individuals who had indicated they were not engaged in regular exercise. The EHI and the EAT were mailed to 1,000 individuals, who responded using postpaid business-reply envelopes. No follow-up or additional mailings were sent to non-respondents.

The response rate was 24.7% with 247 replies. Although these individuals had indicated a lack of interest in regular exercise, 135 said that they did engage in exercise and 112 said they did not. There were 125 males, 73 of whom were exercisers and 52 who were not, and there were 122 females, 62 exercisers and 60 non-exercisers. Ages ranged from 21 to 89 years, with a mean age of 48 years for the total sample, 51 years for the exercisers, and 45 years for the non-exercisers. Coefficient Alpha reliability was 0.94 for the total sample.

The factor analysis for the total sample grouped items similarly to the previous two studies. However, items that would likely have little meaning to non-exercisers were not significantly loaded including choosing exercise over social activities, having job difficulties because of exercise and having concerns over body weight interfering with exercise performance. Those who reported exercising in this sample showed similar item groupings, but did not load items relating to "exercise given high priority," "increased tolerance to exercise," and "stereotyped exercise pattern." These exercisers were likely to have recently begun their exercise program, since they previously identified themselves as non-exercisers. Their average total weekly hours of exercise tended to be lower than in previous studies at 7 hours per week, with walking being most common followed by "other." The other exercises were weight lifting, aerobics, cardiac rehab, calisthenics, stairmaster, and other similar types of activities. Average hours of running per week were 0.8. Given the lower level of exercise reported by these individuals, items relating to the priority, tolerance, and pattern of exercise might not be meaningful.

The non-exercisers in this sample reported very nominal engagement in exercise activities with an average total hours of exercise at 1.1. Of this exercise, walking and swimming each were reported at an average of 0.5 hours per week. There were no reports of running or bicycle riding. The factor analysis revealed that while items relating to alterations in "mood" grouped similarly to the previous samples, items relating to "withdrawal/relief from withdrawal" separated into two groupings. One grouping included items concerning thinking about exercise, satisfaction with fitness level and self-esteem. The second grouping included worrying about not exercising and exercising harder. Items that were not significant included: exercising when sick, feeling mentally relieved after exercise, increasing workout intensity/time to increase fitness, exercising alone, exercising regardless of weather conditions and exercising at the same time of day. These items would not be expected to be meaningful to a non-exercising sample.

There were few differences in responses by gender, exercise status, or both. The majority of the responses for all items tended to be "never" or "rarely" for exercisers and non-exercisers. Over 50% of the male exercisers responded "often," "usually," or "always" to feeling mentally relieved after exercise (72.6%); guilty when exercise is missed (50.7%); exercising regardless of weather (50.7%); feeling more confident (64.8%) and attentive (52.9%); and exercising at the same time of day (61.4%). Fewer female exercisers had responses in the "often," "usually," or "always" categories including feeling mentally relieved (73.8%); confident (55.0%); and attentive (60.7%); and exercising at the same time of day (59.0%).

The relationship between total exercise hours per week and the total EHI scores were close to zero and not statistically significant for either exercisers or non-exercisers. There were statistically significant ($p \leq 0.01$) inverse relationships between total EHI scores and television viewing ($r = -0.29$), reading ($r = -0.40$) and gardening ($r = -0.29$). Berggren[28] concluded that there were few behaviors displayed by a non-exercising sample indicative of exercise dependence and that the EHI showed good reliability and validity.

D. Study 4: Exercise Dependence, Eating Disorders and Food Intake

Findings from studies 2 and 3 discussed above led Muhs[29] to suggest that exercise-dependent behaviors would be more likely to occur in younger age groups. Many of the studies listed in the reference section of this chapter have been conducted with individuals under the age of 45. Older adults who exercise for long periods may be involved in less-intense activities such as walking, and the primary motivators for their exercise may be related more to health promotion than fitness or body shape.[27] Eating disorders also appear to be more prevalent among college age or younger women.[30] For these reasons, Muhs tested college students using the EHI and the EAT. Several researchers have found patterns of food consumption behavior typical of anorexia nervosa and bulimia;[31-33] however, no studies have been reported that looked at food intake in exercise dependence, so Muhs also examined food intake in her study.

Subjects were college students enrolled in an introductory nutrition course. These students kept 3-day food records, calculated the nutrient contents of the foods and calculated average intakes as a course assignment. Students agreeing to participate in the study provided copies of their 3-day averages and completed both the EHI and EAT. There were 239 completed questionnaires matched with assignments, 78 were from males and 161 from females. Ages ranged from 19 to 42 years, mean of 21 years. Body Mass Index (BMI)[37] was calculated from self-reported heights and weights and ranged from 20 to 39 for the males, mean 25, and from 16 to 33 for the females, mean 22.

As with the previous studies, the Coefficient Alpha reliability was high at 0.95. The factor analysis for the total sample differed slightly from the previous studies by combining the items related to "mood" and "withdrawal/relief from withdrawal." Also grouping into one factor were the items associated with "exercise despite injury, illness, medical advice," "exercise given high priority" and "stereotyped exercise patterns." Both of these combinations seem appropriate given the nature of the items. Items not loading at the 0.40 cut-off level were exercising more than once per day and exercising at the same time of day.

Among the respondents, 73% ($n = 175$) said they engaged in a regular exercise program and 10% considered themselves to be compulsive exercisers. Weight lifting was the most frequent activity followed by walking, aerobics, and running, with most engaging in multiple exercises. Total weekly hours of exercise averaged 7 hours for the total sample, 9 hours for the males and 6 hours for the females. EHI was significantly ($p \leq 0.01$) correlated with total weekly hours of exercise for the total sample ($r = 0.28$), for the males ($r = 0.38$) and the females ($r = 0.47$). There was a strong correlation between EHI and EAT scores ($r = 0.50$, $p \leq 0.01$) for the total sample, males ($r = 0.44$, $p \leq 0.01$) and females ($r = 0.62$, $p \leq 0.01$). No significant correlations were found between

EHI and food intake. However, as might be expected, EAT scores were inversely related to total calories, protein, fat, saturated fat, and cholesterol for the total sample and the females, but not for the males. Of note, the mean EAT score for the females was 14, with the cut-off indicating the potential for eating disorders being 20.

While the average scores on the EHI and the EAT were not high for the total sample, the males, or the females, Muhs found that females who had an EAT high enough to indicate an eating disorder also had significantly higher EHI scores. The males had higher EHI scores than the females, but the EAT scores were low, indicating a lack of eating disorders. There did not appear to be macronutrient consumption patterns related to exercise dependence but, as expected, lower intakes of calories, protein, fat, saturated fat, and cholesterol were seen as EAT scores increased.

Muhs made suggestions for shortening the EHI based on her findings and findings in the previous studies. These suggestions were used as the basis for forming a 30-item version of the EHI (Table 15.2). The following two studies discuss preliminary findings from this questionnaire:

Table 15.2. Thirty-Item Exercise Habits Inventory

EXERCISE HABITS INVENTORY

	Please place an (X) under the column that applies best to each of the statements. The following questions relate to exercise habits and behaviors. All of the results will be strictly confidential. Please answer each question carefully. Thank you.	**ALWAYS**	**USUALLY**	**OFTEN**	**SOMETIMES**	**RARELY**	**NEVER**
1.	I have chosen to engage in my regular exercise routine over social activities with family and friends.						
2.	I have exercised when I had a cold (common cold, flu, etc.) or a long-term illness.						
3.	I feel guilty when I don't exercise.						
4.	I increase my workout intensity or workout time to increase my desired level of fitness.						
5.	I exercise despite an injury or pain in my body.						
6.	When I miss a scheduled workout time, I feel tense, irritable, or depressed.						
7.	I feel that an increase in my body fat would inhibit my exercise performance.						
8.	Some days I feel the need to exercise more than once per day.						
9.	My exercise seems more effective if I do it by myself instead of with a partner.						
10.	I find myself thinking about exercising throughout the day.						
11.	I exercise regardless of the weather conditions such as high heat, rainstorms, and extreme cold.						
12.	I need to workout longer and/or more frequently than others to be satisfied with my level of fitness.						
13.	I use various weight control techniques such as laxatives, fasting, or diet pills to increase my athletic performance.						
14.	My family members or friends have said that I exercise too much or too hard.						

Table 15.2. Thirty-Item Exercise Habits Inventory (Continued)

EXERCISE HABITS INVENTORY Please place an (X) under the column that applies best to each of the statements. The following questions relate to exercise habits and behaviors. All of the results will be strictly confidential. Please answer each question carefully. Thank you.	ALWAYS	USUALLY	OFTEN	SOMETIMES	RARELY	NEVER
15. I have continued to exercise against the advice of a health professional.						
16. When unable to exercise, I find myself worrying more about personal problems.						
17. Exercise helps me feel more confident.						
18. I experience a "high" when I exercise.						
19. Exercise allows me to feel more in control emotionally.						
20. I feel more self conscious about myself and have a lower self-esteem when I can't exercise.						
21. When I don't workout, I feel sluggish.						
22. There is a difference in my mood before and after I exercise.						
23. I would consider terminating a relationship or job if it interfered too much with my exercise.						
24. I am more attentive, alert, or focused after I exercise.						
25. I have difficulties with my family, friends, or job in regard to my exercise routine.						
26. If I miss a workout, I constantly think about exercise.						
27. I would consider refusing a new job, promotion, or any additional responsibilities that would possibly interfere with my exercise routine.						
28. I exercise at approximately the same time of day each day I exercise.						
29. If I accomplish an exercise-related goal, I strive for a harder goal the next time I exercise.						
30. I follow the saying, "No pain, no gain" when I exercise.						

E. Study 5: Initial Test of Revised EHI

Committed exercisers who were members of area exercise facilities were recruited for this study.[34] There were 151 participants, of which 49 were males and 102 were females. Ages ranged from 19 to 54 years with a mean age of 29 years. All but five respondents reported having been regular exercisers for 1 to 40 years with a mean of 9.11 years. They exercised from 2 to 7 days per week with an average of 4 days, and from 1 to 47.25 hours per week with a mean of 8.2 hours per week.

The Coefficient Alpha reliability of the EHI was 0.92. The factor analysis results are shown in Table 15.3. The groupings of the questions remaining after revision are similar to the previous studies.[26-29] An item relating to exercising alone did not load perhaps because this sample was drawn from exercisers who attend exercise facilities. The greatest differences between this sample's

Table 15.3 Factor Loadings for Study 5: the Revised 30-Item Exercise Habit Inventory[34]

		Factor Loadings
Mood[a]		
(24)[b]	I am more attentive, alert, or focused after I exercise.	0.794
(22)	There is a difference in my mood before and after I exercise.	0.779
(19)	Exercise allows me to feel more in control emotionally.	0.743
(17)	Exercise helps me feel more confident.	0.596
(18)	I experience a "high" when I exercise.	0.566
(21)	When I don't workout, I feel sluggish.	0.491
(6)	When I miss a scheduled workout time, I feel tense, irritable, or depressed.	0.452
Withdrawal/relief from withdrawal		
(20)	I feel more self conscious about myself and have a lower self-esteem when I can't exercise.	0.723
(3)	I feel guilty when I don't exercise.	0.651
(16)	When unable to exercise, I find myself worrying more about personal problems.	0.583
(6)	When I miss a scheduled workout time, I feel tense, irritable, or depressed.	0.436
Exercise despite injury, illness, medical advice		
(2)	I have exercised when I had a cold (common cold, flu, etc.) or a long-term illness.	0.778
(5)	I exercise despite an injury or pain in my body.	0.556
(15)	I have continued to exercise against the advice of a health professional.	0.594
Exercise despite interference with work, family, or social life		
(23)	I would consider terminating a relationship or job if it interfered too much with my exercise.	0.775
(27)	I would consider refusing a new job, promotion, or any additional responsibilities that would possibly interfere with my exercise routine.	0.726
(1)	I have chosen to engage in my regular exercise routine over social activities with family and friends.	0.707
Increased tolerance		
(29)	If I accomplish an exercise-related goal, I strive for a harder goal the next time I exercise.	0.631
(12)	I need to workout longer and/or more frequently than others to be satisfied with my level of fitness.	0.630
(8)	Some days I feel the need to exercise more than once per day.	0.609
(10)	I find myself thinking about exercising throughout the day.	0.607
(26)	If I miss a workout, I constantly think about exercise.	0.603
(4)	I increase my workout intensity or workout time to increase my desired level of fitness.	0.526
(25)	I have difficulties with my family, friends, or job in regard to my exercise routine.	0.445
Stereotyped exercise pattern		
(28)	I exercise at approximately the same time of day each day I exercise.	0.742
(11)	I exercise regardless of the weather conditions such as high heat, rainstorms, and extreme cold.	0.637
(4)	I increase my workout intensity or workout time to increase my desired level of fitness.	0.556
Performance concerns		
(30)	I follow the saying, "No pain, no gain" when I exercise.	0.808
(7)	I feel that an increase in my body fat would inhibit my exercise performance.	0.635

Table 15.3 Factor loadings for Study 5: the revised 30-item Exercise Habit Inventory[34] (Continued)

		Factor Loadings
Weight control concerns		
(13)	I use various weight control techniques such as laxatives, fasting, or diet pills to increase my athletic performance.	0.673
(14)	My family members or friends have said that I exercise too much or too hard.	0.596

[a] The factor labels were arbitrarily assigned based on the items included in the factor.
[b] Numbers in parentheses indicate the item number on the questionnaire.

factor analysis and the previous ones were the inclusion of a factor that indicated performance concerns and a factor suggestive of eating disorders.

Total score on the EHI was correlated with hours per week of aerobics ($r = 0.29$, $p \leq 0.01$), and with hours of aerobics and running combined ($r = 0.25$, $p \leq 0.01$), and inversely correlated with hours per week of walking ($r = -0.18$, $p \leq 0.05$). Those who scored one standard deviation above the mean on the EHI reported significantly higher hours of aerobics and hours of aerobics and running combined.

F. Study 6. Comparison of EAT and Revised EHI

In this study (n = 251), 73 male and 178 female college students enrolled in credit-hour recreation or physical education courses participated.[36] The courses included aerobic dance, cross-training, physical education/fitness and weight training. The participants' ages ranged from 19 to 35 years with a mean age of 20.5 years. All but 22 reported that they exercised regularly and 65 stated that they felt a compulsive need to exercise. Also, 219 reported that they exercised outside of class. Most (n = 172) seemed to feel that their intensity of exercise was high and they reported spending from 1 to 55.17 hours per week exercising, with an average of 9.7 hours per week. Walking (mean 3 hr./wk), weight lifting (mean 2.4 hr/wk), aerobics (mean 1.6 hr/wk), and running (mean 1.5 hr/wk) were the most common exercises. The males reported significantly ($p \leq 0.01$) greater mean total hours per week of exercise and weight training, while the females reported significantly greater mean weekly hours of aerobics. The males also had a significantly higher mean body mass index (BMI) at 24.82 ± 3.45 compared with the females (mean = 22.07 ± 3.19).

The Coefficient Alpha reliability for the EHI was 0.95. Table 15.4 shows the five-factor solution of the factor analysis, which consolidated items related to exercise causing difficulties with work, family, and friends. Also, items relating to stereotyped schedule and increasing priority were combined into one factor. The factor analyses for the males and females separately showed few differences. The males had a seven-factor solution with the item "I feel that an increase in my body fat would inhibit my exercise performance" being the sole one to load in factor seven. For factor six, exercising at the same time of day loaded along with striving for a harder goal once the initial goal had been reached.

For this study, EHI items were scored in the same manner as the EAT items[14] with "never," "rarely," and "sometimes" being scored as "0," "often" as "1," "usually" as "2," and "always" as "3," in addition to scoring items from "never" as "0" to "always" as "5." The total score was calculated by adding all the item scores. For the total sample, males and females, EHI score was significantly ($p \leq 0.01$) correlated with EAT score, weekly hours of running and total hours of weekly exercise. Examining the data using t-tests showed no significant difference between the males and females on mean EHI scores; however, the females had a significantly higher mean EAT score, although the mean at 8.6 was lower than the cut-off of 20 used to predict presence of disordered eating behavior.

Table 15.4. Factor Loadings for Study 6: the Revised 30-Item Exercise Habit Inventory[35]

		Factor Loadings
Mood[a]		
(24)[b]	I am more attentive, alert, or focused after I exercise.	0.780
(19)	Exercise allows me to feel more in control emotionally.	0.773
(22)	There is a difference in my mood before and after I exercise.	0.770
(18)	I experience a "high" when I exercise.	0.723
(21)	When I don't workout, I feel sluggish.	0.644
(17)	Exercise helps me feel more confident.	0.623
(20)	I feel more self conscious about myself and have a lower self-esteem when I can't exercise.	0.452
Withdrawal/relief from withdrawal		
(3)	I feel guilty when I don't exercise.	0.689
(20)	I feel more self conscious about myself and have a lower self-esteem when I can't exercise.	0.636
(16)	When unable to exercise, I find myself worrying more about personal problems.	0.631
(9)	My exercise seems more effective if I do it by myself instead of with a partner.	0.616
(6)	When I miss a scheduled workout time, I feel tense, irritable, or depressed	0.614
(7)	I feel that an increase in my body fat would inhibit my exercise performance.	0.574
(10)	I find myself thinking about exercising throughout the day.	0.510
(26)	If I miss a workout, I constantly think about exercise.	0.475
(21)	When I don't workout, I feel sluggish.	0.466
(12)	I need to workout longer and/or more frequently than others to be satisfied with my level of fitness.	0.450
(8)	Some days I feel the need to exercise more than once per day.	0.430
Exercise despite interference with work, family. or social life		
(25)	I have difficulties with my family, friends, or job in regard to my exercise routine.	0.830
(27)	I would consider refusing a new job, promotion, or any additional responsibilities that would possibly interfere with my exercise routine.	0.809
(20)	I have continued to exercise against the advice of a health professional	0.722
(23)	I would consider terminating a relationship or job if it interfered too much with my exercise	0.718
(14)	My family members or friends have said that I exercise too much or too hard.	0.659
(13)	I use various weight control techniques such as laxatives, fasting or diet pills to increase my athletic performance.	0.645
(26)	If I miss a workout, I constantly think about exercise.	0.461
Exercise given high priority		
(2)	I have exercised when I had a cold (common cold, flu, etc.) or a long-term illness.	0.697
(5)	I exercise despite an injury or pain in my body.	0.635
(1)	I have chosen to engage in my regular exercise routine over social activities with family and friends.	0.620
(11)	I exercise regardless of the weather conditions such as high heat, rainstorms, and extreme cold.	0.607
(12)	I need to workout longer and/or more frequently than others to be satisfied with my level of fitness.	0.529
(8)	Some days I feel the need to exercise more than once per day.	0.522
Increased tolerance		
(28)	I exercise at approximately the same time of day each day I exercise.	0.748
(29)	If I accomplish an exercise-related goal, I strive for a harder goal the next time I exercise.	0.691
(4)	I increase my workout intensity or workout time to increase my desired level of fitness.	0.590
(30)	I follow the saying, "No pain, no gain" when I exercise.	0.403

[a] The factor labels were arbitrarily assigned based on the items included in the factor.
[b] Numbers in parentheses indicate the item number on the questionnaire.

It has been suggested that a marker for exercise dependence could be the continuance of exercise even when it interferes with medical, occupational, family, or social life.[2–8] For this reason, the items that grouped under the factor heading of "difficulties with friends, family, job" were added to form a separate score. There were no differences in the mean scores for this variable between the males and females. However, the marker variable was significantly related to the EHI scores ($r = 0.74$) and the EAT scores ($r = 0.54$) for the total sample.

To examine the EHI in greater depth, cluster analysis was conducted choosing a two-sample solution. Discriminant analysis was conducted to determine the variables that maximally separated the two clusters. Cluster group 1 contained 52 of the respondents and cluster group 2 contained 190 respondents, with the remaining nine excluded due to missing data. Results of t-tests showed that mean EAT scores, EHI scores, and marker scores were significantly higher for cluster 1 at $p \leq 0.01$, while mean total weekly hours of running and mean total weekly hours of exercise were higher at $p \leq 0.05$. There were no differences in the gender makeup of the two cluster groups. Individual items from the EHI and EAT as well as the total scores were entered into the discriminant analysis. Also entered were hours per week of individual exercises and total weekly hours of exercise. The variables that maximally separated the two cluster groups were the EHI score, "withdrawal/relief from withdrawal" items, "exercise given high priority" items, "difficulties with friends, family, job" items, EAT score, "mood" items, and "increased tolerance" items, respectively. The 52 individuals in cluster group 1 had significantly higher means for all the variables. In addition, chi square analysis indicated that cluster group 1 mmberswere significantly more likely to say that they felt a compulsive need to exercise.

Individual EAT items that were more likely to be answered as "often," "usually," or "always" in cluster group 1 were generally related to body weight. For example, cluster group 1 members were more likely to say they were terrified of becoming overweight, were aware of the calorie content of foods, were preoccupied with thinness and with body fat, and were trying to burn calories with exercise. In terms of gender, females were more likely to respond that they were terrified of becoming overweight, felt guilty after eating, were preoccupied with thinness and food, were eating diet foods, felt uncomfortable after eating sweets and were engaging in dieting behaviors.

Overall, the studies cited and the preliminary findings from testing the revised EHI suggest that the EHI has promise as an instrument for identifying exercise dependence. Exercise dependence may be more common among younger adults, particularly college students. Also, exercise dependence may have a relationship with eating disorders, especially among female college students.

IV. RESEARCH NEEDS

While the Exercise Habits Inventory described in this chapter consistently displayed high internal consistency and reflected diagnostic criteria for exercise dependence, additional testing is needed before validity can be ascertained. The EHI should be compared with other commonly used instruments for identifying exercise dependence, as was done in Kirkby and Adams' study.[21] It would be logical to assume that, as hours of exercise increase, so would scores on the EHI; however, in the studies described above, this was not always the case. It is possible that using a simple measure of reported hours of exercise is not sensitive enough to identify commitment to exercise. Several questionnaires are available for measuring physical activity beyond estimations of weekly hours of exercise[37] and these should be tested with the EHI. A better measure of commitment to exercise may provide more insight into the relationship of habitual exercise to exercise dependence. Also, exercise dependence in relation to type of exercise and in comparison between competitive athletes and non-athletes needs to be studied.

Questions about the nature of exercise dependence, as a primary, secondary, or variant syndrome, require additional study. To answer these questions, the EHI should be tested with individuals undergoing treatment for eating disorders to better understand their perceptions about exercise.

Further study comparing the perceptions of males and females toward exercise and eating would also help to more clearly define exercise dependence.

A scoring system for the EHI is needed. Because there are no physiological markers for the syndrome and because the syndrome is not clearly defined, determining a cut-off for exercise dependence is difficult. In Study 6, cluster analysis identified a group of people who were differentiated primarily on the basis of their EHI scores. Their mean EHI score was 1.5 standard deviations from the mean score for the total group, which might provide a basis for developing a cut-off. Further testing with larger samples is required before this can be determined.

Development and testing of the EHI presented some intriguing insights into the nature of exercise dependence. There were indications that males and females have slightly differing perceptions about exercise, with males perceiving exercise more as a means to increase fitness and females seeing it more as a means to reduce body weight or fatness. This finding, along with the relationship of the EHI with the EAT in several of the studies, suggests some overlap between exercise dependence and eating disorders, or that exercise dependence is a variant of eating disorders. Weekly hours of running tended to have a positive relationship with EHI score while hours of walking did not, although total weekly hours of exercise tended to be positively related to EHI score for college students. This suggests that there may be exercises of choice for individuals who are exercise dependent, and that these exercises may be ones that are associated with weight loss or loss of body fat. In addition, there were suggestions that older adults have different reasons for engaging in prolonged exercise. It is possible that, like anorexia nervosa and bulimia, exercise dependence occurs more frequently in younger adults. More study of both college students and young adults not attending college is needed, along with pre-college-age teenagers.

Perhaps the most important question about exercise dependence is whether it causes harm. Regular exercise is a positive, health-promoting behavior. Does increasing the pattern of regular exercise to a level that some might think of as excessive constitute a problem requiring intervention? If the exercise pattern is used as an excuse for avoiding difficult work, family, or social situations, is it as dangerous as using drugs or alcohol for the same reason? Certainly, continuing exercise against the advice of a health professional is an indicator of dysfunction, but does using exercise to achieve a "runner's high" in an otherwise healthy individual give reason for concern? These questions cannot be answered until a way to identify exercise dependence is developed and the nature of exercise dependence is defined.

V. SUMMARY

Even though there are many observations and anecdotal accounts of individuals who exercise when medically or otherwise contraindicated, there is no real consensus about the existence of primary exercise dependence. Likewise, although excessive exercise is a diagnostic criterion for several eating disorders, there is insufficient information regarding the relationship between exercise dependence and anorexia nervosa. Our inability to confirm the existence or the nature of exercise dependence is at least in part due to the lack of valid, reliable methods for measuring the disorder. Using proposed diagnostic criteria and other observations from the literature, an Exercise Habits Inventory was constructed and tested in a series of studies. The resulting 30-item questionnaire showed high internal consistency and reflected the criteria of exercise dependence. Other results from the validation studies suggest that males and females differ in their perceptions about exercise and eating, younger as opposed to older adults are more likely to display signs of exercise dependency, and exercise dependency may be related to eating disorders in females but not males. Further testing of the Exercise Habits Inventory is needed before we can answer the questions of whether exercise dependence exists, how it relates to eating disorders, and whether exercise dependence should be considered a health concern.

REFERENCES

1. American Psychiatric Association. *Diagnostic and Statistical Manual of Mental Disorders.* 4th ed. American Psychiatric Association, Washington, D.C., 1994, 539.
2. Morgan, W.P. Negative addiction in runners, *Physician Sportsmed*, 7, 57, 1979.
3. Dishman, R.K. Medical psychology in exercise and sport, *Med. Clin. N. Am.*, 69, 123, 1985.
4. De Coverley Veale, D.M.W. Exercise Dependence, *Br. J. Addiction*, 82, 735, 1987.
5. Stoll, O. Endogenous opiates, runner's high, and exercise addiction. *Leipziger Sportwissenschaftliche Beitraege*, 38, 1, 1997 as summarized by Stoll in http://www.uni-leipzig.de/~asp/endoengl.htm (July 12, 1999).
6. Davis, C., Kennedy, S.H., Ravelski, E., and Dionne, M. The role of physical activity in the development and maintenance of eating disorders. *Psych. Med.,* 24, 957, 1994.
7. Hauck, E.R. andBlumenthal, J.A. Obsessive and compulsive traits in athletes. *Sports Med.*, 14, 215, 1992.
8. Eisler, I. and le Grange, D. Excessive exercise and anorexia nervosa. *J. Eating Disord.*, 9, 377, 1990.
9. Kaye, W.H., Weltzin, T.E., Hsu, L.K.G., Bulik, C., McConaha, C., and Sobkiewicz, T. Patients with anorexia nervosa have elevated scores on the Yale-Brown Obsessive-Compulsive Scale. *Int. J. Eat. Disord.,* 12, 57, 1992.
10. Yates, A., Leehey, K, and Shisslak, C.M. Running — an analogue of anorexia? *N. Eng. J. Med.*, 308, 251, 1983.
11. Owens, R.G., and Slade, P.D. Running and anorexia nervosa: An empirical study. *Int. J. Eat. Disor,.* 6, 771, 1987.
12. McDonald, K. and Thompson, J.K. Eating disturbance, body image dissatisfaction, and reasons for exercising: Gender differences and correlational findings. *Int. J. Eat. Disord.,* 11, 289, 1990.
13. Krejci, R.C., Sargent, R., Forand, K.J., Ureda, J.R., Saunders, R.P., and Durstine, J.L. Psychological and behavioral differences among females classified as bulimic, obligatory exerciser and normal control. *Psychiatry,* 55, 185, 1992.
14. Garner, D.M., Olmsted, M.P., Bohr, Y., and Garfinkel, P.E. The Eating Attitudes Test: Psychometric features and clinical correlates. *Psych. Med.*, 12, 871, 1982.
15. Dewsnap, P.A. Exercise dependence (Letter). *Br. J. Add.*. 83, 446, 1988.
16. Richert, A.J. and Hummers, J.A. Patterns of physical activity in college students at possible risk for eating disorder. *Int. J. Eat. Disord.,* 5, 757, 1986.
17. Kennedy, C.D., Ravelski, E., and Dionne, M. The role of physical activity in the development and maintenance of eating disorders. *Psych. Med.*, 24, 957, 1994.
18. Brewerton, T.D., Stellefson, E.J., Hibbs, N., Hodges, E.L., and Cochrane, C.E. Comparison of eating disorder patients with and without compulsive exercise. *Int. J. Eat. Disord.,* 17, 413, 1995.
19. Davis, C., Brewer, H., and Ratusny, D. Behavioral frequency and psychological commitment: Necessary concepts in the study of excessive exercising. *J. Behav. Med.*, 16, 611, 1993.
20. Szymanski, L.A. and Chrisler, J.S. Eating disorders, gender-role, and athletic activity. *Psychology,* 27, 20, 1990.
21. Kirkby, R.J. and Adams, J. Exercise dependence: The relationship between two measures. *Percept. Mot. Skills*, 82, 366, 1996.
22. Imm, P.S. and Pruitt, J. Body shape satisfaction in female exercisers and nonexercisers. *Women Hlth.,* 17, 87, 1991.
23. Hailey, B.M. and Bailey, L.A. Negative addiction in runners. A quantitative approach. *J. Sport Beh.,* 5, 150, 1982.
24. Blumenthal, J.A., O'Toole, L.C., and Chang, J.L. Is running an analogue of anorexia nervosa? An empirical study of obligatory running and anorexia nervosa. *J. Am. Med. Assoc.*, 252, 520, 1984.
25. Yates, A., Shisslak, C.M., allender, J., Crago, M., and Leehey, K. Comparing obligatory and non-obligatory runners. *Psychosomatics*, 33, 180, 1992.
26. Wanetka, M.J. The development of a valid questionnaire to assess exercise dependence. Unpublished Masters Thesis, University of Nebraska, Lincoln, NE 1995.
27. Brown, T.M. Exercise dependence and eating disorders. Unpublished Masters Thesis, University of Nebraska, Lincoln, NE 1995.

28. Berggren, J.J. Comparison of exercisers and non-exercisers in relation to scores on the exercise habit inventory. unpublished master's thesis, University of Nebraska, Lincoln, NE 1996.
29. Muhs, S.R. Exercise dependence and its relationship to eating disorders, and food consumption patterns of college students. Unpublished master's thesis, University of Nebraska, Lincoln, NE 1996.
30. Fredenberg, J.P., Berglund, P.T., and Dieken, H.A. Incidence of eating disorders among selected female university students. *J. Am. Diet. Assoc.*, 96, 64, 1996.
31. Hetherington, M.M., Altemus, M., Nelson, M.L., Bernat, A.S., and Gold, P.W. Eating behavior in bulimia nervosa: Multiple meal analyses. *Am. J. Clin. Nutr.,* 60, 864, 1994.
32. Johnson, C. and Tobin, D. The diagnosis and treatment of anorexia nervosa and bulimia among athletes. *Athletic Training*, 26, 119, 1991.
33. Stoner, S.A., Fedoroff, I.C., Andersen, A.E., and Rolls, B.J. Food preferences and desire to eat in anorexia and bulimia nervosa. *Int. J. Eat. Dis.,* 19, 13, 1996.
34. Betts, N.M. Unpublished data, 1997.
35. Robinson, S. and Betts, N,M. Unpublished data, 1999.
36. Kriska, A.M. and Casperson, C.J. A collection of physical activity questionnaires for health-related research. *Med. Sci. Sports Exer.*, 29 (supplement), S5, 1997.
37. Lee, RD and Nieman, DC. *Nutritional Assessment*. Brown & Benchmark Publishers, Madison, WI, p.133.

PART V

Nutritional Knowledge of Athletes

CHAPTER 16

Nutrition Knowledge of Athletes

Patricia Henry

CONTENTS

I. INTRODUCTION

Athletes need and want reliable, accurate information to improve their health and performance. Athletes of every age and level of competition believe that nutrition may give them the competitive edge. Much of the information they receive comes from the electronic and print media, their peers, or coaches, and may or may not be accurate. A majority of the advice is of a general nature and may not take into account the athlete's body composition and age, specific sport, duration, intensity, actual intake, and training or competition needs. To be of maximum benefit, advice should be tailored to the individual athlete.

Individuals involved in sports and fitness do not always realize that there are qualified sports nutritionists and dietitians in the field of sports and cardiovascular nutrition. A registered dietitian (RD) or licensed nutritionist (LN) who has a background in nutrition and exercise is an essential part of the athlete's team.[1] Organizations such as the American College of Sports Medicine (ACSM) and the Sports and Cardiovascular Nutrition (SCAN), a practice group of the American Dietitian Association, are just two of the organizations who do research in this area. Numerous research journals such as *Medicine and Science in Sports and Exercise, Journal of Nutrition, International Journal of Sport Nutrition, Journal of Sports Science,* and *Journal of the American Dietetic Association* are just a few of resources available to athletes, coaches, dietitians, and other professionals interested in nutrition and sports.

0-8493-8199-1/00/$0.00+$.50

Universities and colleges now offer classes specifically in sports nutrition. Degrees are also offered in the field of sports nutrition, either as a specialty or as part of an academic curriculum. A list of colleges and universities offering sports nutrition degrees is available from SCAN.

Intensive nutrition education is needed to combat quackery and fads that are targeted to athletes. To start this process, nutritional knowledge of the athlete must first be explored.

Interest in sports nutrition and fitness over the last 10 years has increased dramatically. Athletes are breaking new records every year and rely on nutrition to help them reach their goals, which makes them the perfect target for "the magic formula or pill."[2] Because of this belief or quest, many athletes fall prey to fads that may hinder their performance, and, in some cases, harm them. Nutrition education is the key to combating this misinformation. Athletes and physicians are often poorly informed about nutrition.[3] Common errors include a disproportionately high intake of protein, vitamins, and minerals in excess of the Recommended Daily Allowances, poorly designed weight-gain or -loss programs, and various food fads. Athletes may be more inclined to eat right if provided with appropriate information. It is important to determine what kind of nutrition education is reaching athletes and how to improve upon this information so that it produces positive changes in eating habits.[4]

II. CHILDREN AND ADOLESCENTS

Children begin their informal nutrition education in early infancy from their parents or care givers usually by role modeling.[5,6] Preschoolers and their parents receive nutrition education primarily through Head Start, Nutrition and Education Training Program (NET), and Special Supplemental Food Program for Women, Infants and Children (WIC).[8] Formal education begins in school, using materials and programs developed by groups funded by the National Institute of Health (NIH), NET, the food industry, private volunteer organizations (such as American Heart Association, American Cancer Society, etc.) and other state and local sources.[7] Information given to child athletes comes from guides published by the organizations such as Little League.[9] Many coaches allow information to be picked up from the parents and caretakers of children. School health programs can help children and adolescents attain full education potential and good health by providing them with the skills, social support, and environmental reinforcement they need to adopt long-term, healthy eating behaviors. Hornick et al.[10] reported that family was the most frequently reported source of nutrition information, followed by the coach or teacher in adolescents. Only 13.5% of adolescents reported that friends were their source of sports nutrition.

Furtado et al.[11] found that nutrition education resulted in improved nutrition knowledge among Little League cheerleaders. This was accomplished by presenting nutrition lessons over a 2-month period to cheerleaders aged 7 to 13. When analyzed by age, the older female cheerleaders' knowledge improved significantly over the younger ones.

Sossin et al.[12] developed a nutrition program for parents, coaches, and 400 children aged 7 to 10 years who played youth soccer. They used a series of nutrition booklets and refrigerator fact sheets highlighting six topics. Participants felt they increased sports nutrition awareness and knowledge and encouraged positive dietary choices by some parents and children.

Blaha et al.[13] examined the effect of nutrition education on weight maintenance of 29 male high-school swimmers. Those in the experimental group participated in a nutritional education presentation with a parent and received printed nutritional information on sport-specific nutritional information, snack ideas, and sample training menus. The results proved that nutritional education had a positive effect on their ability to maintain weight throughout a rigorous season.

Tiilikainen et al.[14] also investigated the effect of parental participation in sports nutrition workshops in young swimmers' food choices in Finland. This study showed that those who had a workshop reported changes in food choices before competition. No changes were reported in food and fluid choices during or after competition or in the timing of intake before competition in either the control or experimental group.

A study done by Chapman et al.[15] looked at 72 subjects and their nutrition knowledge and food choices. Those who received nutrition education showed a significant difference in nutrition knowledge, but no significant improvement in dietary intake and food choices were concluded. They attributed this to the limited duration of the study.

Short et al.[16] looked at 210 adolescent athletes and whether their knowledge or attitudes have an impact on dietary iron intake and iron-deficiency anemia. They concluded that knowledge and attitudes regarding dietary iron were not significantly related to dietary iron intake or hemoglobin status. However, those who had heard about dietary iron cited the classroom as the source of the information.

To determine the impact of a nutrition education program on adolescents' knowledge of sports nutrition and use of ergogenic products, Hornick et al.[17] found that nutrition knowledge did not increase test scores. However, the decreased usage of vitamins, minerals, muscle-building products, protein supplements, amino acids, and salt tablets were reported in adolescents after the education program.

A study of Massachusetts adolescents[18] and their nutritional knowledge and behavior indicated that adolescents have limited nutrition knowledge. The responsibility of teaching nutrition has shifted from the home economics teacher to the physical education teacher. The diet and health curriculum should emphasize practical application including selection of food in restaurants, safe dieting practices, and exercise.

Knowledge of sports nutrition is lacking in some areas. Most high school students agreed that carbohydrates are the most important energy source, liquids are important before, during, and after exercise, and nutritious foods are important every day. However, they lack knowledge in the use of fluids and carbohydrates during and after exercise, and that large amounts of protein are necessary in a training diet.[19]

A study of 943 high school athletes showed females had higher nutrition knowledge scores than males.[20] However, they did not appear to use their knowledge in making food choices. This may be because males have a higher food intake, therefore make more food choices. All perceived parents to be the best source of nutrition knowledge followed by books, magazines, and medical personnel, respectively.

Peron et al.[21] looked at a group of female high school athletes, of whom 92% reported previous enrollment in a nutrition course. They scored higher on "general nutrition" than "nutrition for athletes" portion of a questionnaire. It was noted that they too did not always apply their nutrition knowledge to their food choices.

Providing nutrition education programs for children is only part of the picture. To actually improve eating behaviors, there is a need for innovative outreach strategies that include educational and environmental approaches.[22] Environmental factors such as increased availability and promotion of appealing, convenient foods within homes, schools, and restaurants must be addressed. Adolescents' input is also essential.[23] The American Dietetic Association has released statements on nutrition guidance for child and adolescent athletes in organized sports.[24] The American Academy of Pediatrics committee on Sports Medicine and Fitness released a statement on "Promotion of healthy weight control practices in young athletes."[25]

Computers are another avenue to teach nutrition. In one study,[26] a web page as a medium of communication was effective in increasing awareness of nutrition. Students will access the web sites for information, causing web site visits to have increased from an average of eight per day to an average of 95 per day. This allows students to have online access to nutrition brochures. Computers also have the ability to analyze actual intake of athletes. However, intake must be actual for the information to be useful.

III. COLLEGE STUDENTS

Nutritional knowledge and nutrient intakes of 37 elite female high school runners and 17 female college cross country runners were compared.[27] College runners had greater nutrition knowledge than their high school counterparts, although many misconceptions were evident. Women with more knowledge tended to make better food choices and eat more healthfully.

Shearer et al.[28] assessed the nutritional status and nutritional knowledge of 42 freshman football and basketball players. The study suggested that nutrition education should focus on macronutrient intake to increase intake of complex carbohydrates and decrease intake of simple sugars, fat, and saturated fat.

Bermudez et al.[29] assessed the effect of nutrition education on nutrition knowledge. They found that education provided through small group lectures resulted in a significant improvement in nutrition knowledge for female college athletes, while there was no significant improvement in male college athletes.

Looking at nutrition knowledge and food practices of 115 collegiate athletes compared with 55 non-athletes, results indicate that nutrition knowledge was not related to better dietary practices.[30] Non-athletes and female subjects had significantly higher nutrition knowledge scores and significantly lower dietary intake than athletes and male subjects, respectively.

Reed-Weisner and Read[31] looked at 49 young male athletes and the relationships among demographics, family health history, health belief, and nutrition knowledge. Although university athletes know about choosing low-fat and low-sodium foods, 34% consumed high-sodium and high-fat food three times per week. Additionally 43% scored below 70% correct on the nutrition knowledge test regarding sodium and fat.

By using peer education for university student-athletes, nutrition knowledge was increased.[32] Student athletes were assigned to a peer educator who met with them once a week for 7 weeks. Nutrition knowledge increased significantly. At the same time, selected blood values also responded appropriately.

An earlier study indicated that individualized self education resulted in an increase in nutritional knowledge as compared with group education.[33] Students did better watching a slide show and reading a script as opposed to watching a slide show and listening to someone else explain it.

College football linemen had low nutrition knowledge and food practice as compared with male college students.[34] More than 80% of the lineman believed that vitamins were good sources of energy, and more than 70% believed that bread and potatoes should be avoided when trying to lose weight. They also had a relatively low carbohydrate intake. Should these misinformation and dietary practices continue, cardiovascular risk factors in these athletes will be worsened.

A comparison of nutrition knowledge of female varsity athletes and university students showed the athletes were younger, taller, and heavier than the students but were considerably more active.[35] The athletes used more nutritional supplements (especially iron) and were less likely to exclude red meat from their diets. Both groups had similar knowledge of both general and sports nutrition knowledge.

The United States Military Academy integrated an Introduction to Sports Nutrition Program into the freshman curriculum.[36] It included topics on macronutrient metabolism, vitamin and mineral usage, post-event nutrition, and eating nutritiously on the road. Of the 1,040 students attending the program, 50% voiced a desire to have more information regarding nutrition, 30% felt the class was unnecessary for non-athletes, 18% did not respond, and 2% felt the class and information were boring. No data were reported regarding behavior changes or increase in knowledge.

McReynolds et al.[37] looked at a nutrition education program for women's softball, men's track, and women's track teams. Knowledge concerning a healthy fat intake increased the most. The top five changes that the athletes felt they needed were: decrease fat intake, eat less fast food, increase fruit and vegetables, eat fewer snacks, and decrease total calories, in that order.

Gagliardi and Byrd[38] studied 40 university athletes who were enrolled in a sports nutrition pilot course. Thirteen of the students had previously completed a basic nutrition course. Twenty-five percent were taking vitamin supplements. There was no significant difference in the mean percentage of energy nutrients consumed between men and women athletes. Four of the female athletes were deficient in iron, potassium, and folacin even though the mean energy intake was 2400 kilo calories/day. One male athlete consumed less than 1.5 g/kg/day of dietary protein, while 30% of the men consumed a protein supplement. This research indicated that many university athletes possess inadequate sports nutrition knowledge coupled with poor dietary habits.

A study of changes in nutrition knowledge and dietary intake among university female cross-country runners before and after nutrition education revealed that nutrition knowledge increased for those who had the nutrition education program.[39] Participants seemed very receptive to the topics on nutrition but were especially interested in the topic of amenorrhea.

Looking at 262 varsity athletes regarding the relationship between nutritional knowledge and gender, ethnic background, and year in school, Whitcombe and collaborators[40] found the level of general nutritional knowledge was quite poor. Female athletes scored higher than male athletes. Seniors scored higher than freshmen in both general knowledge and the use of supplements. African-Americans scored lower than Caucasian athletes.

Cherundolo and Levine[41] studied the knowledge, attitudes, and usage patterns among 86 male varsity basketball players. Both the athletes' supplement knowledge and supplement attitude were quite low. As attitudes became more positive or more "correct," supplement usage decreased. The relationship between knowledge and usage was not significant. The reasons cited for supplement use were: sports performance, muscle development, and tiredness/fatigue. This study also cited friends (57%), coaches/trainer (35%), parents (35%), and magazines (28%) as providing the greatest influence on the athletes.

Seventeen surveys of female cross-country and field hockey teams were completed to determine if nutrition course work enhances athletes' knowledge of sports nutrition principles and to identify athletes' resources for nutrition information.[42] Those who had taken a nutrition course were more knowledgeable, especially about fluid replacement, energy foods, and muscle mass. They were least knowledgeable about vitamin supplementation and carbohydrate loading. Textbooks, coaches, and trainers were identified as primary sources for nutrition information. Registered dietitians were used by two of the athletes for recommendations.

Former university athletes were sent a survey on athletic participation and nutrition knowledge and attitudes.[43] Scores on sports nutrition knowledge were higher than general nutrition knowledge. The 40% who had taken a nutrition course had higher general knowledge scores and total knowledge scores than those who had not. All those who had not taken a nutrition course thought one would be helpful to athletes. In looking at the beliefs and perceptions about diet and body image among collegiate male bodybuilders, 60 recreational bodybuilders and 26 competitive bodybuilders, and a control group were analyzed.[44] Of those, 61% agreed that fat loss and 55% agreed that restrictive diets were needed to look better. The competitive bodybuilders were more strongly opinionated when addressing dieting and competition. Sixty-nine percent agreed that bodybuilders would be more successful in competition if they were more careful of watching what they ate and that pressure to alter their diet would help to meet goals for competition. All groups believed that there is an optimal diet, optimal weight, and optimal percent body fat to be more competitive. It is important for health professionals to be aware of the rigorous training and diet practices of collegiate male bodybuilders and to be able to provide accurate information that will help the athletes achieve their goals. However, most athletes believe that unless the information will enhance performance, the bodybuilder might be less motivated to change.

Collegiate female athletes reported that time was the largest obstacle to eating a well balanced diet.[45] This included the time to buy, eat, and prepare food for all collegiate females, athletes, and non-athletes. This study emphasizes the need for readily available healthy food choices for all ages.

In analyzing the diets of 20 male collegiate soccer players, the mean calorie intake was 3748 calories daily with 54% carbohydrate, 29% fat, 13% protein and 4% alcohol.[46] Twenty percent of the players reported using multi-vitamin/mineral supplements and 5% reported using amino acid supplements. Individual athletes, however, did not consume the recommended amounts of specific nutrients.

Athletic departments at colleges and universities are beginning to recognize the importance of sports nutritionists to provide nutrition counseling and education. Sports nutritionists can address issues of weight management, nutritional supplements, eating disorders and body composition.[47]

IV. RECREATIONAL ATHLETES

Grandjean[48] reported that sports nutrition professionals who work with recreational athletes were more concerned with encouraging a healthy diet than improving athletic performance.

As the population ages, more Americans are using activity to stay in shape. A mail survey of 500 subjects, including 200 members of a University Wellness Center indicated that adults who exercised are significantly better informed and had significantly better eating patterns than non-exercisers.[49] This underscores the need to focus nutrition education on those Americans who have not adopted regular exercise. Adults who exercise longer than 20 minutes also scored higher than those who exercised for less than 20 minutes.[50]

A study of female marathon runners and fitness-club members found that the majority obtained their nutrition information from magazines and books.[51] Fitness-club members used books and their fitness club as most useful sources of information while runners used books. Runners also scored higher on nutrition knowledge and sports nutrition in general.

Recommendations for nutrition in older athletes should focus on nutrient requirements for the elderly and the nutrient needs for exercising. Physiological changes such as decreased appetite and food intake, poor dental health, loss of sense of thirst, loss of sense of smell, decreased gut function, and special diets to treat disease states are just a few of the problems. When making recommendations, the following should be taken into consideration:[52]

- the changing needs that occur with aging
- the changing needs that occur with exercise
- the presence of chronic diseases or illness
- what type and level of exercising is occurring

Nutrient intake is often inadequate for vitamin B_6, vitamin B_{12}, calcium, and vitamin D. The elderly population should focus on maintaining energy balance while selecting a variety of foods high in complex carbohydrates. Research indicates that elderly people who use nutritional supplements tend to be more health conscious and physically active than nonusers. Older athletes must also be concerned with adequate fluid replacement. Those who compete in high-intensity endurance exercise may benefit from a 4% to 10% carbohydrate-containing sports drink.[53]

Hermann et al.[54] looked at 24 adults who participated in a 12-week nutrition program that included nutrition education and fitness lessons. At the end of the 12 weeks, nutritional knowledge increased on an average of 12%. Of interest, the overall diet of protein, fat, and carbohydrate did not change but the amount of saturated fat consumed decreased. The adults also increased the number of days per week they exercised as well as the time and intensity of exercise.

A study of 93 elite runners found that most were nutrition conscious and made a special effort to eat well.[55] Many saw themselves as being energy deficient and reported eating less than what was expected. Those most likely to supplement their diets with vitamins are the ones least likely to need supplements. When educated on nutrition, most improved their diet.

A survey of 100 adult runners indicated that while most believed that drinking eight glasses of water per day was recommended, less than half actually reported drinking that much.[56]

Female athletes need to be encouraged to give special attention to water and iron.[57] While iron is not required at increased levels for female athletes, it is frequently limited in the diet of women in general. Female athletes need to understand the importance of fluid balance and how to properly rehydrate during and following exercise. Nutritional advice will serve them well.

V. PROFESSIONAL ATHLETES

In a study that involved 13 endurance cyclists and 14 endurance runners, the gap between perceived and actual nutrition knowledge was identified.[58] Fifty-nine percent felt that their current diet did not meet their goals. Forty-four percent indicated an appropriate carbohydrate range, 22% indicated an appropriate protein range, and 74% identified appropriate fat range. All subjects contacted the dietitian who administered the survey to find out the "right" answers. Five athletes volunteered to complete a 24-hour food recall and 2-day food diary. Results indicated that none of these diets was deemed to be appropriate. Four of the five were not consistent with their previous estimates on intake. Sources of nutrition information were magazines (14), books (7), friends (6), and classes (5). Barriers to changing dietary habits were time, source of food, preferences, and willpower.

Clark[59] looked at the dietary habits of two Olympic female athletic teams — women's soccer and field hockey teams. Supplements were used by 14% of the field hockey team and 100% of the soccer team. Misconceptions on carbohydrates and protein were noted by 100% of the athletes. Disordered eating was identified on both teams. Athletes attended two nutrition education sessions, a grocery shopping tour, and had individual nutrition consults on two occasions. Follow-up phone conversations revealed a positive change in food selection patterns with regard to all food groups and fat.

Nutrition education for professional female basketball players was studied in six players.[60] The following positive outcomes were reported: four players reported thinking about the importance of breakfast and trying to eat a larger breakfast, two reported feeling better and performing better because of an improved breakfast intake; four players reported eating healthier snacks, with one reporting adding a snack helped her have more energy; two improved their intake of fruits and vegetables; four reported drinking more fluids throughout the day and making an effort to bring water bottles to practice; three feeling better because they were distributing their calories better throughout the day, while two reported having more energy because of better fueling patterns; and four reported they now focus more on proper fueling than on dieting to lose weight. Overall, each player reported five to six dietary recommendations that could potentially contribute to better health and performance.

A study of 22 recent dietary intake studies of 50 groups of elite athletes concluded that no special one food helps an athlete to perform better and the most important aspect of the diet is that it follows basic guidelines in healthy eating.[61] Demanding training and travel schedules in addition to a possible lack of nutrition knowledge may prohibit them from maintaining an optimal intake.

VI. SUMMARY

The knowledge of nutrition and its relationship to sports has increased dramatically over the past 25 years. Nutrition education, specifically sports nutrition, is a growing field, and educators must constantly improve their knowledge. Different methods of communicating nutrition knowledge must be considered. The Internet is a potentially powerful tool to provide information, however, accurate information as well as inaccurate information will be available. Athletes, coaches, trainers, parents, teachers, and nutritionists must be able to distinguish between accurate and inaccurate information and present it in a usable format to be used. Time constraints and food availability seem to be the two biggest factors in limiting athletes' food choices.

Studies must be done that explore other factors that affect athletes' nutritional status, such as environment; social, economic, and cultural factors; and specific sports. With all the individual factors, there may never be "one diet for each sport." Athletes will need to be informed where they can find the most accurate information for themselves and their sport. It is also important to remember that, even though the athlete may have the best information available, that information may not be put to use. Athletes must be convinced it will improve their performance or they will not use it.

While females tend to be more knowledgeable about nutrition, they need to ensure adequate caloric intake to assure adequate nutrient intake. Those with inadequate diets must be educated about proper nutrition and the possible use of appropriate supplements. Athletes who choose to make better choices may perform better, but this needs to be studied further. Choosing to make changes is only part of the big picture. Food must be available, education must be done, and athletes, coaches, and trainers must be willing to make changes. Only then will sports nutrition be truly beneficial to the athlete.

REFERENCES

1. Marquart, L. F., Cohen, E. A., and Short, S. H., Nutrition knowledge of athletes and their coaches and surveys of dietary intakes. In: Wolinsky, I., (Ed.) *Nutrition in Exercise and Sport, Third Edition,* CRC Press, Boca Raton, FL., 1998, pp. 559-596.
2. Mullin, K., Practical nutrition education: special considerations for athletes. *Nurse Pract. Forum.*, 7, 106, 1996.
3. Manjarrez, C. and Birrer, R., Nutrition and athletic performance. *Am. Family Phys.,* 28, 105, 1983.
4. Rund, J. S., *Nutrition and the female athlete*, CRC Press, Boca Raton, FL., 1996.
5. Shannon, B., Mullis, R., Bernardo, V., Ervin, B., and Poehler, D.L., The status of school-based nutrition education at the state agency level., *J. Sch. Health,* 62, 8, 1992.
6. Colavito, E.A., Guthrie, J. F., Hertzler, A. A., and Webs, R.E., Relationships of diet and health related attitudes and nutrition knowledge of household meal planners and the fat and fiber intake of meal planners and preschoolers., *J. Nutr. Educ.,* 28, 321, 1996.
7. Sims, L. (Ed.), Nutrition education, *J. Nutr. Educ.,* 27, 228, 1995.
8. Sims, L. (Ed.), Nutrition education, *J. Nutr. Educ.,* 27, 277, 1995.
9. Jobe, F.W. and Moyes, D., *The Official Little League Fitness Guide,* Simon and Schuster, New York. 1984.
10. Hornick, T.M., Kopel, B.H., Hermann, J., and Forbes, S., Impact of nutrition education on adolescents' sports nutrition knowledge and use of ergogenic products., *J. Am. Diet. Assoc.,* 94, A-51, 1994.
11. Furtado, M.M., Keane, M.W., Curry, K.R., and Johnson, R.M., The effect of nutrition education on nutrition knowledge and body composition of Little League cheerleaders. *J. Am. Diet. Assoc.,* 90, A-19, 1990.
12. Sossin, K. and Marquart, L., Community-based sports nutrition program. *J. Am. Diet. Assoc.,* 93, A-63. 1993.
13. Blaha, B.J., Melvin, R.A., and Reid, H.C., Nutrition education and weight maintenance in male high-school swimmers. *J. Am. Diet. Assoc.,* 97, A-71, 1997.
14. Tiilikainen, R., Haapala, I., Mykkanen, H. and Probart, C., Changes in young swimmers' food choices as a result of parental participation in sports nutrition workshops. *J. Am. Diet. Assoc.,* 99, A-55, 1999.
15. Chapman, P, Toma, R.B., Tuveson, R.F. and Jacob, M., Nutrition knowledge among adolescent high school female athletes. *Adolescence,* 32, 437, 1997.
16. Short, J, Mattfeldt-Beman, M, Sawicki, M. and Beeson, R., Dietary iron: adolescent athletes' knowledge, attitudes, and dietary intake. *J. Am. Diet. Assoc.,* 98, A-17, 1998.

17. Hornick, T.M., Kopel, B.H., Hermann, J., and Forbes, S., Impact of nutrition education on adolescents' sports nutrition knowledge and use of ergogenic products. *J. Am. Diet. Assoc.,* 94, A-51, 1994.
18. Plummer, P.F., Assessment of nutrition knowledge and behaviors of Massachusetts adolescents. *J. Am. Diet. Assoc.,* 95, A-53, 1995.
19. Greiger, L., Sports nutrition knowledge survey of high-school health class students. *J. Am. Diet. Assoc.,* 97, A-72, 1997.
20. Douglas, P.D. and Douglas, J.G., Nutrition knowledge and food practices of high school athletes. *J. Am. Diet. Assoc.,* 84, 198, 1984.
21. Perron, M. and Endres, J., Knowledge, attitudes, and dietary practices of female athletes. *J. Am. Diet. Assoc.,* 85, 573, 1985.
22. Neumark-Sztainer, D., Story, M., Resnick, M.D., and Blum, R.W., Lessons learned about adolescent nutrition from the Minnesota Adolescent Health Survey. *J. Am. Diet. Assoc.,* 98, 1449, 1998.
23. Neumark-Sztainer, D., Story, M., Perry, C., and Casey, M.A., Factors influencing food choices of adolescents: Findings from focus-group discussions with adolescents., *J. Am. Diet. Assoc.,* 99, 929, 1999.
24. American Dietetic Association. Timely statement of the American Dietetic Association: nutrition guidance for child athletes in organized sports., *J. Am. Diet. Assoc.,* 96, 610, 1996.
25. American Academy of Pediatrics, Promotion of healthy weight control practices in young athletes. *Pediatrics,* 752, 1996.
26. Schulz, G.K., Latimer, L., Bowers, V., and Zelman, K., A communication initiative to increase awareness of healthy eating behaviors among high school students. *J. Am. Diet. Assoc.,* 99, A-46, 1999.
27. Wiita, B.D., Stombaugh, I.A., and Buch, J.A., Nutrition knowledge and nutrient intakes of female high school and college runners. *J. Am. Diet. Assoc.,* 94, A-89, 1994.
28. Shearer, J.D., Yadrick, M.D., Boudreaux, L.J., and Norris, P.A., Nutritional assessment of college freshman athletes. *J. Am. Diet. Assoc.,* 91, A-110, 1991.
29. Bermudez, M.G., Keane, M.W., Curry, K.R., and Lopez, R., The effect of nutrition education on the nutrition knowledge of college athletes. *J. Am. Diet. Assoc.,* 91, A-47, 1991.
30. Leeds, M.J., nad Denegar, C., Nutrition knowledge and food practices of collegiate athletes compared to nonathletes. *J. Am. Diet. Assoc.,* 91, A-13, 1991.
31. Reed-Weisner, A.K. and Read, M.H., Health beliefs, nutrition knowledge, and nutrient intake of university athletes. *J. Am. Diet. Assoc.,* 90, A-103, 1990.
32. Kunkel, M.E., Bell, L.B., and Luccia, B.D., Effect of peer nutrition education on nutritional status and nutritional knowledge of university student-athletes. *J. Am. Diet. Assoc.,* 99, A-38, 1999.
33. Potter, G.S. and Wood, O.B., Comparison on self- and group instruction for teaching sports nutrition to college athletes. *J. Nutr. Educ.,* 23, 288, 1991.
34. Heredeen, F. and Fellers, R.B., Nutrition knowledge of college football linemen implications for nutrition education. *J. Am. Diet. Assoc.,* 99, A-38, 1999.
35. Barr, S.I., Nutrition knowledge of female varsity athletes and university students., *J. Am. Diet. Assoc.,* 87, 1660, 1987.
36. Walantas, S.D., Implementing a sports nutrition education program for the corps of cadets at the United States Military Academy, West Point, NY, *J. Am. Diet. Assoc.,* 90, A-129, 1990.
37. McReynolds, C.J., Cohen, J.W., Gambrell, K.M., and Dirks, K.R., Nutrition education with Texas A&M University athletes., *J. Am. Diet. Assoc.,* 93, A-56, 1993.
38. Gagliardi, M.J., and Byrd, S., Nutrition knowledge and dietary practices in university athletes., *J. Am. Diet. Assoc.,* 92, A-113, 1992.
39. Keller-Grubbs, G.A., Landis, W., Lowe, J., and Finn, A., Differences in nutrition knowledge among female runners upon completion of a nutrition education program., *J. Am. Diet. Assoc.,* 94, A-86, 1994.
40. Whitcombe, D., Nethery, V. and Bergman, E., Relationship between nutrition knowledge and gender, ethnic background, and year in school in varsity athletes., *J. Am. Diet. Assoc.,* 96, A-87, 1996.
41. Cherundolo, L.A. and Levine, A.M., Knowledge, attitudes, and use of dietary supplements in collegiate division III student athletes., *J. Am. Diet. Assoc.,* 99, A-39, 1999.
42. Tartmella, L.D. and Kemler, D.S., Principles of sports nutrition: does nutrition education enhance athletes' knowledge?, *J. Am. Diet. Assoc.,* 96, A-88, 1996.
43. Kaiser, A.S. and Kunkel, M.E., Nutrition knowledge and attitudes of former university athletes., *J. Am. Diet. Assoc.,* 96, A-86, 1996.

44. Bloyd, D.C., Anderson, S.L., Zager, K. and Welch, P., Beliefs and perceptions about diet and body image among collegiate male bodybuilders. *J. Am. Diet. Assoc.,* 95, A-93, 1995.
45. Linton, V.I. and Brown, L.B., Reported obstacles to eating a well-balanced diet among collegiate female athletes., *J. Am. Diet. Assoc.,* 97, A-71, 1997.
46. Leeds, M.J., Nutritional practices of collegiate soccer players., *J. Am. Diet. Assoc.,* 92, A-55, 1992.
47. Clark, K.L., Working with college athletes, coaches, and trainers at a major university, *Int. J. Sport Nutr.,* 4, 135, 1994.
48. Grandjean, A.C., Practices and recommendations of sports nutritionists., *Int. J. Sport Nutr.,* 3, 232, 1993.
49. Gollman, B.S. and Carlyle, T.L., Nutrition knowledge and eating practice survey of exercising adults, *J. Am. Diet. Assoc.,* 90, A-121, 1990.
50. Day, P.J., Nutrition knowledge among male and female participants of four distinct health/fitness facilities, *J. Am. Diet. Assoc.,* 90, A-18, 1990.
51. Barr, S.I., Nutrition knowledge and selected nutritional practices of female recreational athletes, *J. Nutr. Educ.,* 18, 167, 1986.
52. Sacheck, J.M., and Roubenoff, R., Nutrition in the exercising elderly., *Clinics in Sports Med.,* 18, 565, 1999.
53. Rock, C.L., Nutrition of the older athlete., *Clin. Sports Med.,* 10, 445, 1991.
54. Hermann, J.R., Kopel, B.H., McCrory, M.L., and Kulling, F.A., Effect of a cooperative extension nutrition and exercise program for older adults on nutrition knowledge, dietary intake, anthropometric measurements, and serum lipids., *J. Nutr. Educ.,* 22, 271, 1990.
55. Clark, N., Nelson, M., and Evans, W., Nutrition education for elite female runners., *Phys. and Sportsmed.,* 16, 124, 1988.
56. Cumming, C.M., Brevard, P.B., and Pearson, J.M., Recreational runners' beliefs and practices concerning water intake, *J. Nutr. Educ.,* 26, 195, 1994.
57. Steinbaugh, M., Nutritional needs of female athletes, *Clin. Sports Med.*, 3, 649, 1984.
58. Weitzel, N.L. and Myers, E.F., Reaching the competitive athlete: identifying the gap between perceived and actual nutrition knowledge., *J. Am. Diet. Assoc.,* 95, A-99, 1995.
59. Clark, K.L., Dietary habits of two Olympic female athletic teams., *J. Am. Diet. Assoc.,* 96, A-29, 1996.
60. Clark, N. and Polonchek, J., Outcomes of nutrition education for professional female basketball players., *J. Am. Diet. Assoc.,* 98, A-76, 1998.
61. Economos, C.D., Bortz, S.S., and Nelson, M.E., Nutritional practices of elite athletes., *Sports Med.,* 16, 381, 1993.

CHAPTER 17

Nutrition Concerns, Knowledge, and Recommendations of Coaches and Athletic Trainers

Richard D. Lewis, Jennifer Massoni, and Kimberly Crawford

CONTENTS

I. INTRODUCTION

Dedicated training, expert coaching ,and sound nutrition are three essential components for optimal performance and health of athletes. Some athletic professionals perceive the nutrition component of performance to be less important than the training and coaching constituents, and, for this reason, nutrition education for athletes is neglected.[1] This disregard of nutrition education in some athletic programs occurs despite clear evidence that fluid intake[2] and the energy content of the diet, especially the quantity of carbohydrates,[3] are determinants of peak physical performance.

0-8493-8199-1/00/$0.00+$.50

Nutrition education directed to athletes should at least address these essential principles.[4–8] Athletes often lack the nutritional knowledge to make wise dietary choices and rely on others for advice on diet and nutrition related issues. College and high school athletic programs typically do not employ or consult with a registered dietitian (RD) to provide nutritional guidance to athletes.[9,10] Coaches, athletic trainers (ATs), and certified athletic trainers (ATCs) often play the primary role in delivering nutritional information to athletes, partly because of the extensive hours of contact they have with the athletes.[8,11,12] Providing sound nutrition advice that is individualized and tailored to the specific sport, age, goals, and health status of the athlete requires that both coaches and ATCs be educated about the nutritional requirements and eating behaviors of athletes.[13] Because many young athletes are competing during the pubertal years, coaches and ATCs also need to be aware of the athlete's unique nutritional needs during growth and maturation.[14,15]

Formal nutrition coursework offered to coaches and ATCs during their academic training is limited and much of their nutrition knowledge is acquired outside the classroom through seminars, continuing education, and popular resources.[9,16,17] Fitness magazines, newspapers, and the Internet may provide sound nutrition information, though some nutrition misinformation is also conveyed. The purposes of this chapter are to discuss the delivery of nutrition information to athletes, the nutrition concerns, knowledge, and recommendations of coaches and ATCs, their academic preparation and other sources of their nutrition knowledge. In addition, this chapter will address the academic training of RDs, their role in the sports medicine team, and how they can effectively work with coaches and ATCs.

II. DELIVERY OF NUTRITION INFORMATION TO ATHLETES

Coaches and ATCs believe that the dissemination of nutrition information to athletes is the responsibility of both professions, although both groups recognize the leadership role of the coach in disseminating information to team members.[8,18,19] A survey conducted by Graves et al.,[19] of 303 high school coaches and ATCs indicated that ATCs believe the responsibility to disseminate nutrition information to athletes should be equally shared between coaches and ATCs.[19] Coaches from this same sample[19] and that of Bedgood and Tuck[8] believe that it is their responsibility to take an active part in disseminating nutrition information to athletes. In an earlier nationwide survey, the nutrition background and responsibilities of 170 high school and college ATCs, 348 coaches and 2977 athletes were assessed.[18] Unlike the previous findings, 70% of the ATC population and 50% of the coaches indicated that ATCs should assume the responsibility of providing nutrition counseling to athletes.[18] Half of the coaches in this survey believed that they should provide nutrition information to athletes, although only 27% had ever taken a nutrition course.[18] Seventy-three percent of ATCs had completed a formal course in nutrition, and, in the author's opinion, were more prepared than coaches to deliver nutrition education to athletes.[18]

Coaches and ATCs exposed to nutrition in their academic programs are likely to be introduced to more basic-level nutrition and lack the advanced clinical nutrition training of an RD. Effective nutrition education and interventions targeted to athletes on topics such as dietary strategies for weight loss require the knowledge and skills of an RD with expertise in sports nutrition. There are no published reports identifying the number of athletic programs currently using RDs, but informal surveys indicate that the number of RDs providing services to athletic programs has increased over the last 10 years. Surveys of coaches in the '70s and '80s indicated that only 2% or fewer of coaches relied on RDs for guidance on nutrition and performance issues.[9,10,16] In 1999, one response to a professional sports nutrition Internet listserve indicated that approximately 30 universities and colleges have established sports nutrition programs.[20] Furthermore, professional athletic teams are hiring full- or part-time RDs to provide nutritional expertise to their athletes; the extent to which this occurs, however, is not documented.

III. NUTRITION CONCERNS, KNOWLEDGE, AND RECOMMENDATIONS OF COACHES AND ATHLETIC TRAINERS

Providing nutrition education to athletes at the high school, college, and professional levels often becomes the responsibility of coaches and ATCs.[18] While nutrition may not be the top priority for coaches and ATCs, most are aware of the contribution of nutrition in helping athletes to maintain hours of hard training and to perform at their maximum ability during competition. Misasi et al.[17] surveyed ATCs and had them rank priorities for the responsibilities they assume in their athletic positions. Nutrition was ranked as the third priority behind their primary responsibilities of injury rehabilitation and prevention. In 1984, Parr, Porter, and Hodgson[18] and Graves[19] noted that both high school and college-level coaches, ATs, and ATCs ranked fluid needs, weight management, and nutritional supplementation as the top three nutrition issues. Additionally, coaches identified energy needs and the pre-game meal as important nutrition issues.[18] Much of what is reported in the literature with respect to the nutritional knowledge and recommendations of coaches and ATCs is related to their principal concerns of fluid intake, nutritional supplementation, weight management, the training diet and pre-game meal. Because some of these surveys of high school and college coaches and ATCs are almost 20 years old,[1,9,16,18] there is uncertainty whether the nutrition practices followed by coaches and ATCs today are similar to what we know from the older surveys. What is documented in the literature with respect to coaches' and ATCs' knowledge and recommendations on these major nutrition concerns is discussed below.

A. Fluid Needs

Most coaches and ATs appear to be knowledgeable about fluids and hydration and aid their athletes in avoiding dehydration by encouraging fluid replacement.[1,4,9] Corley, Demarest-Litchford, and Bazzarre,[9] assessed the nutrition knowledge of 105 college coaches, 75 male and 30 female, representing a wide range of athletic sports including swimming, tennis, basketball, gymnastics, track and field, cross-country, football, wrestling, and golf. Overall, 70% of the nutrition questions were answered correctly and questions regarding hydration status and sodium needs had the highest percentage of correct responses. In this study, 88% of coaches recommended fluid intake to prevent dehydration, but only 31% actually monitored hydration status among their athletes. Bentivegna, Kelley, and Kalenak[1] surveyed 75 coaches and ATs involved primarily in football and determined that 70% provided fluids *ad libitum*, 19% encouraged one water break, 7% gave water only on hot days, and 2.5% did not provide water. The high percentage of coaches in this study recommending *ad libitum* fluid intake is consistent with responses from a survey of high school coaches. Almost 80% of high school coaches were under the impression that athletes can rely on thirst to maintain optimal hydration status.[8] Voluntary or *ad libitum* fluid consumption does not adequately replace sweat losses.[21] In contrast, a more recent study of college coaches found that 74% were aware that athletes couldn't rely on thirst as an indicator of hydration status.[9]

These findings imply that coaches are aware of the general need to recommend fluids for athletes, but not all coaches understand that voluntary fluid replacement is not adequate and that athletes need to adhere to specific fluid consumption guidelines as recommended by the American College of Sports Medicine (ACSM).[2] Furthermore, coaches and ATCs may be unaware of the interaction of specific nutrients and their potential impact on hydration status. Sports drinks containing small amounts of sodium and glucose seem to enhance palatability and promote rehydration better than water alone.[21] Coaches and ATCs should encourage athletes to use sports drinks in an effort to replace sweat and glycogen losses. A practice that appears to be common among coaches is the recommendation of high-protein shakes, bars, or supplements to athletes in an effort to enhance gains in fat-free soft tissue.[10] While the protein requirement for some athletes may be higher than the requirement of the Recommended Dietary Allowances,[22] consumption of a well-balanced diet should provide more than adequate protein to accommodate the needs of most athletes.

High protein intakes associated with the use of protein supplements may increase fluid needs and alter hydration status among athletes.[23] Coaches' general knowledge of fluid needs, without an appreciation for the role of other nutrients on fluid balance, may not be sufficient to promote optimal hydration of athletes.

B. Nutritional Supplementation

There is limited conclusive evidence that nutritional supplementation in a healthy individual consuming a well balanced diet will result in improved performance.[8] Athletes who follow chronically energy-restricted diets may consume lower amounts of micronutrients, thus increasing the potential benefits of supplementation. For some athletes, a sudden increase in physical training may transiently elevate requirements for some vitamins and minerals.[24] However, most athletes consuming a variety of foods in proper proportions, as demonstrated by the Food Guide Pyramid, should acquire adequate amounts of most nutrients.[4,24]

The practice of coaches recommending supplements to athletes appears to be higher today than in previous years, however, there are no recent surveys documenting this practice. An informal survey of Division 1 colleges and universities in the Southeast revealed that thousands of dollars are spent each year on nutritional supplements.[25] These funds allotted to nutritional supplements suggest that the practice of athletic personnel supporting supplement use is common. Bentivegna, Kelley, and Kalenak[1] reported in 1979 that 8% of coaches and ATs recommended the use of supplements only during the season and 14% always recommended supplements. Results from a survey by Wolf, Wirth, and Lohman[16] of 137 college coaches in 1979 revealed that 35% of these coaches recommended vitamin supplementation and that 50% of those making the recommendations also provided the supplements to their athletes. In 1994 Baer, Dean, and Lambrinnides[10] surveyed 135 football coaches and found that 65% made recommendations for using vitamin and mineral supplements and approximately 20% recommended protein supplements. In this same study, 30% of coaches recommended protein powder supplements to football players to gain fat-free soft tissue. Additionally, 47% of the coaches indicated that protein was a food group that should be increased in the diet to build fat-free soft tissue.

In the majority of these surveys, the rationale for recommending supplements was unclear. It is the position of the American Dietetic Association that, "The best nutritional strategy for promoting optimal health and reducing the risk of chronic disease is to obtain adequate nutrients from a wide variety of foods. Vitamin and mineral supplementation is appropriate when well accepted, peer-reviewed, scientific evidence shows safety and effectiveness."[26] It is likely that coaches and ATCs recommend supplements to athletes without assessment of their diet or determination of their individual needs. Forty-six percent of coaches reported that their supplement recommendations were based on specific reasons (B-vitamins for energy) rather than individual assessment.[1] According to Wolf, Wirth, and Lohman[16] only 12% of male coaches and 6% of female coaches measured the nutritional health of athletes. Except for two coaches who used dietary surveys, most made conclusions on nutritional health by informal observations.[16]

In a recent review of nutritional supplementation practices of athletes by Sobal and Marquart,[27] it was reported that almost half of the athletes surveyed used supplements. The authors stressed that in order to provide thorough nutrition supplement education to athletes, RDs should conduct an in-depth assessment of an athlete's supplement usage history.[27] The RD's involvement is essential since, according to Bedgood and Tuck,[8] Graves et al.[19] and Sossin et al.,[7] coaches possess little knowledge of nutritional supplementation. A survey of high school coaches indicated that, out of five questions on supplementation, 70% answered all incorrectly.[8] Furthermore, only 17% of high school wrestling coaches reported that they were knowledgeable regarding vitamin supplements.[7] Athletic trainers appear to be somewhat more knowledgeable regarding nutritional supplements than coaches.[19] Sixty-four percent and 49% of ATs and coaches, respectively, correctly responded to nutritional supplement questions.[19] Because of coaches' minimal knowledge of nutritional supplements, it is to their advantage to consult with an RD when considering supplement recommendations to athletes. The RDs' academic training provides them with the background to adequately review the scientific and lay literature and make sense of the many complicated nutritional supplement issues.

C. Weight Management

For most sports, including football, gymnastics, swimming, cross-country running, and wrestling, management of the athletes' weight and body composition is a major concern.[10,13,18,28,29] Coaches and ATCs are important sources of information to high school and college athletes with respect to weight control and body composition.[30] Eighty-two percent of a group of teenage wrestlers indicated that coaches were the main source of weight-loss information.[30] Only 16% of coaches recommended that athletes consult with nutritionists for weight-management issues.[31]

In general, little is known about the knowledge and recommendations made by coaches and ATCs regarding weight management. Griffin and Harris[31] reported that 66% of high school coaches described their knowledge of obesity and weight-control issues as above average, although they tended to actually possess little knowledge. Results from several surveys, including that of Griffin and Harris,[31] suggest that recommendations made by some coaches for weight management are appropriate.[7,9] Increasing exercise,[7,9,31] gradual dieting,[31] consuming fewer snacks,[7,32] and eating smaller meals[7,9,32] are strategies recommended by coaches for promoting weight loss. While these are sound recommendations for weight management often employed by RDs, individualized guidance and monitoring of athletes is needed. Furthermore, unrealistic body weight and fat percentage goals are often imposed on athletes. The possibility exists that the combination of unrealistic weight and body fat goals for athletes, with little or no guidance on nutrition and dietary management, could contribute to inappropriate weight-loss behaviors.

The ACSM recommends in its position stand on the "Female Athlete Triad" that if weight or body composition guidelines must be used, a range of values should be employed instead of single values.[33] Furthermore, number five of the position stand states, "All sports medicine professionals, including coaches and trainers, should learn about preventing and recognizing the symptoms and risks of the triad. All individuals working with active girls and women should participate in athletic training that is medically and psychologically sound. They should avoid pressuring girls and women about losing weight. They should know basic nutrition counseling and medical and mental health evaluation."[33] Accurate assessment of an athlete's need for body weight or composition intervention is essential in lessening the risk for disordered eating behaviors. Griffin and Harris[31] reported that high school coaches recommended weight loss strictly on appearance, without the use of anthropometric data. Approximately 50% of male and 36% of female college coaches predicted the optimal weight for an athlete based on preseason appearance.[16] Only 24% of the coaches utilized body composition measurements.[16] Coaches and ATCs should include thorough assessments of body weight and composition prior to establishing goals for weight management. They should communicate realistic body weight and composition goals to athletes and make appropriate referrals to RDs. Ongoing dietary assessment and follow-up counseling strategies are needed to achieve positive results.

D. The Training Diet and Pre-Game Meal

Helping athletes consume a balanced diet is a priority of coaches and ATCs.[18] In a recent roundtable discussion on the impact of sports medicine on coaching,[4] a high school basketball coach stated: "We encourage our athletes to eat breakfast and to take in enough calories throughout the day, but we can't control the types of foods that they are eating." Coaches encourage athletes to eat regular meals in an effort to keep their energy levels up and improve the quality of their diet.[4] Unfortunately, coaches are unlikely to monitor the type or amount of foods consumed and may be unaware of the recommended training diet composition best suited to benefit athletes.[4]

Bentivegna, Kelley, and Kalenak[1] and Corley, Demarest-Litchford, and Bazzarre[9] reported that only 22% and 20% of college coaches, respectively, identified the recommended energy distribution for carbohydrate, fat, and protein. The majority of coaches and ATs surveyed indicated that the correct distribution of macronutrients for a weight-maintenance and -training diet is 45% carbohydrate, 45% protein, and 10% fat.[1] Thirty-five percent of the coaches reported that they "had no idea" what the recommended distribution of calories should be.[9] Based on a more recent survey, seven wrestling coaches recommended that their wrestlers should not limit their intake of breads, rice, and potatoes. These coaches' recommendations are consistent with the 1995 Dietary Guidelines, which recommend eating a variety of foods emphasizing increased consumption of grains, vegetables, and fruits, and a decreased intake of fat.[34] The macronutrient composition resulting from adherence to these guidelines is approximately 55% carbohydrate, 15% protein, and 30% fat. Overall, coaches desire that athletes consume a balanced diet. There is still some question, however, regarding the ability of most coaches to make the appropriate macronutrient recommendations for a balanced diet.

Little information is available that describes the recommendations by coaches or ATCs regarding the pre-game-meal composition. Of 100 college coaches surveyed by Corley, Demarest-Litchford, and Bazzarre,[9] approximately 50% assume the responsibility for planning pre-game meals, however, 82% had never taken a nutrition course. Wolf, Wirth, and Lohman[16] revealed that coaches' most preferred pre-competition foods were pancakes, dry toast, eggs, and fruit.[16] Only 13% of coaches, primarily football, identified steak and other high-protein foods as essential to the pre-competition meal. While specific pre-competition foods were not identified, Bedgood and Tuck[8] reported that 89% of coaches recommended low-fat foods. From an ATC's perspective, pre-game meals should be composed of high carbohydrate, low-fat, easily digestible foods,[35] a diet composition consistent with current sports nutrition guidelines and 1995 Dietary Guidelines. The perspective of this ATC, combined with a report by Graves et al.[19] that ATs had more correct responses to questions on the pre-event meal, suggest that ATs may be better prepared than coaches to provide guidance on the pre-game meal. Both coaches and ATs, however, are aware of the recommended time frame for consuming the pre-event meal. Eighty-six percent of coaches and ATs[1] and 58% of coaches[9] recommended that the pre-game meal be consumed 3 or 4 hours before competition.

Increasing carbohydrate intakes to 55–70% of total caloric intake for the training diet or the pre-event meal can be difficult for some athletes. Besides focusing on a balanced diet with emphasis on breads, grains, fruits, and vegetables, athletes can boost their carbohydrate intake by supplementing their regular diet with sports drinks and energy bars during practice and competition. Coaches and ATCs should encourage athletes to follow these higher-carbohydrate-intake guidelines by having the RD provide practical and appealing ideas for incorporating these foods and beverages into a busy schedule.

IV. ACADEMIC BACKGROUND OF COACHES AND ATHLETIC TRAINERS

Physical conditioning, teaching, motivating, and helping athletes perfect their skills are a few of the many roles assumed by coaches. The main responsibilities of ATCs are the prevention and rehabilitation of injuries, including providing guidance on strength and conditioning.[19] The academic backgrounds differ between these professionals, but one commonality is the fact that nutrition education is limited within both curriculum pathways.

A. Academic Background of Coaches

Most athletic coaches pursue higher levels of education and have earned at least a master's degree.[35,36,37] There is no systematic governing body like the National Athletic Trainer's Association

(NATA) Board of Certification (NATABOC) for trainers that certifies coaches in all sports, however, some areas such as swimming or strength and conditioning strongly encourage certification. Furthermore, coaches are not required to accumulate hours of clinical or practical experience as part of their academic training. The most common academic path for coaches is to obtain a degree in physical education.[9,37] Richardson[37] and Corley, Demarest-Litchford, and Bazzarre[9] reported that approximately 83% and 72% of college coaches, respectively, had graduated with a physical education degree. Seventeen percent had graduated with degrees in education, guidance and counseling, or administration, with 10%, 13%, and 20% of Division I, II, and III coaches, respectively, earning their Ph.D. in physical education.

Course work typically offered as part of the curriculum for a bachelor of science degree in physical education emphasizes health and wellness, human anatomy, physiology, kinesiology, physical activity, theories of learning, education, administration, and psychology for various age groups. Some undergraduate or graduate physical education programs offer specific concentrations in teaching, athletic administration, exercise science, or coaching. Additional course work may include organization and administration of health education and promotion, current trends and issues in health, science research methods, sport administration, comparative education, sport facility management, financial principles in sport, special topics in sport administration, sport marketing, and legal aspects of sport. Nutrition education within a physical education curriculum is minimal, as most physical education degree programs do not offer a class in nutrition. Course offerings such as health education and exercise science provide some basic nutrition principles, but this is limited. In two surveys of college coaches, only 18%[9] and 39%[18] had completed a college-level course in nutrition. A sample of 135 high school coaches revealed that 33% had completed a course in nutrition or had exposure to nutrition issues through continuing-education programs.[10]

While certification is not systematically required by the coaching profession, several sports encourage certification for coaches.[38,39] For example, the American Swimming Coaches Association (ASCA) offers five levels of certification, with level five reflecting the most advanced level of education.[39] The top 2% to 5% of swimming coaches are certified in level five. To become certified, swimming coaches must be ASCA members, and for each level of certification are required to complete classes at local clinics or through home school and must pass an exam. As part of the ASCA certification process, coaches are required to obtain 50 CEUs over a 3-year period to maintain their certification level.[40] The continuing-education programs are sources of nutrition information related to swimming performance and health. Strength and conditioning coaches also have an option for certification and can become Certified Strength and Conditioning Specialists (CSCS).[39] This is a rigorous certification program that includes training in anatomy, exercise physiology, biomechanics, and nutrition issues, and requires coaches to pass a national examination.[39] The CSCS program provides coaches with nutrition knowledge they may not get from a coach's typical physical education curriculum.

Excluding their academic preparation, and, for some coaches, certification, much of a coach's experience in a sport is typically derived from his or her own past athletic participation or experience as a graduate assistant. Richardson[37] reported findings from a 1978 survey of 1706 coaches and found that 65%, 89%, and 69% of coaches from Divisions I, II, and III, respectively, had participated in their coaching sport during their undergraduate years in college.

B. Academic Background of Athletic Trainers

Before athletic trainers can practice, they must obtain their certification credential by NATABOC. Two different routes can lead to certification of athletic trainers: 1) completion of a baccalaureate or post-baccalaureate program from an accredited college or university including clinical experiences; or 2) completion of a baccalaureate degree from a non-accredited program and completion of an internship program. Once students have met one of the above requirements they are eligible to sit for the national exam administered by NATABOC.

A typical baccalaureate curriculum includes one introductory nutrition class, anatomy, exercise physiology, kinesiology, chemistry, health education, and psychology. Parr, Porter, and Hodgson[18] reported that 73% of NATA-certified ATCs have had one formal nutrition class. Additional course work also includes pharmacology, first aid, and cardiopulmonary resuscitation (CPR).[41] The NATA organization requires that advanced athletic training course work include prevention of athletic injuries, recognition and management of acute athletic injuries, rehabilitation of athletic injuries, therapeutic modality evaluation of injury, and health care administration. The academic pathway for athletic trainers often includes specialization in related areas through post-baccalaureate training. According to George,[35] over 70% of NATA members have earned a master's degree in related fields such as health, physical education, or exercise science and 32% have taken post-graduate nutrition classes.[18] Foster and Leslie[42] reported that greater than 50% of 154 ATCs were teacher-certified and had obtained a master's degree or higher. Advanced teacher certification may be beneficial since 69% of 101 ATCs reported that they spend 30% of their professional time in clinical instruction. Those students who attend an accredited program must complete a minimum of 800 athletic training hours under the supervision of a NATABOC certified trainer. Athletic training students attending a non-accredited program must complete an internship to obtain certification.

The focus of the internship is to provide practical, hands-on experiences for prevention, evaluation, treatment, and rehabilitation of injuries.[41] Typical settings that provide clinical experiences include a primary setting (the athletic training room), a secondary setting (athletic practice and game coverage), and an allied health setting (sports medicine clinics, summer sports camps, sports performance facilities, and hospital settings). Training in nutrition education and counseling strategies are typically not incorporated into these clinical experiences. Students attending a non-accredited program completing the internship route must obtain a minimum of 1500 athletic training hours, 500 of which must be supervised by a NATABOC certified trainer.[41] It is noteworthy that, by 2004, all students must graduate from an accredited program to sit for the NATABOC examination.

Successful completion of the national exam is the final step to certification. The exam focuses on subject matter from five domains of athletic training that are categorized as prevention of athletic injuries; recognition, evaluation and immediate care of athletic injuries; rehabilitation and reconditioning of athletic injuries; health care administration; and professional development and responsibility.[41]

Surveys of ATCs have been conducted to assess their selected route to NATABOC certification. Of 183 entry-level ATCs with 108 males and 75 females, 45% had completed the NATA-approved undergraduate program, 35% selected the internship route, and 19% completed the NATA-approved graduate program.[36] When asked how effective the program was at preparing these entry-level ATCs for professional practice, ATCs who had completed the NATA-approved graduate program were the most satisfied.[36] Seventy percent indicated that they had accrued over 1800 hours of clinical work experience during their professional preparation, well beyond the minimum requirement.

Misasi et al.,[17] reported that 42% of 90 ATCs from Division I, II, III, and National Association of Intercollegiate Athletics (NAIA) colleges and universities had completed the NATA curriculum program and 47% had chosen the internship route to certification. The majority of the 69 ATCs had earned a master's degree, while six had prepared at the doctorate level and two had other degrees.[17] Certified athletic trainers were asked to reveal whether their academic or clinical program prepared them to provide nutrition counseling.[17] Seventy-eight percent of ATCs believed their academic program prepared them, while 62% indicated that the clinical component of the program prepared them for nutrition counseling. It is of interest, however, that 83% of ATCs suggested that more emphasis should be placed on nutrition during academic preparation. Of those who indicated that additional nutrition course work would be helpful, 70% reported that nutrition course work should be incorporated equally within the academic and clinical setting components of the program. Additional nutrition education is not common for most programs and most ATCs will possess the minimal nutrition background required by the NATABOC. However, some states require that students pursuing certification as an athletic trainer take an additional nutrition course as part of their internship program, in addition to the base NATA requirements.[19]

Like many other health professionals, the ATC is required to complete continuing education units (CEU) throughout their careers. Minimum requirements include the completion of eight CEUs every 3 years that can be achieved by:

1. attending symposiums, seminars, workshops, and conferences
2. speaking at clinical symposiums
3. taking post-certification education classes at a college or university
4. completing CPR certification

While the extent to which nutrition is offered through continuing education is unclear, 74% of ATCs indicated that they had participated in nutrition training through continuing education.[17] In addition, 91% of the same sample noted that they would participate in continuing-education nutrition workshops, seminars, or classes, suggesting that having knowledge in the area of athletic nutrition is a priority for ATCs.

A majority of ATCs believe that their clinical and academic programs prepare them to provide nutrition education to athletes.[17] However, formal nutrition coursework and training is limited in most baccalaureate curriculums. Like coaches, some ATCs may gain additional nutrition training by obtaining the CSCS credential.[39] The structure of the ATC's academic program is founded primarily on exercise science, with special emphasis on exercise physiology and biomechanics. The only nutrition class that is required in core curriculums of ATC students is generally taught at an introductory level and provides only an overview of basic nutrition principles. Certified athletic trainers have a desire to gain more nutrition knowledge and would pursue future training regarding nutrition in the form of workshops, seminars, or classes.[17] Continuing-education classes taught by RDs would aid ATCs in gaining more nutrition education following the completion of their degrees.

V. OTHER SOURCES FOR NUTRITION KNOWLEDGE

Coaches and ATCs may lack extensive formal training in nutrition, but they do possess some knowledge of nutrition gained from a variety of other experiences and resources. The majority of coaches surveyed over the years identified professional journals,[8,16,19] popular magazines,[8,16] textbooks,[9,19] and newspapers[8] as major sources of nutrition information. Interestingly, while coaches identified journals and popular magazines as sources of nutrition information, 69% of the sample of coaches indicated that they rarely read anything related to nutrition. Corley, Demarest-Litchford, and Bazzarre[9] also reported that only 2% of coaches consulted RDs for dietary guidance, while 17% relied on physicians' advice. Graves et al.[19] identified the physician as the major resource person for nutritional information by 68% and 76% of coaches and ATs, respectively. Coaches and ATCs report that professional journals, textbooks, and popular magazines are important sources of nutrition information, but the extent to which these athletic professionals use these resources is unclear. Furthermore, with the current advances in communications technology, it seems likely that the Internet is a major source of sports nutrition information. The use of an RD as a nutrition resource for athletic departments has been limited, but as more high schools and colleges implement interdisciplinary sports-medicine programs, the number of coaches and ATCs utilizing RDs should increase.

VI. HOW REGISTERED DIETITIANS WORK EFFECTIVELY WITH COACHES AND ATHLETIC TRAINERS

Coaches and ATCs are exposed to limited nutrition training and can benefit by consulting with or including an RD specialized in sports nutrition as part of the sports-medicine team.[9,18,16,19,43,44] Registered dietitians have the depth of nutrition training and knowledge necessary to address the pervasive misinformation present in athletics. Even in 1979, Bentivegna[1] recognized this issue and concluded that high school coaches need training sessions in nutrition and the sessions should be taught by nutrition experts. Lombardo[43] also recognized in 1985 that the use of an RD was essential to educate athletes about nutrition performance issues. Berry, in a 1999 article, states that the combination of an RD and an ATC is ideal for delivering accurate and useful nutrition information to athletes.[44] The inclusion of an RD will enhance the sports-medicine team by reinforcing sound nutrition recommendations and helping athletes deal with misinformation.[44]

A. Academic Background of Registered Dietitians

The academic and clinical training required to become an RD provides the knowledge and skills necessary to offer effective nutrition services to athletes. Graduation from an accredited undergraduate or graduate dietetics program is the first step to becoming an RD. Programs must be accredited by the Commission on Accreditation Approval for Dietetics Education (CAADE). Core courses founded in the sciences and introductory and advanced classes in nutrition are reviewed and approved by CAADE. Some of the preliminary science classes include inorganic and organic chemistry, biology, physiology, microbiology, and biochemistry. Required introductory and advanced nutrition classes include macronutrients, micronutrients, clinical assessment, lifecycle nutrition, medical nutrition therapy, nutrition support, food service management, sanitation, quantity meal preparation, and community nutrition. Following the completion of the didactic program, all students must successfully complete a dietetic internship and pass a national exam.

The dietetic internship requirement can be completed by participation in a CAADE-accredited Dietetic Internship or a CAADE-Approved Pre-professional Practice Program (AP4). Dietetic internships and AP4 programs provide students with practical and applied nutrition experiences within the following areas: health promotion, clinical nutrition, food service management, and public health. A minimum of 900 hours under the supervision of an RD is required to satisfy the internship and AP4 requirement.[45] The internship program prepares the dietetic intern to assess body composition, dietary intakes, and biochemical and clinical indices of nutritional status. Furthermore, interns are exposed to food service management and menu planning services that provide them with adequate skills to plan affordable, nutritious, and palatable meals. Within the outpatient and public health setting, interns are able to gain experiences counseling patients within the various stages of the lifecycle. In addition, they learn the value of teamwork and networking to provide nutrition education effectively to the public. An intern can choose to specialize in a variety of fields within the core of dietetics including clinical, wellness, food product development, sports nutrition, teaching, research, or private practice.

A minimum score of 75% must be earned on the national exam to obtain the RD credential. Categories included on the exam reflect the academic and clinical experiences of the RD. They include normal nutrition (addresses the biochemical and physiological aspects of nutrition), community nutrition, medical nutrition therapy, food science, food service operations, marketing, management, and a miscellaneous category that encompasses topics such as research, education, statistics, and counseling. The exam serves to standardize the knowledge base of the entry-level nutrition professional, which has been founded upon the basic and applied sciences.

B. Model Sports Medicine Programs that Use Registered Dietitians

Most major universities have comprehensive sports-medicine programs typically comprising a director of sports medicine, team physicians, ATCs, a physical therapist, sports psychologists, orthopedic surgeons, and exercise scientists. Some sports-medicine programs also include as part of the team an RD with expertise in sports nutrition. Many of the high school, college, and professional sports nutrition programs that exist today were initiated by RDs volunteering their services. Table 17.1 provides the responses to a question posted on a sports nutrition listserve.

Table 17.1 University Sports Nutrition Services[1,2]

Student Health Services RD:*

- Brown University
- Columbia University
- Cornell University (another RD also provides services)
- Florida State University
- James Madison University
- Kansas State University
- Michigan State University
- Mississippi State University
- New York University
- Penn State (1/2 paid by student health services and 1/2 by nutrition department)
- Syracuse University
- University of California, Davis (peer counselors and MD with nutrition specialty are also available)
- University of Illinois (private practice RD also provides services)
- University of Iowa (1/2 time is paid by the athletic department)
- University of Kentucky (1/3 time is paid by the athletic department)
- University of New Hampshire
- University of Pennsylvania
- University of South Florida
- University of Virginia
- West Chester University
- Western Michigan University (some money from individual team budgets)
- Yale University

Volunteer Graduate Students:

- Colorado State University

Funded Graduate Students:

- Central Washington University (release time from graduate assistantship)
- University of Georgia (1/3 funded by athletic department)
- University of Massachusetts, Amherst (10 hours/week funded by grant)

RD paid by Athletic Department:

Full-time	Part-time
Georgia Tech	Arizona State
North Carolina State University (1/2 time paid by athletic department and 1/2 from dining services)	Ohio State University
	San Diego State University
	Stanford University
Penn State University (PhD RD 75% by athletic department and 25% by nutrition department)	University of Arizona
	UCLA (22% of salary)
University of Nebraska-Lincoln (intern also provides services)	University of Colorado
	University of Massachusetts, Amherst
University of North Carolina	University of Montana
University of Oregon	University of Tennessee
University of Washington	

Habash, D., Ph.D., R.D., Personal Communication; responses posted on the Bunnyfox Sports Nutrition listserve to the question: "How many colleges or universities support sports nutritionist for their athletes?" bunnyfox @ concentric.net, 1999.46.

[1] These are categorized based on the area of the university that funds the sports nutritionist.

[2] Some of this information is based on second-hand responses.

* Most student health services dietitians work full-time with student health services while providing part-time services to athletes.

"How many colleges and universities actually support sports nutritionists for their athletes?"[46] The majority of universities providing sports nutrition services to athletes utilize RDs employed by student health services. In some cases, sports nutrition programs are staffed by graduate students, faculty members at the university or a sports nutritionist (RD) in the community. Programs such as Colorado State University's utilize volunteer graduate students, while the University of Georgia has an athletic department-funded graduate student program for the delivery of sports nutrition information.[46] Pennsylvania State University formalized one of the early sports nutrition programs in 1985 with a graduate assistant assigned the responsibility of a part-time sports nutritionist (RD).[47]

Since then, this position has become one of the first full-time funded sports nutrition positions in the country. Georgia Tech, Nebraska, North Carolina, North Carolina State, Oregon, Penn State, and Washington all offer full-time sports nutrition positions funded by the athletic departments.

For those RDs providing services to athletic departments, a considerable amount of time is spent interacting with the staff on the sports medicine team. Table 17.2 describes some of the athletic personnel with whom the RD may interact and the purpose of the interaction. Below are listed six strategies that an RD can employ to facilitate these interactions and the success of the program:

1. Communicate regularly with coaches, ATCs, and athletes. Long working hours often limit the time that coaches and trainers have available, especially while their sport is in season. Communicate with ATCs during the times of day when they are least likely to be working with athletes, primarily mid-morning, when athletes are in class. When communicating with coaches, ATCs, and physicians, use the traditional methods of telephone and fax.[47] E-mail communication should be encouraged. Hand delivering dietary analysis, medical reports, progress notes, or body composition analyses, while not time efficient, provides opportunities for the RD to communicate in person with the athletic staff.
2. Be open to coaches', trainers', and athletes' opinions on nutrition issues. Immediate dismissal of their ideas or concerns may result in a lack of trust of the RD's expertise or suggestions.
3. Be flexible when scheduling appointments with the athletes. ATCs typically refer and schedule athletes for nutrition counseling, and often the only times available are early in the morning or evening. Work around the athletes' limited time. Establish office hours in the training room or rehabilitation facility to create a convenient location for counseling athletes and interacting with trainers.
4. Increase visibility by attending sporting events,[47] creating a newsletter, presenting seminars, and offering programs in the community. Attend practice sessions on a regular basis and introduce yourself to coaches and trainers.
5. Enhance credibility by staying abreast of current sporting events and athletes' performance. Prior to one-on-one counseling with athletes, become knowledgeable of their performance from the previous week. Keep up with an athlete's team and personal performance by attending sporting events and paying attention to the media, radio, local university newspapers, and the Internet World Wide Web (www).
6. Finally, careful budget management is important. The RD must manage the budget by assessing the financial and material resources available when deciding which services will be offered. Careful planning of available resources will help set priorities for services provided such as individual counseling, group presentations, shopping tours, and supplement reviews. A variety of nutrition services offered by sports nutrition programs to athletes are listed in Table 17.3. All of the services listed involve, in some way, input or significant interaction with coaches and ATCs. The most frequently provided services include individual counseling, group presentations for athletes or sports-medicine-team members, supplement reviews, newsletters, diet analysis, and body composition assessment.

VII. SUMMARY

Good nutrition is essential to maximizing performance in athletes. Coaches and ATCs recognize this fact, and, when surveyed, have identified specific priority areas including fluid needs, nutritional supplementation, weight management, the training diet, and the pre-game meal.[18,19] The responsibility for disseminating nutrition information to athletes is shared between coaches and ATCs.[8,18,19] There is limited documentation of the use of RDs in high school and college sports-medicine programs, but, based on informal surveys, the number of RDs delivering nutrition information to athletes appears to be increasing.[20]

Table 17.2 Personnel with whom a Registered Dietitian may Interact

Position or Title	Interaction Purpose
Director of Sports Medicine Team (usually the head trainer or physician)	Establish protocols, schedule special topics seminars, collaborate publications, athlete referrals, supplementation evaluation, newsletters and conferences, discussion of research
Team Physicians	Make and accept referrals; participate in policy development, for example, helping establish an eating disorders protocol
Coaches	Make referrals, schedule team presentations; discuss progress of individual athletes; discuss issues of nutrition and performance
Athletic Trainers	Make and accept referrals for one on one counseling, discuss pre- and post-game meals for eating on the road, address supplementation issues; schedule body composition assessments; follow-up with individual athletes.
Sport Psychologists; Counselors from university health services	Make and accept referrals; meet with individual athletes and eating disorders committee meetings
Sports media personnel	Provide printable nutrition information, WEB sites, newsletters; provide radio and television interviews.
Food Service Personnel	Plan training menus, guide food service director in menu selection, provide educational materials at training tables.

Modified from Clark, K.L., Working with college athletes, coaches, and trainers at a major university, *Int. J. Sport Nutr.*, 4, 137, 1994.47

TABLE 17.3 Sports Nutrition Services Commonly Provided to Athletes and the Sports Medicine Team

Counseling
Dietary analysis of meals and meal plans
Body composition analysis
Group presentations for athletes
Sports nutrition newsletters
Supplement reviews
Eating Disorders Committee participation
Managed care for athletes with eating disorders
Presentations to the sports medicine team
Influencing food service management
Provide educational materials
Research studies
Shopping tours

Surveys, some of which are almost 20 years old, have demonstrated that coaches and ATCs do possess some nutrition knowledge. ATCs seem to have more nutrition knowledge than coaches and much of the expertise attained by coaches and ATCs is limited to more-general concepts.[9,18] For example, coaches are aware of the athlete's need for fluids to prevent dehydration, but they may not know the strategies for monitoring fluid intake or guidelines for fluid replacement.[1,2,9] While coaches and ATCs may be able to offer athletes general nutrition information, the extent to which they can provide in-depth assessment and counseling on issues related to guidelines for fluid replacement, nutritional supplementation, and weight management is uncertain.

The academic training of coaches and ATCs often extends beyond the baccalaureate degree with a significant number of ATCs and coaches pursuing M.S., Ed.D., and Ph.D. degrees.[18,35,37] Even with advanced training, only one introductory nutrition course is included in the curriculum for ATCs[41] and there is no mandatory nutrition course requirement for coaches. Continuing-education programs as part of certification requirements,[17] popular resources,[8,16,19] and years of experience of working with athletes have provided coaches and ATCs with significant exposure to nutrition principles. In many of the surveys and reviews, coaches and ATCs have expressed a strong desire for exposure to more nutrition education. It is anticipated that with the incorporation of the interdisciplinary sports medicine approach into more athletic programs in the 21st century,[48] coaches and ATCs should have more contact with RDs, providing another significant source of nutrition information. The requirement by NATOBOC that all ATCs enroll in an accredited program by 2004, along with the requirement for CEUs, should offer ATCs opportunities to enhance their nutrition knowledge.

Coaches and ATCs spend hours in close contact with athletes and are in an obvious position to provide leadership in disseminating health and training information. Some of the major health and performance issues confronting athletes and coaches are fluid and hydration status, nutritional supplementation, weight management, the training diet, and the pre-game meal. The training and rehabilitative responsibilities of coaches and ATCs limit their time and ability to provide the individualized nutrition care needed by many athletes. Registered dietitians have the expertise to address these issues, and, most importantly, the knowledge and training to conduct in-depth nutrition assessments. All professionals working in the area of sports medicine need to understand their distinctive roles and work collectively as one unit to facilitate the best performance, health and nutritional care of athletes.

REFERENCES

1. Bentivegna, A., Kelley, E. J., Kalenak, A., Diet, fitness, and athletic performance, *Physician Sportsmed.*, 7, 99, 1979.
2. Convertino, V. A., Armstrong, L. E., Coyle, E. F., Mack, G. W., Sawka, M. N., Senay L. C., Jr., Sherman, W. M., American College of Sports Medicine position stand. Exercise and fluid replacement, *Med. Sci. Sports Exerc.* 28, i-vii, 1996.
3. McArdle, W. D., Katch, F. I., Katch, V. L., Optimal nutrition for exercise and training, in: *Sports and Exercise Nutrition,* Lippincott, Williams and Wilkins, Philadelphia, 1999, p. 194.
4. Gatorade Sports Science Institute, The impact of sports medicine on coaching and sport in the 1990s, *Sports Sci. Exchange Roundtable*, 7, 2, 1996.
5. Oppliger, R. A., Case, S., Horswill, C. A., Landry, G. L. and Shelter, A. C., Weight loss in wrestlers, *Med. Sci. Sports Exerc.*, 28, ix, 1996.
6. Gatorade Sports Science Institute, Methods of weight gain in athletes, *Sports Sci. Exchange Roundtable*, 6, 1, 1995.
7. Sossin, K., Gizis, F., Marquart, L. F., Sobal J., Nutrition beliefs, attitudes, and resource use of high school wrestling coaches, *Int. J. Sport Nutr.*, 7, 219, 1997.
8. Bedgood, B. L., Tuck, M. B., Nutrition knowledge of high school athletic coaches in Texas, *J. Am. Diet. Assoc.,* 83, 672, 1983.
9. Corley, G., Demarest-Litchford, M., Bazzarre, T. L., Nutrition knowledge and dietary practices of college coaches, *J. Am. Diet. Assoc.,* 90, 705, 1990.
10. Baer, J. T., Dean, D. J., Lambrinnides, T., How high school football coaches recommend their players gain lean body mass, *J. Strength Con. Res.*, 8, 72, 1994.
11. Slavin, J. L., Calorie supplements for athletes, *Physician Sportsmed.*, 14, 201, 1986.
12. Wiita, B. G. and Stombaaugh, I. A., Nutrition knowledge, eating practices, and health of adolescent female runner: A 3-year longitudinal study, *Int. J. Sport Nutr.,* 6, 414, 1996.
13. Storlie, J., Nutrition assessment of athletes: A model for integrating nutrition and physical performance indicators, *Int. J. Sport Nut.*, 1, 192, 1991.
14. Perron, M., Endres, J., Knowledge, attitudes, and dietary practices of female athletes, *J. Am. Diet. Assoc.,* 85, 573, 1985.
15. Kemper, H. C. G., Post, B., Twisk, J. W. R., Rate of maturation during the teenage years: Nutrient intake and physical activity between ages 12 and 22, *Int. J. Sport Nutr.*, 7, 229, 1997.
16. Wolf, E. M. B., Wirth, J. C., Lohman, T. G., Nutritional practices of coaches in the big ten, *Physician Sportsmed.*, 7, 113, 1979.
17. Misasi, S. P., Davisa, C. F., Morin, G. E., Stockman, D., Academic preparation of athletic trainers as counselors, *J. Ath. Train.,* 31, 39, 1996.

18. Parr, R. B., Porter, M. A., Hodgson, S. C., Nutrition knowledge and practice of coaches, trainers and athletes, *Physician Sportsmed.*, 12, 127, 1984.
19. Graves, K. L., Farthing, M. C., Smith, S. A., Turchi, J. M., Nutrition training, attitudes, knowledge, recommendations, responsibility, and resource utilization of high school coaches and trainers, *J. Am. Diet. Assoc.*, 91, 321, 1991.
20. Sports Nutrition Listserve., bunnyfox@concentric.net.
21. Murray, R., Fluid needs of athletes, in: *Nutrition for Sport and Exercise,* 2nd ed., Bering, J.R. and Steen, S.N., Eds., Aspen Publishers, Inc., Gaithersburg, 1998, chap. 8.
22. National Academy of Sciences, Protein and amino acids, in: *Recommended Dietary Allowances*, National Academy Press, Washington, D.C., 52, 1989.
23. Snyder, A. C., and Naik, J., Protein requirements of athletes, in: *Nutrition for Sport and Exercise*, 2nd ed., Bering, J.R. and Steen, S.N., Eds., Aspen Publishers, Inc., Gaithersburg, 1998, chap. 3.
24. Keith, R. E., Vitamins and physical activity, in: *Nutrition in Exercise and Sport,* 2nd ed., Wolinsky, I. and Hickson, J.F., Eds., CRC Press, Boca Raton, FL, 1994, chap.8.
25. Lewis, R., personal communication, 1996.
26. American Dietetic Association, Position of the ADA: Vitamin and mineral supplements, *J. Am. Diet. Assoc.*, 96, 73, 1997.
27. Sobal, J., and Marquart, L. F., Vitamin/mineral supplement use among athletes: A review of the literature, *Int. J. Sport Nutr.*, 4: 320, 1994.
28. Fogelholm, G. M., Koskinen, R., Laakso, J., Rankinen, T., Ruokonen, I., Gradual and rapid weight loss: Effects on nutrition and performance in male athletes, *Med. Sci. Sports and Exerc.,* 25, 371, 1992.
29. Rosen, L.W., McKeag, D. B., Hough, D. O. and Curley, V., Pathogenic weight-control behavior in female athletes, *Physician Sportsmed.,* 14, 79, 1986.
30. Lakin, J. A., Steen, S. N., Oppliger, R. A., Eating behaviors, weight loss methods, and nutrition practices among high school wrestlers, *J. Comm. Health Nurs.*, 7, 223, 1990.
31. Griffin, J. and Harris, M. B., Coaches' attitudes, knowledge, experiences, and recommendations regarding weight control, *The Sport Psychologist*, 10, 180, 1996.
32. Weissinger, E., Housh, T. J., and Johnson, G. O., Coaches attitudes, knowledge, and practices concerning weight loss behaviors in high school wrestling, *Pediatrics*, 5, 145, 1993.
33. Otis, C. L., Drinkwater, B., Johnson, M., Loucks, A., and Wilmore, J., American College of Sports Medicine position stand. The Female Athlete Triad, *Med. Sci. Sports Exerc.* 29, i-ix, 1997.
34. United States Department of Agriculture and United States Department of Health and Human Services, Nutrition and your Health Dietary Guidelines for Americans, *Home and Garden Bulletin,* 4th ed., no. 232, 1995.
35. George, F. J., The athletic trainer's perspective, *Clin. Sports Med.*, 16, 361, 1997.
36. Weidner, T. G., Vincent, W. J., Evaluation of professional preparation in athletic training by employed, entry-level athletic trainers, *J. Ath. Train.*, 27, 304, 1992.
37. Richardson, H., Academic preparation of athletic coaches in higher education, *J. Phys. Educ. Rec.*, 52, 44, 1981.
38. The American Swimming Coaches Association., http://www.swimmingcoach.org.
39. National Strength and Conditioning Association., http://www.nsca-cc.org.
40. The American Swimming Coaches Association., Personal communication. 1999.
41. National Athletic Trainer's Association Board of Certification — Online Documents. Site accessed 01/10/00. http://www.nataboc.org/standards.html
42. Foster, D. T., Leslie, D. K., Clinical teaching roles of athletic trainers, *J. Ath. Train.*, 27, 298, 1992.
43. Lombardo, J.A., Sports medicine: A team effort, *Physician Sportsmed.*, 13, 72, 1985.
44. Berry, L., ATC + RD = Healthy Athletes., *Training and Conditioning*., Dec, 27. 1999.
45. American Dietetic Association. Accreditation/Approval Manual for Dietetics Education Program. *Commission on Accreditation/Approval for Dietetics Education of the American Dietetics Association.* 4th ed. Chicago IL Page 11, 1997.
46. Habash, D. personal communication responses posted on the Bunnyfox sports nutrition listserve. 1999.
47. Clark, K., Working with college athletes, coaches, and trainers at a major university, *Int. J. Sport Nutr,* 4, 135, 1994.
48. Gatorade Sports Science Institute, University sports medicine teams: An interdisciplinary approach, *Sports Sci. Exchange Roundtable*, 4, 3, 1993.

Part VI

Summary

CHAPTER 18

Nutritional Applications in Exercise and Sport

Ira Wolinsky and Judy A. Driskell

CONTENTS

I. INTRODUCTION

This volume focuses on nutritional applications in exercise and sport and, as such, does not discuss nutrient-specific metabolism, per se. The field of sports nutrition is in its infancy and is a rapidly growing area of practice. The field has grown rapidly due to an increasing number of health professionals, athletes (both professional and recreational), coaches, and trainers concerned about the impact of nutrition on performance. However, nutrition misinformation may be widespread in this group. With the increasing popularity of sports and exercise, greater numbers are actively involved in exercise programs to enhance health and well being, and for rehabilitative purposes. Increasingly, participation in these activities starts at an early age, as young as 5 years, and continues into the later years, greater than 80 years of age. With the widening age range of active individuals, it is important to recognize the variation in their nutritional needs so as to not only meet the needs of the normal physiological processes but also that of exercise, physical activity, sport, disabilities, and lifestyle.

II. LIFE CYCLE NUTRITIONAL CONCERNS OF ATHLETES

For some women, the physiological stress of pregnancy may be combined with that of exercise or sport. For healthy women experiencing normal pregnancy, regular exercise is not contraindicated,

0-8493-8199-1/00/$0.00+$.50

except under specific circumstances. The benefits of exercise during pregnancy include weight control, reduction in risk of hypertension, promotion of psychological well being, and maintenance of healthy bones, muscles, and joints. But, without adequate energy and nutrition to compensate for the increased caloric needs required for pregnancy, as well as physical activity, it is reasonable to expect that this exercise might compromise fetal growth and the mother under certain conditions, unless protective compensatory adaptations develop. Resuming or initiating a moderate level of physical activity 6–8 weeks postpartum may improve maternal cardiovascular fitness and not adversely affect lactation — either quantity or immunological properties.

The number of children participating in athletic activities is increasing. Regular physical activity in children is associated with improved strength, maintenance of healthy body weight and composition, and cardiovascular fitness. Children who are physically active or participate in sports are likely to become physically active adults. Adult health risks associated with inactivity may decrease in this group. Whereas $\dot{V}O_{2max}$ is recognized as the single best indicator of aerobic fitness in adults, this is not necessarily so in children, where a modified physical work capacity equation (PWC_{195}) may be a more accurate predictor. Both aerobic and anaerobic activities are safe and beneficial for children under supervised conditions. Optimal duration and intensity of physical activity for children is not known. Many children participating in competitive or high-level individual sports train up to 16 hours per week with no apparent problems. Excessive mechanical loading should be avoided. Non-anemic iron deficiency, or sports anemia, has been, to date, reported in child athletes. Usually, endurance-sports training, thought to be a factor in this type of anemia, is not included in childhood athletic activities. But as elite athletes become younger and participate in more-intensive training, the likelihood of seeing sports anemia in childhood exists. Use of dietary supplements or ergogenic aids should not be necessary in the active or athletic child who consumes a recommended dietary intake.

Adolescence is a time of rapid growth and development, exerting a profound effect on energy and nutrient needs. Estimates are that more than half of adolescents in the USA participate in competitive athletics. Strenuous physical activity or sport places stress on adolescents by increasing the already high nutritional demands of rapid growth. If dietary intake is not sufficient to meet the challenge, sports training can potentially negatively impact growth and biological maturation of the adolescent athlete. Reports indicate that adolescent athletes have only a poor knowledge of general nutritional principles or sports nutrition concepts. This group is a challenge to the nutrition educator. Adolescents are at high risk for nutritional deficiencies, especially iron and calcium. It is difficult to comment on the adequacy or inadequacy of energy in adolescent athletes, since data are sparse and conflicting. Inadequate energy intakes would, however, be expected to be accompanied by marginal intakes of macro- and micronutrients. Of particular concern are adolescent female athletes in sports that emphasize leanness or weight-dependent sports. These women place themselves at risk for micronutrient deficiencies with ill health sequels.

Over the next decades, the proportion of the population 65 years old and over is expected to reach 20%. Most of the elderly can expect an increased proportion of abdominal fat, reduced lean body mass, and reduced bone mineral density. Physical exercise can modify many of the aging-related physiological and metabolic changes and improve quality of life factors of the older adult, even the frail elderly and the "very old" elderly. But, many older adults do not engage in regular physical activity — 18% of men and 30% of women aged 50–59 years. These percentages increase with age, reaching 40% in men and 62% in women aged 80 years plus. At least one-third of the elderly population has self-reported limitations due to chronic conditions, while more than 50% report at least one disability. Some of the physiological changes associated with aging are also related to inactivity. While there is meager information as to nutritional needs during aging, aside from lower energy requirements, the overall health benefits attributed to regular physical activity in aging include better functional capacity, less physical and musculoskeletal disability, less medical care, lower body weight, better cardiovascular fitness, and improvement in psychological aspects.

III. GROUP-SPECIFIC NUTRITIONAL CONCERNS OF ATHLETES

This section of the book deals with groups of athletes with special problems and needs. Within each group, they may occur at any point during, or over, the entire life cycle.

Dietary habits of Olympic athletes have always been of abiding interest to health professionals, athletes, and the public. Olympic hopefuls strive for top physical condition and work toward that goal in diverse ways, some good, some not so good. The diets of elite athletes are as varied as the athletes themselves and a variety of eating patterns are employed. Trial and error is the method used to determine the best nutrition program for the athlete's needs. Recent decades of research indicate that the nutritional needs of athletes do vary from those of non-athletes. Research has indicated, for example, that elite athletes may be "energy efficient," i.e., expending less energy than estimated by indirect methods, that some female athletes have energy requirements that are lower than their non-athletic peers. We look to the future for more research on elite athletes, an area of sports nutrition still in its infancy, indeed.

More and more people, including athletes, are becoming vegetarians, both for informed and uninformed reasons. There are many types of vegetarians, ranging from selective to strict vegan. Most vegetarians appreciate the alleged health benefits of vegetarian diets, but it should be borne in mind, the more restrictive the diet, the more difficult it will be to meet nutrient requirements. On the other hand, if appropriately planned, vegan diets, although restrictive, can provide adequate nutrition even for competitive athletes. A main concern for athletes is to obtain enough high-quality protein to meet their increased needs. This is of lesser concern to the lacto-ovo vegetarian than to the vegan.

Each year in the USA alone, as many as 2–3 million athletes with physical disabilities compete in recreational and organized sports. The health and nutritional concerns of competitive athletes with cerebral palsy and spinal cord injury (wheelchair athletes) are discussed in this book. The limited mobility of these athletes often places them at higher risk for cardiovascular disease, obesity, osteoporosis, and malnutrition. Currently, there are no reference standards for the assessment of arthropometrics, hardly any research on the relationship between nutrition and performance, and quality strength and conditions. More research attention should be given to this very dedicated group of athletes.

The impact of an exercise program on the health of many individuals with chronic disease or conditions is often a positive one. It can confer health benefits to individuals with diabetes mellitus, hypertension, and coronary artery diseases. Regular aerobic activity coupled with sound nutrition can usually slow the disease progression and even partially reverse it, depending on such factors as, among others, intensity, frequency, and duration of the training. In some cases, however, exercise can worsen some chronic medical conditions. Professional advice should be sought in each case.

IV. THE SPORT

This section of the volume discusses the practicalities of competitive sport.

It is important that athletes choose the proper fuel for optimal performance. Training tables, both at home and on the road, must supply, not only the fuels needed by the exercise bout, but also the nutrients required by the body for health. Because athletes have a high requirement for carbohydrates and have a difficult time making wise food choices, they need to learn strategies to eat better while traveling. It is important for them to learn that the food guide pyramid can be used as a guide in making food decisions as well as a menu guide for the training table. If athletes have a nutritious training table during the season and on the road, it will help them eliminate nutrition pitfalls. It is helpful to the athlete to have good nutrition role models in their parents, coaches, and trainers.

A discussion of the practical issues of athletes eating on the road and the design and implementation of programs for feeding these athletes in travel situations is included in the volume. The logistics of travel, morale, fatigue, food economics, and nutrition, as components of the substrate for a winning team, are discussed. The applied sports nutritionist can be an invaluable asset to athletic administrators and the team in striving to ensure that the team is fed nutritious diets in an efficient and cost-effective manner on the road.

Food and beverages consumed prior, during, and immediately following an event can exert significant impact on the athlete's ability to perform and to recover following performance. Generally, pre-event meals should be high in carbohydrate to maximize liver glycogen stores, consumed 1–4 hours prior to event, be composed of safe foods on the bland side so as to not produce or increase intestinal motility. The total calorie content of the meal should be under 1000. Fiber content should be low to minimize defecation; adequate fluids must be consumed pre-event. In general, small pre-event meals should be consumed prior to competition or heavy training i.e., the food should be cleared from the stomach and small intestines by the start of exercise. Appropriate pre-event nutrition can positively impact endurance performance. Eating during high-intensity short-term events is not practical and probably not necessary. Consumption of carbohydrates and fluids during prolonged events can be beneficial. Following exercise or the event, consumption of adequate carbohydrate, protein, and replacement fluids is important to replenish glycogen stores, promote net protein synthesis, and restore fluid and electrolyte balance. Beverages that induce a diuretic effect and facilitate body water loss are contraindicated, therefore, beverages with alcohol or caffeine are not recommended for rehydration.

There can be enormous pressure on young athletes to be successful in performance and to achieve an ideal body weight. Many cases of eating disorders may go unnoticed in the athletic world because there is often not a clear line between healthy and unhealthy eating. Disordered eating may be defined as eating or not eating in response to an external cue rather than an internal one. Anorexic nervosa, bulimia nervosa, binge-eating disorder, and muscle dysmorphia are among disordered eating behaviors to be found among athletes. Muscle dysmorphia is a relatively new term used to describe individuals who are pathologically preoccupied with being fit and muscular. It is not an eating disorder per se, but, rather, a psychiatric disturbance involving body image. Eating disorders in athletes have been found to be higher in aesthetic and weight-dependent sports than in endurance, technical, and team sports. Athletes with eating disorders are at a greater risk for injury and illness than their not-disordered colleagues. The sports nutritionist is often the person in the athlete's life with the ability to identify and intervene when a potential eating disorder exists.

The occurrence of recreational drug use among athletes appears to be similar or even greater than in non-athletes in high school, college, and professional sports. This includes use of alcohol, amphetamines, caffeine, cocaine, diuretics, marijuana, and nicotine. They may work to improve or hamper performance, and lead to physiological or psychological addiction. These drugs can impact an athlete's nutritional status, including hydration, body weight, and micronutrient status.

We can observe some people who indulge in excessive exercise to the point of injury, even death. Like an eating disorder, excessive exercise can be practiced as a means to control body weight. Although excessive exercise may be often viewed positively, there are habitual exercise patterns that do appear dysfunctional. The best descriptor of disordered exercise patterns may be the term "exercise dependence." It is differentiated from eating disorders but may lead to eating disorders.

V. NUTRITION KNOWLEDGE OF ATHLETES, COACHES, AND TRAINERS

Athletes need and want reliable, accurate information to improve their health and performance. This includes the range of athletes, children, adolescents, college students, recreational athletes, and professional athletes. Much of the information they receive may not be accurate; athletes may fall victim to quackery and fads specifically targeted to this group. With the growth of interest in sports nutrition, different methods of communicating sound nutrition knowledge must be considered. A registered dietitian or licensed nutritionist, with a background in nutrition and physical activity, who can tailor diets to the individual athletes in a specific sport, may one day become an essential part of serious sports efforts.

Where registered dietitians or licensed nutritionists may be limited or lacking, coaches, athletic trainers, and certified athletic trainers often play a primary role in delivering nutritional information to athletes, partly because of the extensive hours of contact they have with the athletes. Though their formal education in nutrition may be limited and their nutrition knowledge shallow, many coaches and athletic trainers may be desirous of more nutrition education. These are two groups warranting attention from nutrition educators.

SELECTED GENERAL REFERENCES

1. Watson, R.R. (Ed.), *Handbook of Nutrition in the Aged,* CRC Press, Boca Raton, FL, 1994.
2. Parizkova, J., *Nutrition, Physical Activity, and Health in Early Life*, CRC Press, Boca Raton, FL 1996.
3. Ruud, J.S., *Nutrition and the Female Athlete*, CRC Press, Boca Raton, FL, 1996.
4. Wolinsky, I., Klimis-Tavantzis, D. (Eds.), *Nutritional Concerns of Women*, CRC Press, Boca Raton, FL, 1996.
5. Wolinsky, I., (Ed.), *Nutrition in Exercise and Sport*, third edition, CRC Press, Boca Raton, FL, 1998.
6. Leutholtz, B.C., Ripoll, I., *Exercise and Disease Management*, CRC Press, Boca Raton, FL, 1999.
7. McMurray, R.G., *Concepts in Fitness Programming*, CRC Press, Boca Raton, FL, 1999.
8. Tarnopolsky, M. (Ed.), *Gender Differences in Metabolism: Practical and Nutritional Implications*, CRC Press, Boca Raton, FL, 1999.
9. Driskell, J.A., *Sports Nutrition*, CRC Press, Boca Raton, FL, 2000.

Index

A

B

C

D

E

F

G

H

I

P

R

S

T

U

V

W

Z